Beyond
Broccoli

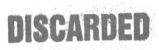

Beyond Broccoli

Creating a Biologically Balanced Diet
When a Vegetarian Diet Doesn't Work

Susan Schenck, LAc, MTOM

Printed in the USA

First Edition, 2011

Published by Awakenings Publications, P.O. Box 558, Concrete, WA, 98237

Editor, Designer, and Production Manager: Bob Avery (bobavery@umich.edu)

Cover design: Brion Sausser (www.bookcreatives.com)

ISBN 978-0-9776795-2-2

Nutrition/Diet   Health   Weight Loss   Raw Food

This book is dedicated to Dr. Stanley S. Bass, who led me down into the rabbit hole of true health understanding.

*To all other Health Warriors
and Truth Seekers around the world who
may come into possession of this book:*

You will always be rewarded for keeping an open mind!

Table of Contents

Part 2: Evolution of the Human Diet

Part 3: Finding Balance in Fats, Carbohydrates, and Protein

Part 4: Morality, Spirituality, and Sustainability of Eating Meat

Foreword

I first met Susan Schenck in the summer of 2009 in New York City, having already been introduced to her 600-page book, *The Live Food Factor*. After a careful reading of the entire book, which I found full of a wealth of valuable information and advocacy of a vegetarian diet, even more so of the vegan diet and lifestyle, I was greatly surprised and impressed by the fact that she also included her personal experience and knowledge about the use of meat and animal foods, as well as her meetings with professional nutritionists who advocated the paleolithic diet for modern living, etc.

This open-minded quality I had rarely seen before of a writer who wrote intensely in favor of a vegan diet and yet had the courage to speak favorably of the use of primitive man's hunter-gatherer diet and the use of animal foods. I know that by this she was opening herself up to hostile attacks and more criticism by vegans, some of whom contributed articles to her book. Her courage and honesty impressed me, and I was immediately drawn to her personality.

During our first conversation, I told Susan about my experiences as a vegetarian (lacto-ovo) for more than 15 years, then as a Natural Hygienist, then about my many fasts totaling well over 1,000 days, one year on a 100 percent vegan diet followed by a two-year extension of the same raw vegan diet, then with my experiment with testing a 100 percent raw diet including raw animal food and meat for over ten years, also pointing out the dangers of heavy fruit eating and high-carbohydrate diet.

I told her about many patients of mine and the near-miraculous results which followed by a strict curtailment of high carbohydrates in the diet. Also about people who develop severe deficiencies in vitamins A, B_{12}, D_3, K, proteins, hormones, etc. on a strict vegan diet lasting two or more years, and then making rapid recoveries in a matter of weeks just by adding a small amount of raw animal foods to their diets. I recommended several writers that she investigate for her future writings.

Susan, after reading your new book in its entirety, I was greatly impressed by the extent and breadth of the research you did on the history of primitive man and the paleolithic diet, wherein you proved the superior health and success man experienced by the use of meat and animal food for almost three million years of history. This is one of the very best I have read on the subject, and I will recommend it highly to all who are instructed in superior health.

Yours for Superior Health,

—Dr. Stanley S. Bass, ND, DC, PhC, PhD, DO, DSc, DD

www.drbass.com

Acknowledgements

Firstly, I owe a most hearty thank you to Bob Avery, who has been the best editor and fact checker an author could wish for, not to mention his work on the layout design, index, and production aspects of this book. His computer and typography skills make my life as an author so much easier. I can just write and let him handle all the technical details of getting the book into publishable form.

He has supported me in this present effort even when he didn't share my opinion on every claim made in this book. Without his own accumulated dietary knowledge base from his many years of personal study, experience, and experimentation in following a raw diet himself — in addition to his technical assistance and guidance — this book couldn't have become what it is.

Great appreciation must also be extended for the enthusiastic support of my friend Guillermo Martin with his expertise in anthropology and nutrition, for helping me with fact checking and for encouraging me to write this book.

Thanks to Brion Sausser for working so hard on the cover and listening carefully to my requests.

Dr. Leanna Palmero, DC, thank you so much for your careful review and suggestions for the book.

Thank you, Payson Stevens, for coming up with the book's title.

I must not forget to thank former vegetarians Lierre Keith and Dr. Ron Strauss, and former vegans, like Paul Nison and Kevin Gianni, who personally encouraged me to move forward despite the controversial nature of this book.

Thank you also to all those who contributed to chapter 5 and to the reviews on the back cover.

I also feel a special appreciation and affection for all bloggers and readers who e-mailed me with words of gratitude and support for addressing this much-neglected but crucially important dietary issue within the alternative health literature.

And to my mostly piscetarian husband: Thank you for supporting my more omnivorous ways despite your own dietary slant.

Most of all I want to thank Dr. Stanley Bass for freely sharing his decades' worth of accumulated knowledge from his academic training and his own independent research, personal experience, and clinical practice based on nutritional principles.

I also owe him an enormous debt of gratitude for offering me personal dietary assistance and research recommendations — in short, for taking me gently down the rabbit hole of holistic nutrition.

Preface

After spending a number of months achieving some success in marketing *The Live Food Factor*, my book on the raw food diet, I yearned to return to writing. I decided to write on calorie restriction (CR). In my never-ending quest for higher levels of health, I had attempted a calorie-restricted diet, prompted by many compelling studies that prove it leads to life extension.

After about five months, I found myself losing too much weight, even though I was reducing my calories by only 20 percent. (The animals in the studies were restricted by 35 to 40 percent!) I didn't like the gaunt look of other CR practitioners (been there, done that as a former anorexic). While I appreciated being thin, I didn't want to look emaciated.

In addition, I had spent over a thousand dollars on my new size 6 and size 4 clothes; I wasn't about to spend more on size 2s and size 0s. Most of all, I didn't want to be so light that osteoporosis was a constant threat. Very thin people have to exercise even more religiously than I do to maintain bone density.

I then noticed something mentioned in the studies and articles about CR: those who practice calorie restriction aren't really restricting their calories after a certain point, because as they lose a lot of weight, their bodies require many fewer calories for maintenance.

I figured that since there is no observation that extremely thin people live longer, there must be another factor. When I read Dr. Ron Rosedale's book *The Rosedale Diet*, in which he explains that his patients achieve all the healthy biomarkers that the calorie-restricted animals do but without feeling constantly hungry, I became very excited.

The key to longevity is not starving yourself into some stick figure, as I had done as a teenager; the key is a moderate-calorie, low-carbohydrate diet (what some may regard as excessively high in fat), balanced with adequate protein and packed with the natural foods which we evolved eating. I would add to Dr. Rosedale's recommendations that we should make the diet mostly, if not entirely, raw.

In this book, I may contradict a few things I wrote in *The Live Food Factor* — but only as they concern meat. (When I say *meat*, I am including fish.) At that time, I sincerely believed what I wrote about the superiority of eating at least a vegetarian, if not vegan, diet.

I have now changed my mind because I know I am healthier including just a few ounces of meat in my daily diet, especially small fish. I know there are others out there like me who could be healthier if they too would just add a little meat to their otherwise vegan diets!

For some, my book on the raw vegan diet was proof of the power of veganism. For me, it was meant to be solid proof, tight proof, of the power of eating raw. As you will note if you read between the lines, I wasn't totally convinced about veganism, though willing to give it a try. I believed with all my heart and mind that it was healthier and morally superior to eat vegetarian, if not vegan. I also thought it was necessary for spiritual evolution.

Upon hearing my radio interviews in which I came out as a nonvegan, some bloggers have commented that you should "never trust someone who changes her mind."

Oh, then perhaps you can't trust Dr. Stanley Bass, Dr. Vivian Vetrano, and Dr. Gabriel Cousens, raw food doctors with their combined 100-plus years of clinical experience! They formerly thought people got enough vitamin B_{12} on vegan diets. After years of observation, they changed their minds.

I guess you can't also trust Victoria Boutenko, who started off vegan but now writes about eating insect eggs and admits to eating chicken eggs as well.

Then there is David Wolfe, a famous raw food advocate. He started his career telling people to eat mostly fruit. (I know someone who had a paid consultation with him.) Now he says to go easy on the fruit.

There are even world famous people, like Albert Einstein and Louis Pasteur, who also revised theories in their fields of study after publishing them one way.

Is it better to remain mired in dogma or to show growth by learning and admitting you may have not been right about everything from the beginning?

I gave the vegan diet six years, more than ten percent of my life. That is a fair shake. In the long run, veganism was a disaster for me, as you will read in this book. As the saying goes, "To admit that you were wrong is merely to admit that you're much wiser today than you were yesterday."

Still, I want to emphasize here that I *do* know some successful long-term vegetarians and vegans. The point of this book is to show that it doesn't work for *everyone*, and *why*. You may be one of those individuals.

Introduction

Though few people are talking or writing about this topic, many people feel they have failed on vegan or vegetarian diets. But the truth is, the diets failed them. These diets are not our biologically natural or evolutionary diets. Vegetarians believe we are biologically herbivores but that some people have adapted to meat.

Actually, the opposite is true: we are omnivores, and *some* of us have adapted to vegetarianism. It might well be that we are evolving towards a vegetarian or even vegan adaptation, but the bottom line is, if the evolution isn't happening in your body, irreversible damage can take place.

The message of my book *The Live Food Factor* was simply, live according to nature's laws, eat raw, and you will detoxify and become much healthier.

The message of this sequel is, include at least a little bit of animal foods in your diet (preferably raw, or only lightly cooked, and at least 5 to 10 percent of your caloric intake), and you will avoid deficiencies. Eat low-glycemic foods to increase your insulin sensitivity.

The Live Food Factor focused on *eliminating excesses* — toxins, bad foods, cooked foods, and too much food — while the present book focuses on *avoiding deficiencies*. Incidentally, these twin aspects of health are considered very important in Chinese medicine and in hygiene.[*]

Regarding the first edition of *The Live Food Factor*, some people lamented that I didn't take a stand on certain issues. One of them was the vegan question. So in the second edition, I allowed the inclusion of a lot more vegan information to satisfy the readers who wanted more structure and guidance. At the time, I felt it must be a workable diet for most people, since holistic doctors like raw food advocate, author, and clinician Dr. Gabriel Cousens, MD, were promoting it.

I have since learned it doesn't fit everyone. A six-year vegan experiment proved it didn't work in my body, and I have reason to believe I am far from alone. I then spent a year being raw vegetarian, adding raw eggs and just a bit of goat cheese to my diet. A year after that, I added just four ounces of clean, non-factory-farmed meat to my daily raw diet, and I cut back on the carbs. To my astonishment, my health really took off, my mental capacities even at times exceeding those of my youth.

Let me make this clear: I did not want to write this book!

I resisted for a year and a half. I was going to make it just one chapter in a different book. But when I quit resisting, the book just flowed, and the information I uncovered was astounding.

I had to speak the truth. I know there are many people who give up on raw when the real root of their health problems is their vegan diets, not the raw food. I know there are many people who feel great on raw vegan diets until two to ten years later, when their stored nutrients are depleted, as for example fat-soluble vitamins.

They have depleted themselves of nutritional reserves, but they can't imagine that the diet which made them feel so great could be the problem. It's not the raw aspect of the diet; it's the deficiencies that arise when we give up the important foods our species evolved on.

So my motive in writing this is to educate people and alert them to possible dangers. If you are doing well on a vegan or vegetarian diet, my hope is that this book will educate you so that you can stop prejudging those of us who are not biologically suited for such a restricted diet.

A word to my vegan friends: I am asking you to become open-minded enough to consider my arguments rationally. If veganism is your philosophy, that is one thing, but don't be duped into thinking it is nutritionally superior in all cases, because it isn't. If it works for you, don't automatically assume that it works for everyone.

Some of you may already know what I am

---

[*]*Hygiene* is the science of human health. You will find that definition listed first in any dictionary. You will often see it referred to as *natural* hygiene, or Natural Hygiene (NH), in the hygienic literature to distinguish it from the medical concept of antiseptic cleanliness more commonly referred to as hygiene these days. Medical/dental hygienic practices arose from the advent of the overly simplistic germ theory of disease. The true science of human health provides a much more comprehensive understanding than that. See *The Live Food Factor* by this author.

talking about. Have you been a raw vegan, a cooked vegan, or a vegetarian and noticed after a few years that you have lost muscle tone? Have your blood tests revealed high triglycerides (which comes from overeating carbohydrates), low levels of vitamin B_{12}, vitamin B_6, zinc, taurine, vitamin D, or vitamin A? If so, you may find that incorporating some raw animal products (often as little as 5 to 10 percent of your diet) can restore your health.

Note that the liver can store vitamin B_{12} for up to a decade, so this deficiency can take a while to show up. Many times, it can take years for one's health to diminish on a diet devoid of animal foods. If you have been vegan for over a decade, your blood panels and vitality show that you are enjoying superior health, and you look and feel great (and I *do* know *some* raw vegans who fit this profile) — then continue enjoying your diet! It obviously works for you.

But if you are judgmental about others who eat animal products, thinking that everyone can and should be vegan or raw vegan, then you need to read on. I know how you feel. I used to think exactly like that.

I had friends who said they would like to be vegetarians, but when they tried, it just didn't work for them. Their health failed. They developed low blood sugar, and they got tremendous gas from trying plant protein in the form of beans.

I would not say anything too strong, because I didn't want to stir up problems with my friends, but inside I would be thinking, "Oh, you could do it if you tried! You just need to get some hemp seeds! You just need to try harder, get your body cleaned out!"

The reasons for veganism and vegetarianism fall into various categories: religious, ethical, health related, environmental, economic, and spiritual. I am here to dispel some of the rationales behind these reasons, most notably the health one. Don't delude yourself into thinking vegetarianism is always more healthful.

If you still feel for moral or spiritual reasons that you wish to remain vegan or vegetarian after reading this book, please do so, but be sure to read the concluding chapters, which will apply to you. Nevertheless, some of your preconceptions will be challenged. In fact, as you read on, you will begin to question whether it is always healthier, better for the environment, or even better for all animals.

Finally, let me make it very clear for the record that I am not funded, sponsored, or in any way supported financially by any meat, dairy, or egg producers. The vast majority of factory farms would find this book harmful to their businesses. I am opposed to their animal cruelty practices for both moral and health reasons, as I discuss at length in this book. The farms that treat animals properly and humanely have such small profit margins that they would not be able to pay me to promote them.

Part 1

The Vegetarian Mystique

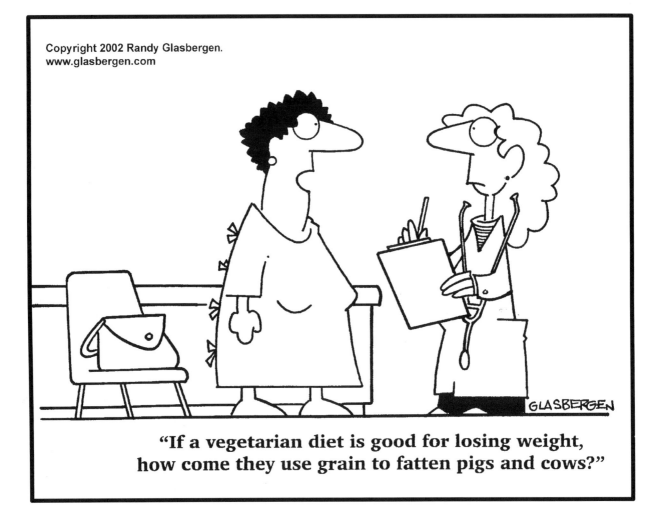

Chapter 1

How a Vegan Diet Compromised My Health

Your body is the only "authority" you can trust unconditionally.

—Konstantin Monastyrsky, *Fiber Menace*

I woke up one morning in January 2009 jumping and shouting for joy. My book, a comprehensive guide to the raw vegan diet, was on the Amazon bestseller list due to an ad campaign I ran.

When it reached number 23 for all genres, I could hardly contain my excitement. Despite a great economic recession, thousands of people were willing to pay $29.95 for my book. I was riding the wave of one of the fastest growing niches in the publishing industry: that of the raw vegan diet category.

People often tell me, "You are so lucky to have so much energy!" I smile, because that is like telling someone who has practiced playing the piano for several hours a day for four decades, "You are so lucky to be able to play music."

I have been a health seeker since the age of 16. Unlike so many people I know, I refuse to get locked into dogma. Show me where I am wrong or some better way, and I will listen eagerly. Seeking energy and health have been my lifelong passions. Nutrition, I have found, is the main key.

Given that half the world's working population earns $2 a day, I count myself lucky that I can wake up every day and ask myself, "What would I like to eat today?" Indeed, I consider myself blessed to have been financially able to experiment with every diet that arouses my curiosity, from Atkins to the Zone, while most people are forced into a sparse diet of beans and rice.

When I found the raw vegan diet, the search ended. *Or so I thought.* I began my raw food journey in 2002, and my health and energy levels at the age of 46 quickly became like those of a child. I had discovered the perfect diet, the best-kept secret to health.

After about six months into my raw vegan diet, I experimented for a few months including raw animal foods. But I really liked the taste of plant foods better, and I got constipated from the dairy. So I dismissed the diet as completely off track.

In addition, all the action was taking place on the vegan side of the raw diet. That's where all the lectures and potlucks were. It was more politically correct. It was more cool and hip. Who wanted to eat dead animals? I love animals, and I hate the abuse they suffer just as much as anybody.

Animals are sentient beings with emotions and, as my thinking went, don't deserve to be eaten. Besides, our teeth are not like those of carnivores. Our digestive tracts are too long for rotting, putrid meat, which is what it becomes when you cook it and then consume it.

I made a commitment to the vegan team. For six years, I was about 95 percent raw (with popcorn and potatoes as my favorite cheats) and about 99 percent vegan (eating only an occasional raw egg yolk to supplement my sublingual methylcobalamin B_{12} vitamins, as well as occasional raw ice cream).

A raw vegan diet is usually restricted to the four "food groups" of fruits, vegetables, nuts, and seeds. Some grains and legumes are OK to eat sprouted, but these tend to be bloating, so for many people they cannot be eaten in as large amounts as when cooked.

You might think, "How can anyone live on such a restricted diet for long?" I did it for six years. I rarely felt deprived.

When people came for dinner, they would get a menu listing what I spent three hours or more preparing: appetizers such as raw nori rolls, soups such as creamy celery cilantro, main dishes such as mock chicken nuggets made of almonds, beverages such as carob mint sesame seed milk, and desserts such as raw carrot cake made with walnuts, dates, and carrots and topped with cashew cream icing.

People always commented that I should open a restaurant, but my passion was research and writing. Because I was a voracious reader, I came to know a lot about the diet and felt it was perfect for everyone. How could I question that a vegan or vegetarian diet could be inadequate for optimal health when even the American Dietetic Association gave the diet its stamp of approval?

It is the position of the American Dietetic Association that appropriately planned vegetarian diets, including total vegetarian or vegan diets, are healthful, nutritionally adequate, and may provide health benefits in the prevention and treatment of certain diseases. Well-planned vegetarian diets are appropriate for individuals during all stages of the life cycle, including pregnancy, lactation, infancy, childhood, and adolescence, and for athletes.[1]

A few years before my book came out, after I had been a raw vegan for several years, my health had begun to deteriorate somewhat. I was continually bloated, sometimes looking very pregnant. I know *now* it was due to my high-carb, low-protein diet. That type of diet doesn't work for my body, though it may for others.

I had tried all the right things: proper food combining, letting my digestive tract heal, drinking green smoothies. But the bloat would pop up nearly every time I ate a meal. Some raw fooders suggest going easy on the nuts to avoid bloat, but it is hard to get enough protein without them.

I eventually gained about ten or fifteen pounds, the amount I initially lost after going raw, and eventually even more. I would get very tired sometimes. This was because of eating too many carbs and releasing too much insulin. The fatigue grew stronger due to a deficiency of vitamin B_{12}. I was also so protein starved that I overate nuts and seeds, which are very high in calories.

Some might say, "Hey, you were postmenopausal, in your 50s, *what do you expect?*" I don't accept that concept. If I am on the perfect diet, I should be able to slow down the aging process. Otherwise, what is the point of being on a particular diet? Why spend so much money on healthful organic produce, why sacrifice some of my favorite treats, why go to the bother of making meals from scratch?

When I had first learned about the raw vegan diet, my first reaction was, "I will collapse from all those carbs and sparse protein!" As soon as I discovered raw desserts and packaged treats, I did. I would eat and then nap. I eventually gained weight. I was challenged several times with, "How can you be a raw fooder? I thought raw fooders were *thin*!"

I once gave a lecture just after eating at a raw food restaurant. My friend told me that my belly was all bloated. She could see a young woman sneering at me and appearing to be thinking, "Who wants to look like that?"

Alsoph Corwin, PhD of chemistry at Johns Hopkins University, may have the explanation for my weight gain.

The body hunger for missing essential amino acids may cause overconsumption of food in an effort to right the deficit.[2]

I'd see photos of myself and be shocked beyond belief at how big I was around the middle. Sometimes I'd go to give a lecture looking very slim and then eat a raw food dinner prior to speaking. Someone might take a photo of me talking, and I wouldn't believe how bloated and large around the waist I appeared. How could I tell people this was a weight-loss or health diet if it wasn't working for me?

Frankly, I was always so bloated that I looked like I was pregnant. If I ate a big salad or a raw gourmet meal, I would sometimes look as if I were five months pregnant, so I had to wear a baggy top. After I lost some weight through a low-calorie raw diet, I still looked pregnant — just three or four months along instead of five.

I discovered that the bloating can have many causes related to overeating carbs. Sometimes it is caused by high insulin levels telling the kidneys to retain sodium and hence water. Furthermore, a high-carbohydrate diet will reduce the secretions of

> *"Why is it so important to eat enough protein? Because your brain senses how much of it your body requires and prompts you to keep eating until you fulfill that need. This is why a diet lacking protein leads to obesity – your brain will always be telling you to eat more."*
>
> *–Arthur De Vany, PhD*
> *The New Evolution Diet*

hydrochloric acid needed to digest protein foods.

If we overeat carbs when not on a low-fat diet, we feed the candida yeast, which adds to bloating. In addition, a raw diet is rich in cellulosic fiber, which humans cannot digest. This doesn't mean we should avoid it, just that it may bloat you if you overeat it. If plant food is all you are eating, you'll likely take in so much cellulose that you will be bloated much of the time.

I was so bloated that I had to wear baggy tops, usually a large size — even though my hips were slim. I went on an anti-candida diet for about six weeks. The bloat left. I finally had a flat stomach, but if I went back to eating lots of fruit (I especially loved fresh orange juice), the bloat would return, even if the fruit was properly combined (eaten alone or with greens). It was the same with a lot of sprouts or a huge plate of salad, but less so.

One day, Aajonus Vonderplanitz (raw meat eater and author of *We Want to Live*) told me, "You are not an herbivore! Your digestive tract can't handle so much cellulose. Man was an ape that traded his gut for a bigger brain." I later learned he was right: I never get bloated with meat or eggs.

My thighs, once huge, firm, and muscular, became droopy skin — especially noticeable in a yoga pose known as the plow, in which the person lies down on the back and bends the legs over the face. This must be from aging, I thought, but that is not good enough.

I have read studies showing that losing muscle with age is unnecessary. According to my research, the effects of aging can be prevented or at least slowed down. Otherwise, there is not as much point in putting time and energy into any health practices.[*]

I knew the culprit was *not* the raw diet!

I was convinced that eating raw, organic foods was the greatest health secret. I had compiled 66 scientific studies in *The Live Food Factor* to prove it.[3] Eating raw changed my life and brought me to a whole new level of health. To this day, I eat at least 85 to 90 percent of my calories from raw foods.

There was something else wrong, but I didn't know what.

I went on a raw version of the Flat Belly Diet. I got rid of my belly by eating at every meal monounsaturated fats, on which the diet is based, but when I wrote about it in my newsletter, I got hate mail. People unsubscribed from my newsletter. They accused me of heresy.

"Eating that much (25 to 50 percent) fat can't possibly be healthy," people scolded. I was a heretic, straying from the essentials of raw foodism by prescribing this diet for women like me who yearned to have a slender waistline.

My memory had also been deteriorating. I'd had an outstanding memory, even graduating magna cum laude from my acupuncture college because of it. I took great pride in the fact that whenever I was talking and digressed, I could always recall what my original point was and get back to it.

I had now lost this ability and felt extremely frustrated. I would go into a room to get something and forget why I went there. If I was dialing a phone number, I could keep only 2 or 3 digits in my head at once before needing to look at the number again. I would go to the food co-op, which I went to regularly at least once a week, and be unable to remember my co-op number. I knew it was really, really bad when I couldn't even remember my husband's cell phone number. There was a moment when *even his name* was on the tip of my tongue!

You can't give me the old line, "Oh, it's just a part of getting older." You see, the whole point of studying and pursuing peak health is that we can extend our health span.

There are records of people living over 100 years in great health.[4] Even in our toxic, polluted environment, we should be able to live much longer than the typical 80 years, and we should stay very healthy if we follow a healthful lifestyle.

Even as soon as my flagrantly pro-vegan book was fresh off the press, I was being prompted to learn about the pitfalls of veganism. A string of coincidences made the message undeniable: my poor memory, my weight gain, and the alarming results of some blood tests.

I started researching weight loss. I couldn't market my book as a weight-loss diet if I was overweight myself. While researching, I wrote an e-

---

[*]See chapter 1 of my earlier book *The Live Food Factor* for ten reasons to eat a high-raw diet, health and antiaging being two.

book with all sorts of weight-loss tips.

I began to catch up on all the Dr. Barry Sears Zone Diet books. As I read *The Omega Rx Zone*, I discovered how important *docosahexaenoic acid* (DHA), an omega-3 essential fatty acid, was to the brain. I also learned from Dr. Nicholas Perricone's books just how vital omega-3 fats were for weight loss. It is the only true weight-loss "silver bullet" he had found.

I grew convinced that pharmaceutical-grade fish oil was the most critical supplement to take. A friend of mine was taking krill oil. I stumbled upon an article by Dr. Joseph Mercola, DO, whose website has a major Internet impact, saying that it was five times more bioavailable than fish oil, so my husband and I experimented with it as well.

After about three weeks of taking a mega-dose of six to nine grams per day of fish or krill oil, my memory improved. My mood improved to the point that initially I was feeling quite blissful. Fish oil increases serotonin. My brain was starving for it! The *eicosapentaenoic acid* (EPA) in the fish is needed by the nervous system for well-being. After about a month, I went down to three grams a day.

I also found keeping the weight off much easier. I was more energetic and could even climb the hill at the daily walk I took much more easily.

Eventually, I had to cut back to about a gram or so a day because any more than that produced gas, perhaps from toxic lipid peroxides. For about a year, I continued to take purified fish oil for the DHA and EPA. At the time, no vegan algae product contained EPA for emotional well-being. I switched later to cod liver oil, since it also contains vitamins D and A, which plant products don't contain.

While studying and researching for the weight-loss book, I came across several tests I felt I should get in order to see how I was doing. I went in for blood tests and found I had high LDL (the "bad" cholesterol) and high triglycerides, both of which are bad biomarkers for heart health. I now know these were from excessive carbs.

I also had a B_{12} deficiency. B_{12} is reliably found only in animal foods. We make some in our digestive tracts and mouths but not much. Some people make enough for themselves; most others, like me, don't.

I realized that this deficiency was not some-thing to mess with, as it could cause permanent damage to the nervous system. So I took bi-monthly injections and proceeded to research how to get it into my diet. I found that liver had the most, and red meat had more than white meat.

For years, I had even been taking sublingual B_{12}. I took the best kind, methylcobalamin, and one of the top brands. This proves that it's always best to get nutrients from food sources, not supplements, in which they are far less bioavailable.

In addition, I had a vitamin D deficiency. D is available in food form only from animals. Contrary to myth, most of us cannot get enough from sunshine alone. I likely had a vitamin K_2 deficiency also. My skeleton was headed for an osteoporosis train wreck!

My hair was falling out a lot (insufficient protein), and my muscles were diminishing, replaced by flab. As we'll see later, I was burning sugar, not fat.

I was stunned to find out about all this. I realized that a nervous facial twitch I had developed must have been caused by the B_{12} deficiency. My liver probably stored enough for just a few years. Once that was depleted in 2006, I began to exhibit some deficiency symptoms.

I was also getting bags under my eyes. I read somewhere that insufficient B_{12} can cause this condition. In addition, I experienced drooling on my pillow while sleeping, another sign of B_{12} deficiency.

Introducing Dr. Stanley Bass

Dr. Stanley Bass, ND, DC, PhC, PhD, DO, DSc, DD, is a hidden gem. He is 93 years old, outliving many vegan leaders in the raw food movement in part because he recognized early on the deficiencies that often arise on vegan diets.

When I told him about my B_{12} deficiency, he related the story of how Dr. Christopher Gian-Cursio, a hygienic doctor, had discovered the need for animal nutrients by observing the effects that strict veganism had produced across three generations in one family of his patients.

Dr. Bass taught me to eat raw egg yolks when I consulted him over the phone. He suggested I eat three eggs a day. In order to be able to consume the whites for their protein, I could do as Dr. Cursio suggested and boil the egg whites for just two minutes, throwing them into water that was already boiling. The yolks would still be raw, folded in with the poached egg white as an omelet. I added chopped onions, tomatoes, and other vegetables to them.

I also included some raw kefir and raw goat cheese once or twice a week.

Dr. Bass had once experimented with raising mice on various diets for four years. He found that the raw vegan mice were killing each other to eat their brains! Those fed raw egg yolks would thrive. He said if people won't eat meat, they should eat three egg yolks a day to get B vitamins, including B_{12}, as well as small amounts of vitamins A and D.

My local doctor had me on bimonthly B_{12} injections for about a year, but the deficiency symptoms still persisted, even when the blood levels checked okay. That may be because blood tests are not the most accurate measurement of B_{12} status: the urine MMA test is better. Meanwhile, I conversed with Dr. Bass from time to time as he dared me to go down the rabbit hole. He gave me a list of books to read that challenged many of my vegetarian beliefs.

Eating Meat Brings Improvement

Let me make clear that I do not particularly like the taste of meat, raw or cooked, with the exception of highly seasoned cooked meat, such as chicken curry and Kentucky Fried Chicken, which has the "secret" ingredient monosodium glutamate (MSG)! I find it bland, tasteless, and as far as culinary factors go, a waste of calories.

I would often look back at my experience of having tried raw meat for a month with great disgust. *What was I thinking? How could I have done that?* Eating meat after a few years of vegetarianism seemed like cannibalism or vampirism.

☞ Even after the B_{12} tests, I refused to eat meat for a year. I resisted, as I was disgusted by the idea of eating meat after 6 years without it.

I was afraid of spiritual devolution. There are so many vegetarian books that make it seem as though you can't possibly be part of the spiritual scene if you are still eating meat.

Most of all, *I didn't want to be a hypocrite*, not practicing what I preached in my book.

Desperate situations make us do things we thought we'd never do. I remember the one and a half years I worked at multi-level marketing (MLM) full-time. Making cold calls every morning, I was sure that if I put in the time and money, I could be one of the few who make it work, living forever on residual income. After using up nearly all my savings, I realized the MLM stood for Many Losing Money.

I began to realize the problem was not with *me* but with the *industry*. It is set up so that only one in a hundred really makes good money, because you need a steady hundred in your downline. I knew a few could make it work. Those people were usually charismatic leader types who had vast social connections and had the luck to hit upon a new, fast-growing company that was destined for stability. At that turning point, I realized that trying to succeed at MLM was for me like putting a round peg into a square hole.

I had that same epiphany one day with diet. It wasn't that I was not trying hard enough, not detoxifying enough, or lacking discipline; it was that I simply had a biological need for meat (especially small, oily fish) for optimal health. The vegetarian diet did not suit my body's constitution any more than MLM suited my personality.

I went to Whole Foods to get clean meat, the flesh of free-range animals fed their natural, organic diet, without having been tortured with hormones, antibiotics, and steroids. Afraid someone might recognize me, I made sure my cloth grocery bag was lying over the tell-tale meat package. When I got home, I marinated it overnight to kill any parasites — and ate it raw!

So, after about a year of being raw ovo-lacto vegetarian (vegan plus eggs and some dairy), I began to eat raw, wild fish and free-range, organic-fed chicken, both marinated in lemon juice in order to kill any parasites. My health and energy improved.

I hadn't eaten meat in over six years, and I never thought I would again. My intuition eventually sent me the message to try red meat. I ate some dehydrated, free-range, pasture-fed buffalo. Eating three or four ounces of that every day alleviated my B_{12} deficiency symptoms, but they are still there to some degree. I may have permanently damaged my nervous system.

A funny thing happened when I resumed eating meat, just three to four ounces a day. My appetite lessened, and my blood sugar became more stable.

I had been diagnosed twice in my youth as being hypoglycemic. Both times I had the whole fasting glucose study done. Even after those tests, I remained in deep denial because of my fondness for carbohydrates, which I considered the fun foods. Yet I couldn't deny it: I felt great with just a little meat (usually fish) in my diet once a day — and not even every day. Sometimes I just ate a few eggs.

When I added meat to my diet, my B_{12} stabilized. I no longer needed injections. I kept a food journal, simply writing down what I ate and noticing how I felt each day. I noticed I was less hungry and more productive when I ate meat or two to three eggs at breakfast time. My blood sugar stabilized, and I wouldn't crave food all day.

Other Benefits

Other benefits have accrued since I started including animal foods in my diet. Blood tests showed my *high-density lipoprotein* (HDL) got higher, and my triglycerides and *low-density lipoprotein* (LDL) got lower. HDL is supposed to be high. Pamela McDonald, author of *The Perfect Gene Diet*, explains.

> HDL provides our body with a natural artery-cleaning service. You simply cannot have too much of this good type of cholesterol.[5]

I am almost never hungry. On a high-carb raw vegan diet, I was frequently hungry. But when I eat fewer carbs and incorporate more animal protein, I find I never get hungry. It is easier than ever for me to eat a high-raw diet because I have so little interest in food, especially the cooked carbs that used to tempt me.

Another great benefit: My food prep time is less than it's ever been! I no longer crave complicated recipes with intense, stimulating flavors.

Furthermore, I am saving money because I no longer need to buy so many supplements. I was always taking things as a vegan and vegetarian because these diets are low in certain nutrients, as I will point out later in the book. I now get every-

thing from nutrient-rich, wild meat and cod liver oil in addition to mineral-rich plant foods. For the most part, I use supplements only as needed.

Best of all, my brain is sharper than it's ever been. The real improvement occurred when I got my carb intake down to 100 grams a day or less. My brain worked better than it ever had in my life. When I curb my carbs, I am clear, sharp, focused, and my memory is better than ever.

If I make a mental note of a page number (not having a book marker handy), I often even recall the exact page numbers where I read things. This is quite a turnaround for someone who couldn't remember her husband's cell phone number!

Whenever I go a week or more eating 100 grams of carbs a day (or less), I read faster than I have ever read in my life, and I often find I get bored with "soft," or light, reading material. I find myself often preferring science, college textbooks, and things that used to be a chore to plow through. Things that were once very challenging for me to understand are much clearer, as my mind is now performing at a higher level.

I usually refrain from writing about what I eat because it changes all the time. But after much experimentation and especially after building back my muscles and replenishing my fat-soluble vitamins, I found I don't need to eat meat every day.

Presently, I eat two or three eggs for breakfast nearly every day with chopped vegetables (no bread, potatoes, bacon, etc!), four ounces of raw liver every week or two, and about three ounces of fish three times a week. The best fishes are wild salmon and small, oily fish like sardines, herring, or mackerel. Where I live, it is hard to find those small, oily fish *raw*, but the canned ones have been steamed at about 130° F, so at least toxic by-products are not being formed. The fish keeps me mentally sharp and very happy.

I also enjoy a very large vegetable salad every night, using only vinegar as dressing and adding avocados and olives for flavor and healthful fats. I enjoy fruit in moderation, especially apples, berries, and mangos. I drink blended greens with lemon juice, ginger, and stevia added to reduce their bitter taste rather than making fruit smoothies.

Chapter 2

Vegetarian Myths Dispelled

The great enemy of the truth is very often not the lie — deliberate, contrived and dishonest — but the myth — persistent, persuasive, and unrealistic.   —President John F. Kennedy

There are some common misconceptions in the vegetarian community we will briefly address here. Some of these issues will be fleshed out in more detail later in the book.

Myth #1: We should emulate the diets of our mainly vegetarian primate cousins.

The most relevant difference between man and other apes is man's relatively larger brain. Our brains are believed to have evolved precisely because we ate animal products rich in DHA, a critically important fatty acid which chiefly comprises brain tissue. To maintain our brains, we need to continue eating this crucial fat.

When man split off from chimpanzees, he traded an energy-intensive digestive tract with the ability to digest cellulose for an energy-intensive brain. In other words, more energy was required to maintain this larger brain endowed with advanced, forward-looking frontal lobes. The energy used for the brain had to be subtracted from elsewhere, and it came at the expense of the digestive tract.

We then began eating energy-dense food that didn't require such intensive digestion. For example, a cow has to devote so much energy to digestion that it has four stomachs! More energy is directed there than to the cow's brain.

The area between the chest and legs of a gorilla is much bigger than it is in man. The gorilla has a larger digestive tract equipped to break down cellulose, a dietary fiber. A chimpanzee is somewhere in between a gorilla and a human, having more intelligence than a gorilla, but less ability to break down cellulose. A chimp also eats more meat than a gorilla but less than a man.

Myth #2: Apes and chimpanzees are strict vegetarians.

Chimpanzees were once thought to be vegetarians. Jane Goodall, who studied them extensively, proved that this was not the case. We now know that 8 to 10 percent of their diet comes from animal foods: insects, bird eggs, and even meat. Flesh is thought to be about 1 to 3 percent of their diet.[1] Some say it is as high as 5 percent.

H. Leon Abrams, Jr., MA, EDS, Associate Professor Emeritus of Anthropology at the University of Georgia and well-known nutritional anthropologist, relates the diets of monkeys and apes.

> Rather than being herbivores, these animals are now recognized as omnivores, and the reason that they do not eat more animal food than they do may be the result of a limited ability to provide it in great abundance. But in seeking the animal foods that they do consume, monkeys and apes are most likely driven by a basic need to meet nutritional requirements that are available only from animal protein.[2]

Abrams points out that golden marmosets in zoos were not breeding until given animal protein. Baboons often kill hares and gazelles. He claims that gorillas in the wild eat birds, rodents, and *even small antelopes*. In captivity, they prefer meat to their usual diets of fruits and vegetables. Orangutans eat insects, birds, and squirrels, while gibbons consume birds, small antelopes, and rodents.

> Apparently, all primates have a basic and fundamental physiological need for at least a minimum amount of animal protein.[3]

Myth #3: We haven't adapted to meat.

The first homo genus, *Homo habilis*, was a meat eater 2.6 million years ago. Some vegetarians familiar with this fact will claim that we were originally frugivores in Africa but have been "eating against our nature for millions of years." Clearly they do not understand the principles of evolution: 2.6 million years is plenty of time to adapt! What we *haven't* adapted to are grains and high-carb diets.

Some speculate that our primate ancestors were frugivores over 5 million years ago, though others claim the African savanna was actually lower in plant life than the forests and arid regions. Even if the frugivore concept is correct, our digestive tracts have changed so much in 5 million years that one could very easily argue we are no longer adapted to primarily fruit diets.

Empirical observation indicates that this is the case. Our digestive tracts have grown shorter, our brains bigger. We need more protein and essential fats than a frugivorous diet provides. Most of us cannot tolerate the high carbs of a grain- and legume-based vegetarian diet, let alone a frugivorous diet high in sugar.

Myth #4: Vegetarianism is no fad — it has been around for thousands of years.

It takes about 40,000 years (2,000 generations) for our genes to make major changes. From an evolutionary stance, *agriculture is a fad*. Even modern-day cooking is a fad, an experiment that has sacrificed our health. While it is true some people can live long lives on vegetarian diets, it can be speculated that many of those same people would have lived significantly longer and with better health had they included at least some quality meat, especially organ meats and seafood, rich in nutrients not found in plant foods.

Veganism has gained popularity in less than 100 years, really gaining momentum only in the last 40. Many of the dangers have already been noticed, but the full impact of this experiment's deficiencies will not be known for decades when long-term vegans get older. Some doctors believe that each generation of vegans grows more nutrient deficient.

Myth #5: We are not fast runners, so could not catch potential prey.

Our ancestors eating natural diets were able to run so long that they exhausted the deer they were chasing.[4] Humans are not as fast as most animals, but their endurance is far greater. They can chase a herd until the slowest or weakest animal must rest. Native Americans chased down animals on foot. The Tarahumara of northern Mexico chased deer through the mountains until the animals collapsed from exhaustion.[5]

Humans are excellent runners because they do not get overheated while running, due to less body hair and to their ability to sweat. In fact, some an-

thropologists believe that these changes evolved in order to enable man to hunt down animals.[6]

Additional changes that enabled us to run faster and longer than other primates include a more balanced head, shorter forearms for balance, longer legs to take huge strides, an enlarged heel bone, as well as larger surface areas in the hip, knee, and ankle joints for better shock absorption, larger buttocks for stabilization in running, and larger vertebrae and disks relative to body mass for shock absorption.[7]

Myth #6: We don't have claws, strong jaws, and sharp teeth like predators.

According to Harold Hawkins, author of the textbook *Applied Nutrition*, 20 of our 32 teeth are of the meat-eating type. Even if that weren't the case, man has been a toolmaker since the dawn of the homo line. He is able to create tools because he has hands with dexterous fingers. In fact, even other primates have been known to make tools! Tools eliminated the need to evolve sharp teeth, claws, and strong jaws.

Furthermore, man began cooking meat long before he began cooking plant material. This enabled the meat to be chewed more easily. Oral features were also influenced by the larger brain, which needed more space, and the development of language, which required a flexible oral system: flexible jaws, tongue, and esophagus. Bipedal posture also influenced the human head shape.

Myth #7: Paleo man may have eaten meat, but it shortened his lifespan.

In reality, scientists do not have any way to determine how long paleo humans lived. Dr. Staffan Lindeberg, MD, PhD, at the University of Lund, Sweden, explains that paleo man may have lived as long as Westerners do today. If a fossil skeleton is that of a child or young adult, the age can be estimated relatively accurately. If older, osteologists often estimate "40 years or older," having no way to determine more precisely. An adult skeleton could be 40, or it could be 90. There are not a great number of these skeletons around for scientists to do a comparative analysis.[8]

Scholars cite agriculture as the culprit for most

diseases. Using epidemiology, anthropology, and archeology, experts have found that pre-agricultural man had greater health than modern man, busting the myth that paleo man was malnourished and ill.[9]

Myth #8: A diet low in saturated fats and cholesterol is more healthful.

The very foundations of the vegetarian diet's health benefits have now been proven false, which will be explained later. We need adequate amounts of saturated fats and cholesterol to have healthy brains and nervous systems. Diets too low in these necessary fats can actually impair the brain and nervous system.

Myth #9: Meat is toxic and causes cancer.

This is true only for modern, factory-farmed meat, which is full of pesticides, hormones, steroids, and antibiotics.

The types of meat can also be important. For example, consumption of processed meats and overeating of red meat can increase the chances of colorectal cancer, while eating fish decreases that risk.[10]

In one study, it was found that a high intake of red meat and processed meat increased mortality rates from cancer and cardiovascular disease, while consumption of white meat was associated with lower rates of cancer. In other words, go easy on eating mammals, and avoid nitrate-cured meats like hot dogs, cold cuts, bacon, ham, and deli meats.[11]

Modern meats also contain much more saturated fat and omega-6 fat than wild meats. Wild meats eaten by our hunter-gatherer ancestors were very low in fat, and the fat they did have was extremely healthful, rich in omega-3 fats.

Furthermore, the claim that vegetarians have lower cancer rates has not held up to scrutiny. A 1994 study comparing vegetarians with the general population found that although vegetarians have slightly lower cancer rates in some areas, the cancer rate of vegetarians is actually *higher* in other areas: endometrial, prostate, brain, malignant melanoma, uterine, cervical, ovarian, Hodgkin's disease.[12]

Even so, meat cooked at high temperatures and dairy are prime promoters of prostate cancer. Their consumption results in the production of dihydro-

testosterone, a carcinogenic form of testosterone, in the prostate.

Researchers at the Cancer Research UK Epidemiology Unit at the University of Oxford stated in their article about vegetarian and vegan diets, "Studies of cancer have not shown clear differences in cancer rates between vegetarians and nonvegetarians."[13]

Myth #10: Meat is overstimulating, which is why you feel more energized after eating it.

You experience sustained energy with meat because it stabilizes your blood sugar. Carbohydrates stimulate insulin release, which can result in a quick boost followed by a sudden drop in energy.

Red meat also contains carnitine, which improves your mitochondrial metabolism and function, giving you more even energy.

Myth #11: Our digestive tracts are like those of herbivores.

The human digestive tract is like that of the omnivorous pig, not like that of a ruminant or herbivore. The human and pig digestive systems are very similar. That's why pigs are typically used for dissection in biology classes. Their digestive systems include all the same organs that we have: the esophagus, the stomach, the liver, the gallbladder, the spleen, the pancreas, and the small and large intestines. The functions of the organs are the same as well.

Pigs do best on a human paleolithic diet of vegetables, fruit, meat, and a small amount of potatoes. They experience better insulin resistance, lower blood pressure, and less inflammation.[14]

Unlike cows, we have only one stomach. Our digestive tract is intermediate in length between that of a carnivore and that of an herbivore, as Ruth F. Rosevear, LD, NC, explains.

Our digestive tract is 68 percent omnivorous. To find this out, divide the length of the spine into the length of the intestines. In an herbivore like sheep, the result is 26; in a carnivore, seven. Man is in the middle with 13 times the length of the spine. Most physiology books will show how a dog has short intestines, the cow a long intestine, and man a middle length.[15]

Technically, we are not omnivores because

omni- means everything, and we cannot digest most grains very well.[*]

Myth #12: You can get all the nutrients you need from a diet of plants alone.

This is a dangerous belief since it doesn't apply to everybody. We now know that most plant sources of B_{12} are only B_{12} analogues and can actually increase your need for B_{12}. Analogues are similar enough to compete for the same receptor sites as the truly usable B_{12}, creating a situation in which you have less metabolically available B_{12}. There are a few seaweed sources of small amounts of B_{12} but only if they are truly raw.

True vitamin A is found only in animal foods. Most people are not efficient in converting beta-carotene into vitamin A, besides which, to consume sufficient amounts would mean eating or juicing a vegetable diet very expensive in time and money.

It is also difficult to get enough DHA, zinc, B_6, CoQ_{10}, taurine, carnosine, and carnitine from a plant-only diet. Some of these nutrients can be synthesized in the body, but the conversion is often not efficient.

Myth #13: We can supplement for whatever animal food nutrients we cannot get from plants.

New nutrients are still being discovered from time to time.[16] There could be many nutrients found only in animal foods that are critical for some people and which have not yet been discovered or developed into supplements. Many vegans ruined their nervous systems and brains before B_{12} and DHA were discovered. Nutrition is a relatively new science. The first vitamin was discovered as recently as 1912. The importance of omega-3 fats was identified only in the 1970s. The glycemic index was first formulated in 1981.[17] There are too many issues and nutrients we still don't know about. Relying on pills is too simplistic.

Furthermore, nutrients work together synergistically. For this reason, it is always better to get them from whole foods in the proper ratios and bal-

ances that humans evolved eating.

Finally, synthetic vitamins are often not assimilated properly by the body. I was taking sublingual B_{12} and yet developed a B_{12} deficiency. Even after taking B_{12} injections for a year, I still had some deficiency symptoms. It wasn't until I started eating meat again that I returned to peak health.

Myth #14: A vegetarian or vegan diet will help you lose weight.

This is not true for people who are not carb types[†] and don't digest carbs well. They might actually gain weight on these diets. Their triglycerides can also become elevated.

For most people, our pancreases have not evolved to tolerate diets as high in carbs as modern-day omnivorous diets, let alone vegetarian diets. Young people appear to get away with it, but they often find themselves with a midlife spread by their 40s.

Some people do lose weight on raw vegan diets. But after a while, one can even gain weight. To get enough protein, a person will eat so many nuts and seeds that he gets sleepy, because these foods are so high in fat. Another factor is that nuts can be hard to digest, even if soaked, increasing fatigue. The extra fat calories from all the nuts and seeds add fat to your body. This is especially true for women, who put on weight more easily than men. Nutritionist Natalia Rose agrees.

> The raw food community comes out hailing the virtues of raw oils and coconut butter — some even promote the fiction that they can eat as much of it as they want and not gain weight! I quickly realized that by and large it was the men in the movement that were praising these fatty substances. Men metabolize fats much more easily; it's a more complex issue for women.[18]

Some people gain weight on vegetarian, vegan, or even raw vegan diets. This is because when you overeat carbs, your body secretes excess insulin. Insulin is a hormone, a metabolic instigator, and one of its messages to the body is "*store fat!*"

When you eat carbs without dietary fat in your

[*]For more information, see "The Biological Case for Omnivorism" on page 53.

[†]See chapter 10.

body, you may find this to be less of a problem. If you go on Doug Graham's 80/10/10 diet of 80 percent carbs (mainly fruit, because it takes too many greens and vegetables to get enough calories), 10 percent protein, and 10 percent fat, your insulin levels won't remain high for long.

The issue I had with that diet is that it simply wasn't enough protein and fat to sustain my health for the long term. It makes a great cleanse; most people can go on it for as long as three months without problems, but I have encountered at least a dozen people who lost teeth or got several cavities from eating so much fruit.

Researchers found that even though the omnivores ate more carbs, they had fewer AGEs because they ate less fruit!

In my own case, I became fatigued on a low-fat diet — my skin grew dry, my energy plummeted, and my brain didn't function. I was not getting enough protein and essential fatty acids.

When you are relying on sugar instead of fat for fuel, you crave carbs. As you eat them, your blood sugar rises, especially if the carbs are cooked, because cooked carbs are absorbed more quickly than the same carbs raw.

On such a diet, you tend to get hungry all the time because you are burning sugar, not fat. This is why so many vegans lose muscle and get flabby. Note that this applies less to younger people, as they can switch quickly from burning sugar to burning fat on an as-needed basis. It may not apply at all if you are a carb type.

However, when you are burning fat, as you do on a low-carb diet, you don't feel hungry when you go several hours without eating. This is because your body simply taps into its fat reserves and burns those for fuel. Another factor in the lack of hunger is that your blood sugar remains stable. You are burning fat because you are on a low-carb diet that doesn't spike your insulin levels.

Many trials have been carried out in the last decade comparing the weight loss and health effects of low-fat vs. low-carb diets. The low-carb dieters in general lost more weight and had much healthier profiles of HDL, blood pressure, and triglycerides. Their risk of heart attacks decreased. The head of one such trial was a vegetarian for 25 years and hoped to prove the opposite, proclaiming it a "bitter pill to swallow" when he saw that those on the Atkins Diet fared much better than the low-fat dieters.[19]

Myth #15: A vegetarian ages more slowly and looks younger.

Eating fruit and cooked carbs leads to higher blood sugar levels. When our blood is bathed in glucose sugar, it reacts with, and attaches to, the proteins of which our tissues are composed to form advanced glycation end products (AGEs), which age us. The results of glycation,[*] the bonding of sugar to protein, show up on our skin as well, producing wrinkles.

Fructose (fruit sugar) consumption results in much, much more glycation than glucose. In one study, researchers compared 19 vegetarians with 19 omnivorous people and found that even though the omnivores ate *more carbs*, they had fewer AGEs because they ate *less fruit!*[20]

Furthermore, the dipeptide *carnosine* is found only in meat. Carnosine suppresses AGE formation, glycation, cross-linking, and protein oxidation.[21]

Myth #16: If a diet makes you feel good the first year or two, it will be good for a lifetime.

This seems very rational. After all, a year or two is a long time. But the body can store B_{12} in the liver, as well as fat-soluble vitamins, like A and D. Deficiencies of these vitamins can take years, or even a decade, to show up.

---

[*]*Glycation* is the product of the nonenzymatic reaction between a sugar and the free amino group(s) of proteins.

Myth #17: Vegetarians live about 7 to 9 years longer.

Studies have shown that many of the health benefits attributed to vegetarians were actually because these folks are more health conscious. They get exercise regularly, don't smoke, and take supplements. For example, in a study done by Dean Ornish, a group was instructed to exercise a minimum of three times a week, use stress management for an hour a day, eat a vegetarian diet, and attend group support sessions twice a week. The control group were told nothing. The experimental group's progress was attributed to the diet, although the participants were adding all those other health-promoting activities too!

A study on California Seventh-Day Adventists showed a similar result.

Choices regarding diet, exercise, cigarette smoking, body weight, and hormone replacement therapy in combination appear to change life expectancy by many years. The longevity experience of Adventists probably demonstrates the beneficial effects of more optimal behaviors.[22]

Adventists consider health a virtue and strive toward it. Diet is only one component of a multitude of health factors that also include a strong social support system.

Another study of 34,000 Seventh-Day Adventists who were vegetarians found them to be healthy and have a low mortality rate. But when compared to other groups of people, such as Mormon high priests who also have healthful lifestyles but include meat in their diets, there was no benefit in being vegetarian. The decrease in mortality rate was found to be from the healthful lifestyle.[23]

Other studies show that while a vegetarian diet may moderately decrease the risk of ischemic heart disease, it has no overall benefits when compared to diets of health-conscious omnivores.[24]

A study done in Germany found that health-conscious people live as long as vegetarians and even have about a 10 percent lower mortality rate on average. Vegetarians showed a slightly higher (4

percent) rate of death from cancer, although the death rate from circulatory or ischemic heart disease was a tiny bit lower in vegetarians.[25]

One study found that in Europe, those in countries eating the most animal products have the healthiest people. There were no significant benefits to being a vegetarian as opposed to a health-conscious nonvegetarian. The study indicated that it is ample consumption of fruits and vegetables and not the exclusion of meat that makes vegetarians healthy.[26]

> *It is the ample consumption of fruits and vegetables and not the exclusion of meat that makes vegetarians healthy.*

Walter Willet, MD, professor of epidemiology at the Harvard School of Public Health, stated that "low intake of red meat does not seem to be an adequate explanation for the general good health of vegetarian populations." He felt it was a higher intake of fruits, vegetables, fiber, antioxidants, and phytochemicals that added to their good health.[27]

One study that reviewed the data from five studies to compare the death rates among vegetarians, vegans, and omnivores discovered the following: a 20 percent lower mortality rate from ischemic heart disease among those that occasionally ate meat, a 26 percent rate lower among vegans, and a 34 percent lower rate for those who ate fish but not other meat. But other causes of death did not show significant differences.

There were no significant differences between vegetarians and nonvegetarians in mortality from cerebrovascular disease, stomach cancer, colorectal cancer, lung cancer, breast cancer, prostate cancer, or all other causes combined.[28]

A study in Japan found benefits to flesh consumption.

Nutrient intakes in 94 Japanese centenarians investigated between 1972 and 1973 showed a higher proportion of animal protein to total proteins than in contemporary average Japanese. ... High intakes of milk and fats and oils had favorable effects on 10-year (1976–1986) survivorship in 422 urban residents aged 69–71. The survivors revealed a longitudinal increase in intakes of animal foods such as eggs, milk, fish, and meat over the 10 years.[29]

It was also found that in Okinawa, the region

of Japan with the highest life expectancy, the proportion of energy from proteins and fats was significantly higher than that of Akita Prefecture, where the life expectancies were much shorter. Intakes of carbohydrates and salt were also lower in the Okinawan.[30]

Finally, Dr. Russell Smith, a statistician, analyzed all the existing studies on vegetarianism in 1991, including the Kahn and Snowden study.

> In effect the Kahn [and Snowden] study is yet another example of negative results which are massaged and misinterpreted to support the politically correct assertions that vegetarians live longer lives.

When all of the data are taken into account, the actual differences of heart disease between vegetarians and nonvegetarians in these studies were hardly a significant amount.[31] Snowden calculated risk ratios and concluded that coronary heart disease mortality increased as meat consumption increased, but the rates of increase were insignificant at 0.04 percent for males and 0.01 percent for females.

Dr. Smith suspected that many studies were left unpublished because they showed the inferiority of a vegetarian diet, and those who ran the studies had hoped to show the opposite. He also found that as animal food consumption increased in several of the studies, mortality decreased! In other words, the vegetarians lived *shorter* lives than people who included meat in their diets.

The yearly all-cause death rate of vegetarian men is slightly higher than for omnivores (0.93 percent vs. 0.89 percent) but a lot higher in vegetarian women (0.86 percent vs. 0.54 percent). Every year, vegetarian women die at a rate of 0.32 percent higher than that of omnivores![32]

Myth #18: Eating meat is unnatural and disgusting, chosen only by conditioning.

Babies have been known to love meat. In fact, Guy-Claude Burger was the modern promoter of the Instinctive Diet,[33] a diet in which people use their instincts to decide what to eat. He fed his day-old newborn meat that was pre-chewed in his wife's mouth. The infant chose to eat it and slept peacefully through the night. Its stools were normal.

Eating preferences are personal and can change. For years I hated fish. When I tried it fresh from the ocean, I tolerated it but didn't love it. Once

I tried raw seviche, I became hooked.

Some people love hot dogs and processed meat, but those with more refined tastes enjoy wild game infinitely better than factory-farmed meat.

I know plenty of people who hate eating vegetables, while they are a favorite food for others. I know more who cannot stand durians, a smelly fruit, while others adore them.

Even though liver is one of the world's greatest super foods, many people have not cultivated a taste for it. Natto, a fermented Asian soy dish with a very strong odor, is likely the only plant food with significant levels of vitamin K_2, critical for the bones. It is so stinky that the Japanese restaurants that serve it have a separate room for people who order it. Healthful foods are not always the best tasting, especially when our tastes have been so corrupted by diets high in sugar, salt, and food additives.

Tastes also change with time and circumstances. When I had been a vegan for several years, I would wonder how I could have ever eaten meat, but after a few weeks of eating it again, I wondered how I could have ever thought that this was unnatural. I grew up absolutely despising the taste of fish. Now I eat small, oily fish because they are crucial for my brain and well-being.

In *The Butcher and the Vegetarian*, vegetarian-raised Tara Weaver takes us on her journey of eating various kinds of meat for the first time. Her descriptions indicate a very innate, primal love of meat, like having "died and gone to carnivore heaven." She also noted that nothing she ever cooked elicited as much excitement from guests as her meat dishes, though her vegetarian dishes were tastier. "No one oohs and ahhs over vegetarian food — certainly no one ever claps."[34] She attributes that to a primordial memory of our ancestors having gathered around the kill from the hunt.

Myth #19: We all need to become vegetarians for global food sustainability.

Agriculture is what is destroying the planet. It destroys the topsoil. It creates deserts. Agriculture, which accelerated with the use of petroleum fuel, created overpopulation, which is destroying the land and creating the extinction of numerous species.

Suppose we remove all animals' habitats and

put domesticated animals in zoos so they wouldn't go extinct, and use all land for crops to feed people. It might feed everyone for a time, but everyone would have poor health because our bodies evolved with dependencies on certain nutrients found in animal products, as we shall see in chapter 6.

Most of us need to eat low-carb diets for peak health. On a high-carb, vegetarian diet, many of us would see our health and our brains deteriorate, and our life spans would greatly decrease. It would be very unsustainable to each individual. To a large degree, this is what happened in India. They now have a large population of undernourished people with short life spans.

Myth #20: You can't reach high spiritual planes when eating flesh.

This is a very subjective experience. If someone feels that way, it may be true for him. He may then decide that his spiritual growth is more important than peak health. Yet there have been numerous great spiritual leaders throughout history who ate meat. Didn't Jesus even multiply the fish? Why would he do that if he thought it was unspiritual to eat them?

Myth #21: We can all reach peak health as vegetarians.

Many people — perhaps a majority — are sensitive to excess carbs. We evolved eating low-glycemic, low-carb diets. Nondairy animal products are the only foods with almost zero carbs. There appear to be different metabolic types, as we shall see. Some people do thrive on vegetarian and even vegan diets.

Myth #22: A high-protein diet is bad for the kidneys and creates osteoporosis.

First of all, a high-protein diet is not recommended. Eating 15 to 30 percent of one's calories in protein, depending on your metabolic type, is considered *adequate* protein, not *high*. Second, a low-protein diet may be called for in kidney disease, but if one is healthy, kidneys are not harmed by protein, especially if it is not cooked.

Studies have shown that an adequate protein diet is great for the bones, in fact necessary for strong bones. After all, they are partially composed of protein. Some studies that showed protein was bad for the bones were using unnatural foods, such as whey powder.[*]

---

[*]See chapter 16.

Chapter 3

Origins of Vegetarianism and Veganism

As yet I have not found a single group of primitive racial stock which was building and maintaining excellent bodies by living entirely on plant foods. I have found in many parts of the world most devout representatives of modern ethical systems advocating the restriction of foods to the vegetable products. In every instance where the groups involved had been long under the teaching, I found evidence of degeneration in the form of dental caries, and in the new generation in the form of abnormal dental arches to an extent very much higher than in the primitive groups who were not under this influence.

—Dr. Weston Price, *Nutrition and Physical Degeneration*

As previously mentioned, I am defining a vegetarian as one who doesn't eat any flesh foods other than eggs. Dairy might also be included. Vegetarianism thus defined has been fairly widespread for a few thousand years, but that's just a blink of the eye in our human evolutionary history.

Origins of Vegetarianism

Eastern Origins

The concept of *ahimsa* (nonviolence to, and the sacredness of, all living creatures) began thousands of years ago in India in the religion of Hinduism, which has a number of gods that are represented by animal images. The cow is especially revered and allowed to go anywhere it wants.

Once while in India, I was waiting for my train at the station and got annoyed that someone had rudely bumped into me. When I turned around to give the person a dirty look, I laughed when I saw that it was a cow!

I adore India. I have been there three times. There are few places in the world where you can go to a small city and see such diverse life on the streets: cows, pigs, goats, monkeys, and the occasional elephant! Nowhere is there a country that so loves animals. The people even dedicate temples to the animals and offer them food.

But did the citizenry's vegetarian diets develop out of reverence, or did they arise from sustainability issues?

Rudolph Ballentine, MD, the medical director of the Himalayan International Institute of Yoga Science and Philosophy in Honesdale, Pennsylvania, is the author of *Diet and Nutrition* and *Transi-tion to Vegetarianism*. He feels that vegetarianism in India developed as a result of overpopulation.

The majority of his practice has involved treating both vegans and vegetarians. He found that for most people, eating a broad vegan diet is not sufficient.

I don't think even a well-balanced vegan diet is going to be sufficient for most people. Ideally, you can argue that it could be if you include a source of B_{12}, if all the food is grown organically in mineral-rich soils, and if you lived in an environment without the pollution and psychological stresses that increase your needs for certain nutrients, such as B vitamins and C and many trace minerals. But even then I still think a high percentage of people wouldn't do well on a vegan diet and could benefit from some milk, eggs, or fish.[1]

Referring to the traditional Hindu system of medicine practiced since the first century AD, Ballentine continues further.

The ayurvedic scriptures don't teach a vegetarian diet. They talk about the use of all kinds of animals: birds, fish, mammals — nothing is omitted. India did not become vegetarian because of a spiritual awakening or for personal health reasons, but because of environmental pressures. It became both uneconomical and unsanitary to raise animals in so crowded an environment.[2]

Anthropologist K. N. Nair concurs.

The avoidance of cattle slaughter originated in the Vedic period (1200–900 BC). The strategy adopted was to restrict animal sacrifice to ceremonial occasions and the entertainment of guests and to make the cow a sacred animal. The sacredness of the cow was ensured by emphasizing the importance of milk in the diet, the cow's divine origin, the belief in the transmigration of the soul, and the cow's role in helping humans along the path to salvation.[3]

Anthropologist Marvin Harris concurs that the cow became sacred in India not because of spiritual reasons (though this was the argument used to convince the masses), but because of economics and overpopulation. Cows are needed by farmers as plow animals. Slaughtering cows would not enable people to have enough for their farms. Others use the cows to sell milk. These cows don't compete with humans for food, as they eat roughage people cannot digest.

Cow love is an active element in a complex, finely articulated material and cultural order. Cow love mobilizes the latent capacity of human beings to persevere in a low-energy ecosystem in which there is little room for waste or indolence. Cow love contributes to the adaptive resilience of the human population by preserving temporarily dry or barren but still useful animals; by discouraging the growth of an energy-expensive beef industry...[4]

Harris explains that people in India refuse to eat their cows during famines because when the famine is over, the people will then have no animals to pull their plows and will thus be condemned to poverty.

While in India, I noted that the Sikhs, Muslims, and Christians (all three of whom *do* eat meat) were often healthier looking than the Hindus. Of course, most of the Hindus, who make up the majority of the Indian population, are very poor. They are eating a barely sustainable diet of mainly lentils and rice. They are extremely underweight and have short life spans.

At the same time, the middle and upper classes are often overweight due to their high-carb diets, especially because their food is mostly cooked.

Nutritional anthropologist Dr. Leon Abrams discussed the nutritional problem in a 1967 *Natural History Magazine* article.

The greater percentage of the population, who subsist almost entirely on vegetable foods, suffer from kwashiorkor [protein-calorie malnutrition], other forms of malnutrition, and have the shortest life span in the world. ...

In my extensive travels over the world, I have noted that those countries whose populations subsist primarily on a vegetarian diet, such as India, exhibit the highest degree of general debilitated health, stunted growth, and the highest death rates at an early age.[5]

It is evident that a high-carb diet is not nearly as healthful as one that includes meat. India has the world's largest vegetarian population. One study found that although the omnivorous people in the northern India area of Punjab eat 17 times more animal fat than those in the Southern city of Madras, they have a seven times lower rate of heart disease.[6]

Despite eating a high-cholesterol, highly saturated-fat diet, and despite smoking more than the southerners, the Punjabi lived on average *eight years longer*.

Western Origins

One of the early Westerners to embrace vegetarianism was Pythagoras in sixth century BC Greece. He was a great philosopher and mathematician and also adhered to a belief in the transmigration of souls. If one ate an animal, he risked "cannibalism" since the creature could be the reincarnation of a human. During the Middles Ages, if a Christian advocated vegetarianism, he risked being accused of this pagan belief called *metempsychosis*.

In the eighteenth century, George Chayne was one of the first animal rights activists, followed by Jeremy Bentham, who in 1789 published "An Introduction to the Principles of Morals and Legislation," which introduced the concept of meat eating as violence.

At the other extreme of the debate was 17th century philosopher René Descartes, who insisted that animals were mere machines. When people reacted with great sympathy to an animal's crying out with pain, his response was that people (themselves animals) were simply responding with a mechanical reflex.

In the US, the vegetarian diet was popularized by health reformers like Rev. Sylvester Graham, who founded the American Vegetarian Society and invented graham crackers. Dr. John Harvey Kellogg, MD, followed him as a vegetarian advocate and invented corn flakes.

The vegetarian movement grew faster in the 1970s after author Frances Moore Lappé's book *Diet for a Small Planet* was released. This book argued that we could feed the world if we stopped raising cattle, overlooking the fact that cattle in nature do not eat the same plant foods that humans eat, which would eliminate much of this advantage.

The study "Vegetarianism in America," published by the magazine *Vegetarian Times*, shows that 3.2 percent of US adults, or 7.3 million people, follow vegetarian-based diets.

It seems that most vegetarians and vegans are young people aged 20 to 40 who are inspired by sustainability, ecology, spirituality, and morality. Better health is thought to be a mere side benefit for many of them. I have observed that many of them give up after five to seven years when they develop deficiencies, experience too much candida or bloating from all the carbs, or lose too much muscle mass.

The Rise of Veganism

I spent a whole month as a vegan one day. Seriously, after all the debates involving intestine-length, canine teeth and gut pH, one fact remains that usually quiets most vegans: there has never, in the history of man, been a society, race, or nation that has survived, let alone thrived, without consuming animal products.[*]

Veganism is a new, stricter version of vegetarianism that prohibits not only meat, but also all animal foods, including eggs, dairy, and gelatin capsules. Even the use of nonconsumable animal products, such as leather, is shunned by some. The word "vegan" was coined in 1944 by British carpenter Donald Watson, founder of the now-worldwide Vegan Society.

According to a 2008 survey, about a million people in the US are abandoning animal products.[7] Under the influence of books like *Vegan: The New Ethics of Eating, Animal Liberation, Diet for a New America, Diet for a Small Planet, Vegan with a Vengeance, Skinny Bitches, The Kind Diet*, and *Fit for Life*, those people are suddenly rejecting all animal foods with no thought whatsoever that it could be detrimental to their health. Indeed, it is promoted as the opposite.

The diet is touted as good for weight loss and health while being likewise kind to animals, eco-friendly, sustainable, and planet saving. Yet for most people, the nutritional deficiencies that result can be profound. For many, it is a stealth factor that may take a decade or more to show up.

For some unfortunate people, by the time they realize it was the lack of animal food, the deficiencies have already created permanent damage. Even without deficiency symptoms, the foods that often replace the protein sources of the vegan who eats cooked foods (grains, legumes, and soy) are toxic and damaging in themselves.[†]

I *do* admire the vegan spirit. As passionate as I am about health and love to teach peak health to everyone who is interested, they are equally passionate in their true compassion for other creatures and feel their mission is to get others to see the light about animal suffering. Veganism has become part of their identity, their *raison d'être*. At the root of veganism is a yearning to see the end of fear, pain, and suffering. Who could be opposed to that?

Many of us have seen glimpses of the movie *Meet Your Meat*, which exposes the cruelty of factory farming, or we've read bits and pieces of the book *Slaughterhouse* and have sworn off animal products forever.

Gary Steiner, a professor of philosophy at Bucknell University and author of *Animals and the Moral Community: Mental Life, Moral Status and Kinship*, makes a plea.

How can intelligent people who purport to be deeply concerned with animal welfare and respectful of life turn a blind eye to such practices? And how can people continue to eat meat when they become aware that nearly 53 billion land animals are slaughtered every year for human consumption?

The simple answer is that most people just don't care about the lives or fortunes of animals. If they did care, they would learn as much as possible about the ways in which our society systematically abuses animals, and they would make what is at once a very simple and a very difficult choice: to forswear the consumption of animal products of all kinds...

---

[*]From *The Primal Blueprint: Reprogram Your Genes for Effortless Weight Loss, Vibrant Health, and Boundless Energy* by Mark Sisson.

[†]See chapter 15.

We have been trained by a history of thinking of which we are scarcely aware to view nonhuman animals as resources we are entitled to employ in whatever ways we see fit in order to satisfy our needs and desires.[8]

Indeed, this is a very complex issue. While most people can agree that we need to treat animals much better than we do, most vegans are unaware that forsaking all animal foods may lead to serious health consequences down the road. Some people cannot thrive on a 100 percent vegan diet. No other primates are vegans. Throughout the vast majority of human history, such a diet never existed for us.

The fact is there are many nutrients found only in animal products. Even if you were to take supplements to compensate, how do you know that there are not as-yet-undiscovered nutrients in animal foods? Researchers are always finding new nutrients.

Even assuming that we have already discovered every important nutrient, a highly dubious supposition, taking synthetic supplements for those nutrients our diets need is never as good as getting those nutrients from whole foods, with all the accompanying cofactors present in proper balance. Much of the time supplements are toxic, and much of the ingredients aren't even absorbed.

Besides, if there are important nutrients that one cannot find in the plant kingdom, doesn't this offer a hint that we evolved eating animal products?

Mahatma Gandhi devoted much of his life to veganism but failed to make the diet work for him. In 1929, he and 22 companions embarked on a plant-only diet. The diet worked well for a time but failed to provide adequate long-term sustenance. They had to add goat milk to their diet.

In 1946 Gandhi declared, "The crores [multitudes] of India today get neither milk nor ghee nor butter, nor even buttermilk. No wonder that mortality figures are on the increase, and there is a lack of energy in the people. It would appear as if man is really unable to sustain life without either meat or milk and milk products."[9]

Former vegetarian Robert Crayhon declares, "Saying that we should eat no animal products is wrong. It is people abuse."[10] This may especially be true if the person did not choose the diet, as in the case of infants, children, and the elderly.[11] There are numerous studies of pregnant or lactating mothers with babies who lack adequate B_{12} and DHA for the brain.

If our health is less than optimal on a vegan diet (and for most people, it eventually is), then at some point we must ask, what is more important to us, our brains and bodies, our children's brains and bodies, or the life of an animal?

The vegan utopia may be unattainable for many of us. Consuming animal products is the way of this world, at least at this point in time — the way of nature. Why resist? Animal cruelty is appalling, admittedly, but there are humane and sustainable ways of animal husbandry.

People have eaten eggs throughout history. People, even vegetarians who would not intentionally eat a living creature, have consumed insects and insect eggs unwittingly.

Insect eggs are often found in raw psyllium or bran. I used to find little worms in my bran or psyllium husk that I kept for fiber and colon cleansing. Someone told me to keep them in the freezer so the eggs wouldn't hatch. I also recall eating a candy bar in Mexico decades ago. I bit into it and saw a tiny worm squiggling around. This explains why most nuts you buy have been heated to kill the insect eggs.

Many of the vegans I have come across feel that it is their life's mission to push themselves and others toward ethical and compassionate eating. I think most are very confident that their health will in no way suffer.

I wonder if they would still refrain from at least eating eggs if they realized that some long-term damage to their brains and nervous systems could result. I wonder if they would eat a vegan diet if they were pregnant, or feed their kids a vegan diet during the critical years that their brains are developing, if they knew it could potentially damage their offspring.

My experience with vegans has shown that many of them are quite dogmatic. It is reminiscent of the dogmatic religious people I used to hang out with in my 20s, who felt that anyone who didn't believe the way they did would perish in hell. When I began to realize that many of the teachings of my fundamentalist religion were flawed, I kept my mouth shut just so as not to lose my social group.

When I began to realize, for example, that the idea of a judgmental, angry, and jealous god didn't jibe with the fact that mere mortal people were able to transcend these frail human traits, my friends didn't get it. I had to keep quiet about my revelations in order to be accepted.

I found the same thing in much of the raw vegan community. I had to shut up if I didn't want to make waves.

Will the Real Vegans Please Stand Up?

When people first get into a vegetarian or vegan diet, they get very excited. It makes a tremendous cleanse the first three months. So does fasting on water — in fact, much more so. I am sure you will agree that living on water as a permanent lifestyle is nutritionally deficient. The same might occur with a vegan or vegetarian diet. But with these restricted diets, the deficiencies can take years or even decades to show up.

It is a good idea to get regular blood tests, as the deficiencies will show up there before you get permanent damage. Vegan diets are especially deficient, as they omit eggs. Eggs contain nearly everything you can find in meat, though you may have to eat a lot of them to get enough of certain nutrients.

Sooner or later deficiencies often manifest. Eventually even the gung-ho leaders feel tempted to cheat, because their brains are starving for saturated fats found in animal foods. Many of them feel guilty and think that their indulgences were merely due to emotional causes or lack of willpower. Few of them reverse their public opinions of the diet, because they truly believe it is the best despite their occasional personal lapses.

Also, they are making a living by selling their books, as well as giving their workshops and lectures. People would unsubscribe from their lists and blackball them if they suddenly came out with, "Hey, I discovered that you now need eggs!" People would be outraged if these leaders mentioned the "M" word approvingly, because, as the chant goes, "meat is murder."

When you are in the vegan movement and have written a book, you become privy to much of this inside information.

According to Dr. Bass, as well as witnesses who have written about this on certain websites, Dr. Herbert M. Shelton, a famous proponent of the hygienic health movement that focuses on eating primarily vegetarian, regularly consumed clabbered goat's milk, so he was not 100 percent vegan as some people presume. He also died of a nervous system disorder, Parkinson's disease, often caused by insufficient B_{12}, although there were likely other contributing factors in his case.

In a published essay, Essene minister Brother Nazariah wrote about the problems he'd had on a vegan diet until he added kefir, yogurt, and eggs.[12] Because he was a leader in the raw food movement, he got close to other leaders who, he says, confided in him about their health problems but would still preach the gospel of 100 percent vegan.

Even the moderator of a raw vegan chat board would tell people, "Don't worry, you're just detoxing," yet confide to Nazariah that he himself had health issues. He claims that one person even died of starvation on a raw vegan diet, as his body began to eat itself, destroying his heart.

Brother Nazariah observed that once people start making a living selling books, supplements, and speaking about the vegan diet, they can't admit that they sometimes cheat and eat cheese or cooked foods. He witnessed several of these leaders doing so, yet they would still claim they had been 100 percent raw vegan for 20 years.

Frédéric Patenaude, owner of www.rawvegan.com, writes after the interview with Brother Nazariah that he himself eats animal products.

> I wish to say that I'm personally not convinced that a vegan diet cannot be healthy. I think it depends on each individual. I personally have found benefits in including some animal products in my diet, and many others have found that too. There are many health benefits in becoming at least mainly vegetarian or even mainly vegan, as well as increasing the amount of raw fruits and vegetables that we eat.[13]

My initial raw food mentor, Bob Avery, also the editor of this book, admits that though he is primarily raw vegan, he occasionally eats raw liver now after developing B_{12} deficiency symptoms more than once. He now also eats raw eggs and has started consuming cod liver oil for vitamin D in the winter months. A noted raw food leader blocked his e-mail address when she discovered that he had been advising a person suffering from a neurological condition to eat a moderate amount of raw fish!

I also heard from my mentor that a prominent leader of the vegan movement, John Robbins, was spotted buying fish at a farmers' market.

Robbins admits that he now supplements his mainly vegan diet with fish. On his site, he says that eating wild fish is not as bad as eating factory-farmed animals. I e-mailed John to ask if he now eats fish. Months later his wife replied, "John suggests you take a look at pages 140–49 in *Healthy at 100*." Coincidentally, I had just read those pages a day before her reply. In his book *Healthy at 100*, he advocates eating fish for the DHA and EPA.[14]

Maybe it's as Brother Nazariah stated in an interview with Frédéric Patenaude: most purported vegans cheat. They feel guilty for it, and some can't go public with their cheating because they make a living off of teaching raw or cooked vegan diets.

But as I found, even that occasional cheat usually isn't enough to provide the nutrition our bodies evolved to depend upon. And other leaders are beginning to catch on. Raw diet author and lecturer Victoria Boutenko now suggests eating insects as our primate cousins do and as most people in Third World countries do![15]

In a book written by Tonya Zavasta, *Raw Foods and Hot Yoga*, Victoria Boutenko also "comes out of the nonvegan closet" by admitting she eats raw eggs. Someone who works for raw vegan leader David Wolfe told me that even David is now telling *some* people to eat krill oil, on an as-needed basis. Furthermore, the Hallelujah Acres raw vegan magazine had an article in which they recommend fish oil for its omega-3s.[16]

Canadian hygienic doctor Ben Kim addresses the issue on his blog.

> Shortly after restoring my health by adding a few clean animal foods to my diet, I discovered that the folks who had originally convinced me to follow a pure vegan diet actually added small amounts of raw, organic cheese and, in one case, organic eggs to their meals. To put it simply, I was astonished that they felt that "sprinkling a little goat's cheese on my salad" was not an important point to share with folks who

are desperate for comprehensive guidance on how to recover from serious health conditions.

To this day I cannot understand how some people can pound home the message of being 100 percent vegan for optimal health while they include small amounts of animal foods in their diets at home. The only explanation that I can think of is that they might feel that by admitting to using small amounts of animal foods, their philosophies are not as tight as they would like them to be.[17]

A blogger named Natasha, who stopped being vegan after the diet destroyed her health, writes about vegans who confessed their cheats to her.

> I received an outpouring of e-mails from fellow "vegan" bloggers who told me in confidence that they weren't really vegan "behind the scenes." They ate eggs or the occasional fish or piece of meat, all to keep themselves healthy, but were too scared to admit to it on their blogs. I even received e-mails from two very prominent and well-respected members of the vegan AR [Arkansas] community. One a published and much-loved vegan cookbook author, the other a noted animal rights blogger, their e-mails detailed their health struggles and eventual unpublicized return to eating meat.[18]

Nonetheless, many leaders are open about their changes. Former raw vegan author Harvey Diamond, who sold millions of copies of *Fit for Life*, which promoted a vegan diet, has since revised his opinion about deleting animal foods from the diet. Raw food advocate Paul Nison now eats some raw dairy and eggs.

Young people on blogs write, "Another one bites the dust!" But what they don't realize is that they are new to the vegan diet and may themselves have challenges down the road.

I want to make it clear that just because man has not eaten a vegan diet throughout history doesn't mean it can't happen now, at least for *some* people, especially with supplements for B_{12}, carnitine, CoQ_{10}, and others. We are evolving, changing creatures. Within a few thousand years, maybe everyone who survives the overpopulation will be vegan or at least vegetarian. But we should monitor where our bodies are now and not push ourselves beyond our current evolutionary stage.

Chapter 4

Can a Vegan or Vegetarian Diet Give You Peak Health?

No society has ever, to my knowledge, sustained itself for long exclusively on plant foods. There may have been traditional cultures whose only animal product consumption consisted of grasshoppers, beetles, grubs, or other insects, but all have partaken of at least a minimal amount of animal foods. —John Robbins, early proponent of the US vegan movement, in *Healthy at 100*

My main motive in writing this book was that I saw so many people who were unable to stick to raw vegan diets. I knew that eating raw was the greatest health secret ever, so *that* part was not to blame. Also, a raw vegan diet, abstaining from all animal products, may be the very best cleansing mechanism that exists.

Periods of meatlessness or sparse eating have been incorporated into many traditional cultures and religions. People have reversed all sorts of diseases on vegan, vegetarian, and raw vegan diets.

Yet I began to realize that vegan diets often led to deficiencies of vital nutrients that the body can stockpile for years. As I researched, I realized even a vegetarian diet that includes only eggs and dairy (but no meat) is not what our bodies evolved on.

We are sold on the vegan diet as sustainable for the planet. *But is it sustainable for our optimal health?* When we first go vegan — especially raw! — we feel so great. A raw vegan diet is the sine qua non of detoxification, and this great feeling can last for *years*. This is because abstaining from animal foods, and especially dietary fat, enables our bodies to cleanse, detoxifying from built-up toxins.

Furthermore, many people come to the vegan diet after years of living on toxic, factory-farmed meat at fast food restaurants, so they experience a dramatic contrast. Over several years, however, it is very common that certain nutrients that these people have stored up begin to deplete. The fact that it is so easy to end up with deficiencies on these diets bears proof that they are not in fact our natural diets.

I once heard Dr. Gabriel Cousens say in a lecture that it is easier to be a vegan now than at any time in history since we now have so many supplements available. But what if there were some critical ingredients in animal products besides B_{12} and DHA that we haven't yet discovered?

We already know that carnitine, rich in red meat, is very hard to get from the plant kingdom. Without carnitine, the mitochondria[*] cannot pump out loads of *adenosine triphosphate* (ATP) for energy.[†] In addition, many people suggest that the need for so many supplements proves that our bodies didn't evolve on vegan diets and aren't quite ready for them.

Those in the vegan and vegetarian movements are so convinced of their dietary perfection that when they have health problems, they cannot imagine it might be the diet that is to blame. The truth is that *these diets are extremely cleansing for the first year or two*, especially because factory-farmed meat is so toxic. On the other hand, deficiencies gradually manifest later.

If you become a raw vegan, you also probably give up grains, beans, and cereals. Just giving up grains alone will lift you to higher health planes than you have ever experienced. And if you're eating raw, your pancreas no longer has to crank out so many digestive enzymes, so you are flying high! As detailed in *The Live Food Factor*, eating raw increases your energy in many ways.[‡]

When health issues pop up, it is hard to connect them to the diet that made you feel so great. No way could any health issues be related to your diet.

---

[*]See page 143.

[†]See page 145.

[‡]"Live Food: Our Biggest Energy Conserver" on page 110 of *The Live Food Factor* lists seven ways that eating raw as opposed to cooked food will conserve energy.

No way, you think.

I recall when I had religiously dogmatic friends who would be elated over their connection to God, love, joy, and peace. Yet they would get depressed because their loved one wasn't accepting the "true religion" and was sure to "burn in hell forever." Or they would become devastated because a loved one died, and there was no way they could communicate with that person until after they died themselves, according to their interpretations of scripture.

I often felt like shaking them and saying, "Just don't be attached to your dogma. Be open to new beliefs, and that will set you free!"

Now it is the vegans (those in poor health) that I wish to awaken from the spell of their dogma. If only they could see that eating animal products is not a crime against animals. If only they could understand it is the way we have eaten for 2.6 million years, and no amount of philosophy is going to change the body's nutritional requirements.

As we will see, a vegan diet often lacks things needed by the brain (DHA, EPA, B_{12}), eyes (DHA, A, B_{12}), nervous system (B_{12}, saturated fats), and bones (D, K_2). I don't know about you, but I consider those to be pretty important organs.

It is not so easy to be a healthy vegan. Raw food researcher and clinician Dr. Gabriel Cousens pointed out in a lecture at Portland, Oregon, in 2004 that it is much easier to be vegan when you start eating that way when young. Hygienic doctor Michael Klaper, MD, has said much the same thing.

As you get older, it is harder for your body to convert the omega-3 fats into DHA, which is critical for the brain and eyes. Many people come into the raw diet at middle age. These people have a harder time converting omega-3 fats into DHA.

Even in a young, healthy person under 30, only 10 to 15 percent of omega-3 fats are converted into DHA. This is why it is so important for many of us to eat foods that already have DHA. These would include fatty fish, certain algae, and eggs from chickens that were fed fish meal and/or flax, chia, or hemp seeds.

Another issue is vitamin B_{12}, which is critical for the brain and nervous system. One British study comparing the effects of vegan to omnivorous diets found low thyroid stimulating hormone (TSH) lev-

els and goitrogenic effects among the vegans. Vegans are especially vulnerable to thyroid damage if they are deficient in zinc and B_{12}, which is common among vegans.[1]

A study from Oxford University shows that vegetarians have more brain shrinkage, due to an insufficiency of vitamin B_{12}.[2] When you are older and more toxic, it is harder to get vitamin B_{12} from soil found on unwashed greens or from the little B_{12} your own body's bacteria supply.

You could fast and purify your body, and it could get easier with time, but you might not be at your peak health and energy level in the meantime. I have seen several raw fooders give up at that point, especially those who switched to raw vegan diets when middle-aged.

Many vegans decide to take supplements for B_{12} and DHA. As stated earlier, scientists are continually discovering new nutrients. What if later they discover additional critical nutrients that are found only in animal products? This is why some prefer to be vegetarians so they can at least eat eggs and some dairy.

Some people will fare better on a long-term vegan diet than others. Some, because of genetics or their age and health status when they start the vegan diet, are better at making the conversions from plant precursors to nutrients such as DHA, EPA, vitamin A, and vitamin K_2.

Some will be savvier about doing research regarding how to get nutrients on a restricted diet. Some will be willing and able to purchase high-nutrient super foods to compensate for not eating fish, liver, meat and eggs. Some will be willing to sunbathe for hours every day to get sufficient vitamin D for robust health, not just enough to prevent rickets.

The nutritional requirements of each individual person should also be considered. Growing infants and children, as well as pregnant or lactating women and the elderly, are best eating at least eggs and dairy, if not clean meat.

Nutritional anthropologist Dr. Leon Abrams declares, "In that no culture has ever existed that was completely vegetarian [he likely means vegan here, since he is no doubt aware of Hindus], and whereas a number that exhibited excellent health, such as the Eskimo, Plains Indians, and Lapps, were primarily meat-eaters, it can only be concluded that humans, though omnivorous, have a basic physiological requirement for animal protein (fish, fowl, meat, eggs, or dairy) for optimal health."

Interestingly, when dentist Weston Price, DDS, was traveling the world examining traditional cultures and their diets in the '30s and '40s, he had hoped to find a healthy vegetarian population.

When he arrived at the Pacific island named Viti Levu, he thought he had found it. Instead, he learned that the islanders ate wild pigs. They also depended very much on seafood, so much so that even when those living inland were at war with the coastal tribes, they traded foods.

Those living in the hills would leave choice plant foods from inland and return later to obtain the seafood left in exchange. They told him they required food from the sea at least every three months.

This was a matter of keen interest, and at the same time disappointment, since one of the purposes of the expedition to the South Seas was to find, if possible, plants or fruits which together, without the use of animal products, were capable of providing all of the requirements of the body for growth and for maintenance of good health and a high state of physical efficiency.[3]

It is now clear to me that maintaining peak health on a vegan diet is difficult for most people. But years ago, even though I had symptoms of deficiency, I was clueless.

Once my raw vegan book was in print, it was time to get busy marketing it on the Internet. I connected with hundreds of people, asking them to join my joint venture campaign. Yet many doctors refused, saying they had valid reasons for being against the raw diet.

In the past, I would have thought, "These guys are brainwashed by the pharmaceutical mafia, and they simply need to read the 66 studies in my book to be deprogrammed." But this time I sincerely wanted to know what their complaints were.

Here's what a business associate of one of the doctors reported.

I asked a few of the main doctors. ... They believe we are supposed to be carnivores, based on our teeth and other physical aspects evolved over time. ...

She went on to say they believe we must have some of the "nonessential" amino acids derived only from meat. They believe a raw diet lacks B_{12}. They claimed a raw diet is dangerous the older one gets because of osteoporosis. So is the lack of hormones from not eating meat.[4]

This person added that she was impressed enough with the first chapter of my book that she decided to go 80 percent raw and eat a bit of cooked or raw meat in addition.

Nutritionist Nora T. Gedgaudas, CNS, CNT, has seen the results.

Far and away, the most damaged and intractably dysregulated brains and nervous systems I have seen or dealt with in my practice have all essentially been vegans, with strict vegetarians a close second — *hands down*. I have numerous other colleagues who have made the same independent observation.

A diet of starch, sugar, lectins, phytates, and common allergens, or food-sensitivity-generating foods, coupled with chronic deficiencies: of numerous critical essential fats (EPA/DHA, healthy saturates), fat-soluble nutrients (preformed A, D, E, and K), amino-acid imbalances, and/or deficiencies and other key animal source nutrients — not the least of which is utilizable B_{12} (and B_{12} analogs from seaweed don't count) — lead to states of over-arousal, anxiety-related disorders, memory problems, cognitive dysfunction, sleep disturbances, brain degeneration, GI [gastrointestinal] disorders and utter metabolic chaos.

It is deeply problematic. These unnaturally restrictive diets, together with other carbohydrate-based diets dysregulate insulin and leptin function to the extreme.[5]

Chapter 12 will go into more detail on insulin and leptin.

What Doctors Say about Veg Diets

I interviewed Dr. Carolyn Dean, MD, ND, Medical Director of the Nutritional Magnesium Association and also author of numerous books, including *The Yeast Connection and Women's Health*. She has a practice in Hawaii and has had many vegetarians and vegans come to her with health problems, such as premature menopause, osteoporosis, loss of gum tissue leading to loss of teeth, and deficiency of adrenal hormones. She believes this is from a lack of quality protein and quality fats to support the hormones and tissues. They are not absorbing enough minerals for the bones and hence get osteoporosis.

☞ You need true vitamins A and D to absorb minerals and proteins, and these are not found in plant products. You can get D from the sun, though as we will see, it is hard for most people to get enough. You can get the precursor to A from plants, but as we will later see, you would need to eat a *lot* of those foods.

She also finds that many of her patients who go on raw vegan diets see their candida yeast infections return. Some of her patients are very emaciated. They do a lot of juicing, and the magnesium creates excessively loose bowel movements, which is not healthy because the nutrients won't all be absorbed.

She tells her patients that "3.2 percent of the American population is vegetarian. If the diet were as beneficial and healthy as claimed, wouldn't more people do it?"

Dr. Dean herself experimented with vegetarianism and raw veganism.

When I tried macrobiotics, in a few weeks I developed fluid in my lungs. I could hear the bubbling through the stethoscope. I was wheezing. My macrobiotic doctor said it was just a healing reaction, a detox, but I was building fluid in the lungs. Within 24 hours of eating free-range chicken, the lungs healed. I needed protein to bind with the fluids.

When she was a 100 percent raw vegan, she felt great until after exercising two hours a day. She felt she required more protein, but it took two to three months to realize it. Her energy was low, her muscles tired. She needed magnesium and realized she also needed more animal fats.

In an interview with Thomas Cowan, MD, who has a practice in San Francisco and is coauthor of *The Fourfold Path to Healing,* he told me he has worked with patients on vegetarian and vegan diets and found them to be deficient in vitamin D, vitamin B_{12}, and often *even their life force.*

We need fats and proteins to build our bodies and plants for vitamins. A vegetarian or vegan diet is good for a detox if you are sick and toxic. You can eat that way for six months.

Women often complain to him, "My belly is swollen, and I can't think properly." They have bloating and gas. He calls this "gorilla syndrome" because the gorilla has a swollen belly from all the plant food and a smaller brain. As we will see later, man traded his longer gut for a larger brain.

He explained that these are usually aspiring vegans who crave meat about every third day and berate themselves for cheating on the vegan diet. They are in a constant battle with themselves, trying to be "good," but instincts take over.

The brain is a completely saturated-fat organ; if you don't eat a lot of saturated fat, you won't have a good brain.

He often sees a pattern in which people "go veg" and eat too many grains. When they realize they are gluten intolerant and have poor thyroid function, maybe from the soy, they "go raw" and overeat nuts. When they get too many antinutrients from the nuts, they overeat fruit, which is largely unripe when harvested and high in sugar.

Dr. Cowan remarked that when the white man came to North America, the topsoil was three feet deep. Buffalo roamed everywhere and fertilized the soil naturally. When agriculture was introduced, the soil was gradually destroyed, even though the food grown was all organic back then.

The fertile plains became a dustbowl, as in the book *Grapes of Wrath.* With agriculture, our diets also degenerated. We traded vitamins, DHA, conjugated linoleic acids (CLAs), good fats, and minerals all for *one* macronutrient: carbohydrates. *The result has been rampant diabetes.*

Dr. Ronald Roth, PhD, sees no advantage to a vegetarian diet.

I have been testing and treating a large number of vegetarian patients over more than two decades. ... Contrary to vegan-based reviews or commentaries, people following a strict vegetarian diet are not healthier than their omnivorous counterparts. In fact, on average, they suffer from as many or more medical complaints as compared to nonvegetarian individuals, who include meat or eggs in their diet.[6]

Australian hygienic doctor John Fielder, DO, DC, ND, posted on his website these observations.

I have seen couples who just could not conceive until such time as they added some form of animal product to their diet. And if they continued this way the children were normal. But if they discontinued the animal product as soon as they conceived, the child was born brain damaged.

The number of brain-damaged children due to the vegan diet I would consider to have been around 3 percent, that is 3 in every 100 births. And there should not have been any. These people were not exposed to chemicals or any other factor that I could find. And they definitely were not involved in the use of social drugs.

The addition of the animal product refers to a vegan diet which includes vegetables and not only fruit. The animal product could be either raw or cooked. It is my own personal belief that if we were able to follow this whole cycle through and observe all its ramifications, as with Pottenger and his cats, we would find that the animal product would produce far superior results if it were raw.[*] ...

I have observed children who have not grown from the age of nine months for the next two years because the parents adopted a fruitarian regimen, and so fed the child. The non-growth of the children was, and is, common where the children are fed exclusively on fruit.[8]

Nutritionist and best-selling author Ann Louise Gittleman, MS, has worked as a nutritional counselor at various centers. She found that vegetarian diets didn't work for many of her patients.

We all know the reasons that show how unsound it is to be eating meat, and on paper I agree with them. ... But in real life I am seeing vegetarian and vegan women who ... have protein deficiencies and fatigue, are losing their hair, and have premature menopause. ...

I think that a strict vegetarian diet (minimal use of dairy products) acts as a good cleansing program for people who come from a diet heavy in animal foods and processed foods, and for a time it is therapeutic. But for some people, when it goes on too long, it seems to backfire.[9]

Dr. James Wilson, ND, DC, PhD, author of *Adrenal Fatigue*, found that vegans have tremendous difficulty recovering from adrenal fatigue. They need more protein and do much better if they can at least include eggs and yogurt in their diets.[10]

Dr. Ron Schmid, ND, is another doctor skeptical of the "veg" diets.

Many individuals have recovered from diseases on vegetarian diets. Most have included dairy foods or at least occasional fish or poultry in their regimens. When well balanced, such natural food diets are far superior to those diets rich in commercial meat, white flour, and sugar eaten by most people. Strict vegetarian diets that exclude all animal foods (known as vegan diets) often result in better health and the alleviation of serious problems. ...

But the success of vegan diets is usually self-limiting. By avoiding all animal foods and animal fats, nutrients essential for development of optimal strength, resistance to disease, and reproductive capacity are lacking. Individuals on strictly vegan diets may thrive for several weeks, months, or even years, but in the vast majority of cases, problems eventually appear.[11]

More Problems with a Veg Diet

A low-fat diet of high fruit is popular among many raw vegans. Fruit is naturally eaten raw and is high in simple carbs and antioxidants. No way can it be as bad as eating cereals and grains. But so many people — and I have come across at least a dozen myself — have gotten cavities or even lost their teeth from eating excess fruit.

In hygiene and in Chinese medicine, the tongue is said to be the only muscle we can see and an indicator of what is happening to the inner muscles of the digestive system. The same can be said about the teeth. If the teeth can't handle a high-fruit diet, what makes people believe their skeletons are in any better shape? Some people think rinsing, flossing, and brushing their teeth is all they need to do. That may help, but I do believe there is a mineral imbalance going on. Remember, our ancestors never used toothbrushes or floss and had perfect teeth! What damages our teeth cannot be good for the rest of our skeletons.

Heed what author Sally Fallon has to say.

Sugar consumption is the cause of bone loss and dental decay. Tooth decay and bone loss occur when the precise ratio of calcium to phosphorus in the blood varies from the normal ratio of four parts phosphorus to ten parts calcium. At this ratio, all blood calcium can be properly utilized.

Dr. Melvin Page, a Florida dentist, demonstrated in numerous studies that sugar consumption causes phosphorus levels to drop and calcium to rise. Calcium rises because it is pulled from the teeth and the

---

[*]Dr. Francis Pottenger ran a ten-year experiment comparing the health outcomes of 900 cats, half fed raw food and half fed cooked food.[7]

bones. The drop in phosphorus hinders the absorption of calcium, making it unusable and therefore toxic.[12]

Thus, sugar consumption causes tooth decay not because it promotes bacterial growth in the mouth, as most dentists believe, but because it alters the internal body chemistry.[12]

Former vegan Gregory Westbrook and his family stayed on an 85 percent raw, 100 percent vegan diet for six years. After some time, they experienced many adverse symptoms, such as extreme fatigue, weight loss, numerous cavities, and more.

The Westbrooks took a survey of people on their Genesis 1:29 diet and found that 49 percent rated themselves as losing health after being on the diet a long time. Typical symptoms included fatigue, loss of libido, loss of muscle tone and musculature, bloating after eating, hair loss, ridges on fingernails (an indication of deficiencies), slumping posture, looking older, cravings, constant snacking, memory loss, inability to concentrate, loss of dental health (including loss of teeth!), lack of ability to lactate, and much more.

These deficiencies spring from vegan diets, not because the person failed to cook his food!

Gregory wrote an e-book about it: *When Hallelujah Becomes "What Happened?" — Crashing on the Vegan Diet*. The family recovered when they introduced clean animal products.

We could do an experiment and put a bunch of people on a vegan diet and make sure they have adequate B_{12}, DHA, zinc, vitamins D and A, as well other things a vegan or vegetarian diet is low in. I would put money on it that after a couple of decades, a significant number of these people would nonetheless have less than ideal health, because other nutrients found only in animal products — ones that we have not yet discovered — would be deficient.

Health researcher Brian White sadly points out in the article "Vegan Centenarians — Where are They?" that there is no record of a strict vegan who lived to be 100, and many in fact die prematurely.[13] Dr. Norman Walker, ND, famous for his juicing, lived to be 109, but he did in fact drink goat's milk.

Someone on an Internet blog told me he knew of a vegan centenarian. I said I would publish it in this book if he would send me more information, but I never got a reply. I suspect he was thinking of a Phoenix online news article about a raw foodist celebrating his alleged 109th birthday, but that man supplements his plant-based diet with occasional fish consumption.[14] Like so many, he may also be exaggerating his age somewhat, but he still looks great for a centenarian.[15]

As I have said, many doctors refused to endorse my book, claiming that they had successfully treated several formerly raw patients who had initially presented with protein, vitamin D, and B_{12} deficiencies. They regained health on prescribed diets that included meat. Yet these deficiencies need not occur on raw diets that include animal products. The deficiencies spring from vegan diets, not because people fail to cook their food!

Vegan diets tend to be low in protein, even more so if raw. A cooked vegan can eat soy, which is full of plant protein, though I do not advise it. Eating soy excessively leads to a whole host of disease conditions, as will be shown later.

A cooked vegan can also eat a higher amount of grains for protein than a raw vegan can, though grains are not conducive to the best health. Grains contain phytates that bind minerals, and cooked grains are full of carbs that spike insulin levels. For many they are also hard to digest.

A cooked vegan can get B_{12} from nutritional yeast, which is not raw and contains mycotoxins.

Nonetheless, a cooked vegan will have other problems from eating too many cooked carbs. When you cook a food, the glycemic index is elevated. Dr. Stanley Bass had this to add.

A primarily carbohydrate diet triggers insulin, which closes cells so fewer minerals can get in. The minerals are wasted in the urine. If you are a raw vegan, the carbohydrates are not absorbed as much, so you are better off. But you are nonetheless very likely eating too many carbohydrates. And you may still be deficient in many nutrients found only in animal products.[16]

You should know that one of my philosophies

is "No dogma!" and this applies to diet. The human body is so wise that it can adapt to almost anything, especially when the power of the mind is harnessed. I do know some successful raw vegans. And I applaud them. I do believe they are a minority.

It helps to start at a young age, as I have heard both Drs. Gabriel Cousens and Michael Klaper say. This is because you can more easily make the conversions: beta-carotene to vitamin A, omega-3s to DHA and EPA, etc.

I would not advise babies or young children to be vegans, as they cannot easily convert beta-carotene to vitamin A. Their growing brains and nervous systems also need high levels of DHA. Their growing skeletons need a lot of vitamin K_2.

I know some vegans who have been successful for decades, but many of them spend a load of money on getting super foods from all over the world in order to get the minerals, proteins, and other nutrients hard to find in the plant kingdom. They are actually leaving more of a carbon footprint and spending more money than if they just bought some local meat and eggs from free-range, organically fed animals.

Again, I am no friend of rigid dogma. I would be the last person to state that absolutely no one can be a successful vegan or vegetarian. After all, I include testimonials of longer term vegans such as Ric Lambart and Annette Larkins in *The Live Food Factor*.[17]

Raw food author Paul Nison has three books in which he interviews long-term raw vegans and includes photos of these very healthy-looking people. So we have living proof that it can be done. Yet I am living proof that some of us cannot achieve peak health on such restricted diets. Raw? Absolutely! Vegan? *No*.

Why Some People Do Better as Vegans Than Others

It is much easier to be vegan if you are not living in a toxic environment and stressed lifestyle, since toxins and stress increase nutritional needs. A retired vegan living in Costa Rica who doesn't smoke or drink will have fewer nutritional demands than a vegan working a demanding job in New York City who drinks a cup of coffee and a glass of

wine a day. But how many of us live in pristine regions with minimal-stress lifestyles?

Even successful raw vegans would be better off to lower their insulin and leptin levels, which comes from eating lower-glycemic diets.* Studies show that low levels of the hormones insulin and leptin correspond to a longer life span and longer health span.

One study was done on two genetically identical African tribes, one living on a lakeshore and its food products and the other, some kilometers away, living on grains and beans on an almost vegan diet.

Compared with their vegetable diet counterparts, both men and women on a fish diet had markedly lower leptin levels, despite having almost identical BMIs [body mass indices]. Although prior studies have consistently reported higher leptin levels in women than in men, women on the fish diet had leptin levels less than half those observed in men on a vegetarian diet.[18]

As for the insulin sensitivity issue, it has been speculated that Northern Europeans can remain free of insulin resistance and diabetes more easily than those of other races because they began milking cows thousands of years earlier.[19] They became adapted to milk sugar and retained the lactase enzymes to digest it.†

There is also some evidence that Asians from certain countries are better at diets with fewer animal products, since their agricultural history is older than that of most people.

Vegan diets may be easier not only for certain races, but also for men. Several of the doctors I spoke with seemed to think women had a harder time with it because of bloating, iron deficiency, and hormonal issues. Pregnant, lactating, and menstruating women have high nutritional needs.

Ann Louise Gittleman found that men in general seem to be able to handle carbs better than women. She says that having more muscle mass and fewer fat cells makes their tissues more metabolically active and enables them to burn up more

---

*This will be discussed later in chapter 12.

†See chapter 18 for more information on the connection between dairy and diabetes.

carbohydrate calories.[20]

In addition, in the luteal phase* of the menstrual cycle, women take much longer to digest carbs, which can lead to bloating.[21]

Women, more than men, seem to have weight issues going vegan. As mentioned in chapter 2, nutritionist Natalia Rose said that some women can actually gain weight on a vegan diet.

In teaching diet workshops, Gregory Westbrook encountered many raw vegan women in whom "metabolism slows down to the point that the person hardly needs to eat any food at all, and it is nearly impossible to lose weight."[22]

Dr. Kathryn Paxton George, PhD, of the Department of philosophy and the University of Idaho, claims vegan diets are only suitable for middle class males.

> The vegan ideal [entails] arguments for ethical veganism based on traditional moral theory (rights and/or utilitarianism) extended to animals. The most ideal lifestyle would abjure the use of animals or their products for food, since animals suffer and have rights not to be killed. The ideal is discriminatory, because the arguments presuppose a "male physiological norm" that gives a privileged position to adult, middle-class males living in industrialized countries.
>
> Women, children, the aged, and others have substantially different nutritional requirements and would bear a greater burden on vegetarian and vegan diets with respect to health and economic risks than do these males. The poor and many persons in Third World nations live in circumstances that make the obligatory adoption of such diets, where they are not already a matter of sheer necessity, even more risky.[23]

There is a great deal of nutritional evidence that infants, children, adolescents, women (especially menstruating, pregnant, or lactating), and the elderly have greater nutritional needs than the average male age 20 to 50.[24] George considers the arguments used by these animal activist males, such as Peter Singer, to be "ageism, sexism, and classism."[25]

She argues that "the best candidates for vegetarianism and veganism are young, adult, healthy males living in industrialized countries" and that these diets "are lower in risk in Western nations when individuals have access to education, medical care, and sufficient resources to buy proper foods and supplements."[26] She emphasizes that in the West, food is often fortified with nutrients such as vitamins B and D, as well as iodine.

Could it be that vegan diets are best suited for Western, middle-class males?† Middle-class people have money for supplements and organic food, whereas lower income folks don't.

I would like to add to that "educated" or "motivated to study," since it takes a certain degree of nutritional knowledge to make sure you prevent deficiencies and keep on top of new research. It also helps to live in a pristine environment and to fast periodically, as these factors reduce one's nutritional needs.

Ironically, most vegetarians and vegans are actually women. I believe this is because men of all cultures are more attached to the manly image of meat, since they were historically the hunters. Women falsely believe this is the key to weight loss, and women are frequently more compassionate toward animals, being more often right-brain dominant.

Why Haven't We Been Warned of the Dangers of Vegan Diets?

Frankly, I was shocked while researching this book about all the deficiencies you can get on a vegan diet. The only one commonly presented is B_{12}. I recently spent two hours scanning the word *vegan* on Google Books. I pored through probably hundreds of books. Most of them warned of B_{12}, but only a few mentioned other deficiencies, such as vitamin D and zinc. *None* of them mentioned EPA or DHA!

Few people are talking about the dangers of vegan (and for some, even vegetarian) diets. Gregory Westbrook lists four reasons why in his e-book *When Hallelujah Becomes "What Happened?"*

---

*The time period from ovulation to the onset of menstruation.

†Of course this is just a generalization. Some men need more zinc than a typical vegan diet provides, and some need more protein. Some also need more B_{12} or other nutrients.

People who don't do well usually quietly drop out. I have met a lot of people who tried it for a year or two and didn't feel good. Their story never gets told.

Some people do really well at first and later when they don't feel so good, they can't believe it is the diet's fault because they have such faith in it. They blame themselves for not being 100 percent, not fasting enough, etc.

Some who don't feel good will cheat and supplement with animal foods but not admit it.

Leaders who have a following will not admit to cheating because they make a living by preaching a contrary message. I can attest to this. After I did a radio show with Kevin Gianni, "coming out" that I ate meat, my book sales for *The Live Food Factor* immediately plummeted by 30 percent — even though it is a book that advocates a raw vegan diet.

I nevertheless decided to press forward with this present book because the truth must be told.

☞ *Vegan and even vegetarian diets aren't for everyone!*

Chapter 5

Vegetarians No More: People Who Went Back to Eating Meat

I was vegan for 16 years, and I truly believed I was doing the right thing for my health. But when I was vegan, I was super-weak. I love animals, and we should not support anything but ethical ranching, but when I eat meat, I feel more grounded. I have more energy.
—Mariel Hemingway, actress, model, and author of *Healthy Living from the Inside Out*

There is a saying in Buddhism, "First there is a mountain, then there is no mountain, then there is." Oftentimes in life, things come around full circle.

First a girl eats meat, and it's from factory-farmed animals, much of it from fast food restaurants. Then she gives it up for a time because her health is poor or she gains an understanding about the cruelty of factory farming. Years later she returns to eating it as a health necessity.

But she has been transformed by her vegetarian experience. She now eats meat *consciously*. She eats only the free range, the organically fed, and, if possible, the more compassionately raised and quickly slaughtered. She eats maybe only half as much meat as before and only meat which is healthful for her body, not the factory-farmed animal that led a tortured life, ate grains instead of its natural food, and was injected with steroids, hormones, vaccinations, and antibiotics.

She might even ingest it with a prayer of thanks to the animal's spirit for nourishing her, recognizing that this is the covenant among all living creatures.

I have found that most of the people who are outspoken about the dangers of vegan or even vegetarian diets are not meat enthusiasts anxious to defend their culinary preferences, but rather those who sincerely delved into a meatless diet themselves. After all, they know better than anyone, having had first-hand experience.

Certain popular media often make meat eaters feel guilty about not eating a "politically correct diet." They are held personally responsible for global warming and world starvation. It's their fault the world is running out of fresh water and the world's fish population is dying.

They bear the brunt of criticism that animals are ruthlessly factory farmed and heartlessly slaughtered. Sometimes they feel this so much that they become vegetarians or vegans until years later when their health has become compromised.

Now let's take a look at some people who reverted to their ancestral, meat-eating roots.

G. Martin

My friend G. Martin from Spain was vegan for three years, during which his six-foot frame got down to an emaciated 130 pounds (59 kg). He ate legumes, fruit, salad, steamed vegetables, and a little bread with olive oil on the bread and salad. His immune system crashed, and he developed all sorts of infections. In retrospect, he thinks his immune system was compromised by a protein deficiency. As a vegan, he especially lacked sufficient *methionine*, an amino acid important for immune cell production and proper nerve function.[1]

G. was diagnosed with a B_{12} deficiency so severe that he suffered from paresthesia (a sensation of prickling, tingling, or creeping on the skin) and limb numbing, so he went in for a series of 10 intramuscular injections of 1000 mg each. He ended up having 10,000 mg of B_{12} injected. That is *five million times* the recommended daily allowance (RDA).

His triglycerides were so high, 375 mg/dl at one point, that the doctor thought he had pancreatitis. The maximum considered to be conducive to health is 150. He was also frequently bloated, describing himself as a "gorilla-like primate with a bulging belly on an otherwise rail-thin body." Added to the health issues were muscle atrophy, fatigue, lack of concentration, and depression.

I felt almost always depressed, in a blue mood, and life seemed not so beautiful as now. I even felt a lot less curiosity for learning, which is a decisive symptom for me not being at my optimum!

A few months after I started to eat fish again, I became a new man, more the one I used to be in my twenties. My muscle mass and my optimism returned, as did my desire to learn and satisfy my innate curiosity. I felt a lot less rigidity in my behavior than when I was vegan, when I tended to be a lot more inflexible and obsessive.

After much research, G. added meat and eggs to his diet. At first, he would sometimes eat over a pound of fish or meat a day. After a while, he didn't feel he needed that much. Now he eats only three or four ounces of animal food a day. He eats a 75 percent raw paleodiet of raw and steamed vegetables, meat (mainly small fish), fruit, nuts, and seeds. He weighs a much healthier 155 pounds (70 kg). He doesn't eat breakfast, just lunch and dinner, so he has a fasting period of 18 hours each day.

I feel really good. Maybe some people can thrive on a vegan diet in the long run. And I gave it a fair try; three years seem like enough to me. I loved it emotionally, and I also adored the textures, flavors, and tastes. But my health is not at its optimum if I go full vegan.

Ann Louise Gittleman

Nutritionist and best-selling author Ann Louise Gittleman relates her own experience as a vegan.

I too was once a committed vegetarian — a vegan who ate only plant foods. But it was not a healthy diet plan for me. I do believe that some people can be healthy on a vegetarian diet, but I do not advocate vegetarianism across the board.

When I was vegan, my body began the slow process of deterioration. For nearly a year, I ate natural, whole foods, avoided all types of animal protein, and worked hard at combining foods to ensure an adequate intake of amino acids. But I was slowly falling apart. My hair started falling out, and my skin erupted. I lost twenty pounds, and I couldn't tolerate any excess stimuli (I became especially sensitive to noise).

Yet I was committed to keeping my body free of animal products. After all, I knew the drill. I could automatically recite how the length of the human intestines and the number of molars versus incisors were physical proof that humans were not designed to be meat eaters. Unfortunately, I was wrong, and my body was protesting with unmistakable signs. ...

The proteins in meat and fish have been a critical part of the human diet for 40,000 years — an eternity for us, but for human genetics, a mere blip in the evolutionary timeline.[2]

Gittleman discusses how she has seen countless women in her practice who prided themselves in being able to live on diets free of animal products, including eggs and dairy. They feel virtuous that they are vegans, yet by nightfall they are wrecks and eat high-carbohydrate snacks, often full of sugar. They experience mood swings, edginess, depression, and physical symptoms, such as water retention, hair loss, fatigue, and a slowed metabolism.

When she convinces them to return to healthful essential fats and animal protein, she notes within weeks their energy soaring, their muscle tone returning, and their metabolism increasing.

Jay Robb

Author and clinical sports nutritionist Jay Robb spent seven years as a vegetarian, occasionally including eggs and dairy with these results.

Not enough protein unless too many starches were consumed, which in turn caused me to become rather corpulent. ... I joyfully spent one year on a 100 percent raw food diet of only organic fruits, vegetables, nuts, and seeds. (Not enough protein, too many carbohydrates, no fat burning.)[3]

He went on to write *The Fat Burning Diet* that promotes a low-carb diet.

Dr. Ben Kim, DC

Hygienic doctor and acupuncturist Dr. Ben Kim, DC, tells his story on his blog at www.drben kim.com.

I chose to adopt a 100 percent vegan diet in the summer of 1999 following a 14-day water fast. I stayed on this diet for close to four years, but I only felt like I was optimally supporting my health for the first two years. The last two years were marked by low energy, constant cravings for some animal foods, skin breakouts, and emotional lows that I had never previously experienced. ...

Why did I stick with this diet for the two years during which I suffered with health challenges? Because

I had faith in the books that I had read on this topic and in the guidance that a few prominent physicians had given me.

Dr. Kim went on to find some online articles that confirmed that his health issues stemmed from deficiencies of nutrients found only in animal foods.

I added organic eggs from free-range birds, cod liver oil, and a small amount of fish to my diet. Over a period of about three months, this minor adjustment to my diet lifted the quality of my health in a significant way. My energy came back, my cravings disappeared, I stopped having skin breakouts, and most notably, I felt physically strong again.

Dr. Kim adds that he knows many very strict vegans who are following this diet for philosophical reasons. After decades on such diets, they have developed health problems.

He respects their choice but with reservations.

I believe that people who choose to be strict vegans for the welfare of animals need to consider this question: Is promoting a 100 percent vegan diet for the welfare of animals a correct moral path if it leads to significant health problems for humans? Personally, I feel bad about an animal being killed to be my food. But if there were no fishermen or farmers around, I believe that I would gratefully sacrifice an animal with my own hands, since I believe that the health of my family requires eating small amounts of animal foods.

Lierre Keith

Author Lierre Keith was a vegan activist for 20 years. She developed a disc problem that she attributes to a lack of good saturated animal fats with vitamins D and A to absorb the calcium. Since she was not a raw fooder, she also included grains and legumes in her diet, foods high in mineral-binding phytates. Sally Fallon offers an explanation.

One of the most common side effects of cholesterol lowering is crippling back pain. The muscles that support our spine require animal foods to maintain their integrity. And the bones in our spine need a good source of calcium, namely dairy products or bone broth, to remain strong.[4]

Lierre's health improved, though she never recovered completely, after her doctor (an acupuncturist) advised her to resume eating meat. After doing five years of research, Lierre became passion-ately convinced that we were meant to eat meat and wrote about it in her book *The Vegetarian Myth*. In this book, she also covers in depth the issues of sustainability, nutrition, and ethics associated with meat eating.

The Westbrook Family

Gregory Westbrook and his family were 100 percent vegan and 85 percent raw for six years. After two years, health problems began to arise, but they had felt so great initially from the vegan diet that they couldn't imagine it was to blame.

His wife Judie experienced excessive weight loss, atrophied muscles, and six cavities. His daughter Sara got 14 cavities. Tim, his son, lost his robust health and grew depressed, with loss of mental capacity and physical coordination. His speech got slower and became slurred. Gregory's weight dropped to 120 pounds, too thin for his 5'7" frame. His cheeks were sunken, his face wrinkled, and he got 10 to 15 cavities *per year*.

Their health improved with eggs and raw goat cheese. It got even better with salmon and turkey, but dramatic improvements came with each family member when he or she worked up the nerve to try red meat despite all the bad press it gets. Red meat was consumed twice a week.

It seemed that there was more power in the red meat than in all the other dairy, eggs, turkey, and fish put together. ...

When I began eating red meat, I began to build serious muscle. I began to feel like doing hard physical work again. ... I was ecstatic to get my youthful vitality back.

It was the red meat that ended his wife's cravings. It was the red meat that brought his son out of depression, with mental capacity and coordination returning in full force.

In researching this phenomenon, we found that there are substances in the red meat that contribute to the brain's ability to process information.

Their story is detailed in the e-book *When Hallelujah Becomes "What Happened?"* The Westbrooks continue to eat a high-raw diet but now supplement it with eggs, dairy, and cooked meat from reputable sources.

Dr. Steve Monkiewicz, ND, PhD, CBT, EFT

My friend Dr. Steve Monkiewicz tells us his story in his own words.

My "journey to raw" was not a short one or an easy one. Being diagnosed with ulcerative colitis was not even enough to move me. No, it took years of experimenting with other things only to wind up in the raw food lifestyle. After almost all the alternative methodologies I tried had failed me, I found the two things that did work: raw food and stress reduction. Actually, it is much more than stress reduction, but in its simplest terms, that is the bottom line.

Emotional reprogramming set the stage for a whole bunch of things, including making the raw food lifestyle more effective. I have known several people who "went raw" without dealing with their emotional issues and came up short in terms of positive results going raw. For optimal effect, I have found both items need to be melded together. That realization got me to thinking: could cooked animal protein be added in modest amounts and be beneficial?

As I got older, I had a taste for the stuff. I have learned that cravings are telling you something. Pay attention. So, I incorporated small amounts of cooked and uncooked animal protein to my diet after being a raw vegetarian for five years. Like others, I noticed an improvement in both my energy and my health. I didn't overdo, but adding a little seemed to have a noticeably positive return.

So I now added some animal protein to my weekly diet. Not with every meal, but maybe three or four times a week. And if I am especially active, I find I have a taste for a little more, *little* meaning maybe a couple of ounces at a time. I am a bit more liberal with that idea if I can get some organic, grass-fed beef, or sushi-grade fish, even cage-free, organic eggs.

Being raw, I feel allowing myself a bit more is natural. Many indigenous people eat animal proteins and suffer little, if any, health problems from it. Then there's the idea of being an omnivore for survival's sake. I feel the wider my food range, the more sensible (from a survival point) and more historically accurate and authentic my food experience is.

There is one more consideration in my mind: By financially supporting the people who produce food that is healthy, natural, organic, and as pure as humanly possible, I am encouraging more people to do the same thing. Let's face it: like it or not, money is a huge motivator. Why not motivate good people to do good things? You vote with your dollar, so I choose to "vote" for those principles. I choose to ignore (as much as possible) the big factory-farming and food-growing conglomerates at the same time. We can follow the money to a healthy, wealthy, and happy life. This is my choice.

Aajonus Vonderplanitz

The story of author and diet consultant Aajonus Vonderplanitz is one of going from eating *rabbit food* to eating *rabbits*!

Vonderplanitz suffered cancer as a child. A vaccination also caused him to become dyslexic and autistic. Yet with great determination to restore his health, he recovered from all of these problems by means of a raw vegan diet, which he followed assiduously. He nonetheless still retained some health challenges.

After remaining raw vegetarian for quite a few years in California, Aajonus biked around North America for three years, living off the land, hoping to learn the truth about optimal health by living in the wild.

He eventually concluded that he'd prefer to starve to death rather than return to Los Angeles, with its pollution and the survival-of-the-fittest rat race. So he began to fast himself into starvation and then unto death.

Coyotes kept waking him up at night. This happened night after night. One night, a coyote rubbed his cold nose on Aajonus's leg and motioned with his head for him to follow. The coyote led him to the pack, and they all killed a rabbit in front of him. A female coyote placed the dead rabbit at Aajonus's feet.

He felt that the coyotes were helping him end his life faster, since at that time he believed that eating raw meat would be toxic. Although Aajonus had not eaten meat in years, it began to taste delicious after only five bites.

Aajonus woke up the next morning after what he describes as the best sleep of his life. He felt strong. He had found the missing link to his health recovery! He peddled back to Los Angeles to spread word of his great discovery. Everyone thought he was crazy. That was in 1976.

People who have seen Aajonus at work no longer think he is crazy. He is respected by medical doctors who have worked with him. He has touched many lives.

In his book *We Want to Live*, Aajonus relates that his teenage son was once brought to a hospital unconscious after a car wreck. Several doctors proclaimed he would probably die, but if he survived, he would be brain dead.

Vonderplanitz relates in mini-novel fashion that when no one was looking, he emptied the drug bottles of antiseizure medications and replaced them with nutritious raw animal foods: honey, eggs, and butter. His son came out of the coma within several days. Aajonus went on to feed him raw meat.

Eventually, his son regained speech and the use of his muscles and brain. Due to the raw meat, the son's muscles did not atrophy as commonly occurs among brain-damaged accident victims.

His son completely recovered and went on to study at a university. Eleven years after the accident, he remained free of any seizures or other complications following an accident from which doctors had condemned him to live the life of a vegetable.

Aajonus has worked with people having all kinds of ailments. In his book, he claims to have facilitated 236 cancer remissions out of 240 cases. He has educated people and assisted them in beating chronic fatigue syndrome, hepatitis C, heart disease, and more.

Ursula Horaitis

Chef Ursula Horaitis has been a partly raw vegan for about 30 years and was more intensely raw for 10 years during her time in California, during which time she ate about 60 to 85 percent raw but included eggs, fish, and occasional dairy. She ate meat, such as lamb, only twice a year for special occasions.

She went 100 percent raw vegan for 18 months, on a low-fat diet (80 percent carbs, 10 percent protein, 10 percent fat) out of curiosity. Her energy level remained high as she worked 14 hours a day at her Good Mood Food Café in California. Nonetheless, she endured many health challenges.

She experienced major hair loss. Her fingernails were not growing. They were constantly infected and sensitive to food acid, including lemon juice, when she prepared food. She lost the nails on her two large toes. She lost four teeth that were constantly infected and became loose after a few months, falling out. She gained 20 pounds from the carbs. She was eating all day long, always craving food.

Now Ursula has gone back to her previous diet and eats about 60 percent raw. She eats a more balanced diet now, including fish and eggs, sometimes cooked, sometimes raw. It took about eight months for her to restore her health (hair and nails) and lose the 20 pounds.

She was influenced by Prof. Brian Peskin, author of *The 24 Hour Diet*, who claims our pancreases are meant to work with a diet of only 20 percent carbs. Ursula now eats mostly that way and feels great: fit and healthy. She utters this warning.

> If one wants to eat a raw vegan diet, it is great, especially for healing from sickness (especially if it is raw). But once well, stay away from too many carbs, and if one is not vegan for ethical reasons, include at least some eggs and fish. Raw eggs are the most perfect protein.

Though Ursula sold the Good Mood Food Café, she still works as a raw vegan chef and teaches classes on raw vegan health. She counsels people on health in her native Germany and worldwide online through Skype video conferences. She also helps restaurants with the new concept of including raw dishes in their menus. She wrote the booklet *The 7 Steps to Natural Health*. She holds lectures about these steps in Europe and America, as well as online through video conferences.

Vegan No More

Kevin Gianni, a high-profile raw fooder who hosts his Internet-based Renegade Health Show, went from raw vegan to incorporating dairy into his diet.

> There have been two times when my vegan, high-raw lifestyle didn't work the way I wanted it to. First was when I encountered digestive issues brought on by a string of failed experiments with super foods and raw chocolate. The second was when I realized I

wasn't making enough hormones to support my body's needs.

After the first instance, I used fermented goat milk to rebuild my gut flora and give me the energy that I needed after battling a gut infection. I tried fermented vegetable products, but none gave me the energy and the relief that I needed. The goat yogurt and kefir did. After a while, I didn't need it anymore and haven't had it in a while. This is relatively unscientific, but it worked. The second example is more science based.

The second instance came after some blood testing. I realized my cholesterol and pregnenolone [a hormone] were very low. My cholesterol was at 110, and my pregnenolone was at 6 (this is lower than that of an 85-year-old). My body was not producing enough cholesterol to produce my hormones!

I began supplementing with pregnenolone and krill oils (I had been using omega 3 oils before — plant based), and my cholesterol (as of last testing) shot up to 145, and my pregnenolone was increased to 70.[*]

These small additions to my diet worked when other vegan or raw options did not. I can't say either way what is good or bad, I just know what worked for me when I had these issues.[5]

The blogger Natasha was "a hardcore, self-righteous, and oh-so-judgmental vegangelical" who "never passed up an opportunity for some preaching." But after 3.5 years of veganism, her health deteriorated. She experienced sugar crashes, mood swings, ravenous hunger, bloating, allergies, feeling cold even when it was very hot outside, depression, listlessness, lower back pain, and more. Her blood tests indicated certain deficiencies despite all the supplements she had taken. This all turned around in two months after reintroducing meat and eggs into her diet.[6]

Other bloggers who have found vegan diets didn't work for them include Raw Model, Debbie Does Raw, Daniel Vitalis, Sweetly Raw, Chicken Tender, the Non-Practicing Vegan, and PaleoSister.[7]

---

[*]Normal levels of the hormone pregnenolone range between 10 and 230 ng/ml.

Part 2

Evolution of the Human Diet

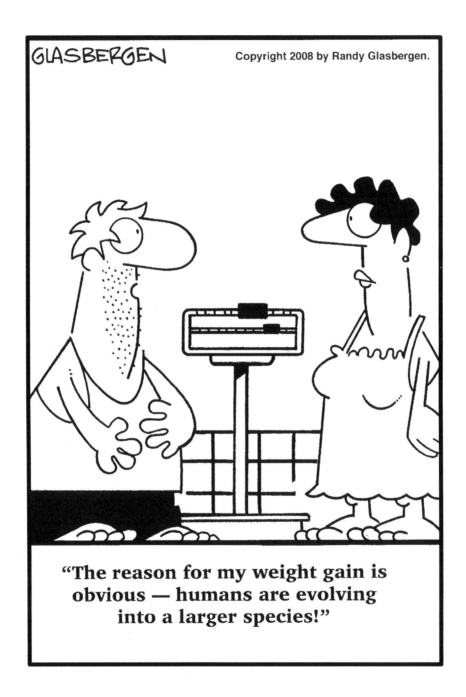

"The reason for my weight gain is obvious — humans are evolving into a larger species!"

Chapter 6

Man's Dietary History

We have 99.995 percent of our genes identical with those of our big game-hunting ancestors. We are they. We have Fred Flintstone bodies living in a George Jetson world. And therein lies the root of our problems. —Drs. Mary and Michael Eades, MDs, *The Protein Power LifePlan*

Vegetarians subscribe to a routine myth that man used to be a fruitarian. I even cited this legend in my book *The Live Food Factor*. It just seemed to make sense: since we originated in the tropics of Africa with plenty of plant life and evolved from mainly vegetarian apes, wouldn't plants be our natural diet? Let's hear from Lierre Keith.

The first myth of the nutritional vegetarians — that we aren't meant for meat — is another fairy tale filled with inedible apples. I try to remember what I believed when I was a vegan. There was a mythic golden age, long ago, when we lived in harmony with the world...and...ate what? Prehistoric paintings of humans hunting left me confused and defensive, but I was unclear on the timeline anyway. Maybe all the hunting happened before the peaceful vegetarian Goddess culture? Or maybe it was after the fall of the peaceful vegetarian...?[1]

In my quest for truth, I spent countless hours on the Internet. I also spent several hundred dollars buying books on Amazon, some out of print. I forked over several hundred more on university-level anthropological textbooks.

I was very surprised to find that the food pyramid that we evolved eating had wild meat at the base. Some anthropologists believe we ate 55 to 65 percent of our calories in raw meat. Some of it may have been cooked, since our ancestors were thought to have taken control of fire as early as 1.4 million years ago.

In fact, *no paleontologist doubts that man's forerunners depended on meat* as a large chunk of their diets. The only points they may disagree about are whether the meat was scavenged or hunted and what the ratio of plant food to meat was.

Why was I surprised? Like so many others, I had been indoctrinated by much of the media to think that meat causes cancer, that animal fats are bad, and that vegetarianism was our optimal diet. I also fell for the vegetarian chart shown in many "veg" books that insists we are herbivores though our digestive systems are so much different from theirs.

Why Study Our Evolutionary Dietary History?

Ronald Schmid, ND, author of *Traditional Foods Are Your Best Medicine*, shows us three ways we can determine the viability of a vegetarian diet.

You can take the practical approach and look at the empirical evidence — based on what we see among the vegetarians we know, and it is plain that some are not doing well. You can also take the analytical approach of a dietitian and examine the nutrients in the diet to see what is missing and look at the problems of absorption, etc. Or you can look at the historical record and ask, what do the diets of traditional indigenous cultures teach us?

Dr. Staffan Lindeberg explains in his textbook *Food and Western Disease* that there are four causes of disease or symptoms from the perspective of evolutionary biology: attack, as with bacteria[*] and viruses; defense, as with a fever, in which your body is heating itself up to limit the cell division of the bacteria and viruses; design error, as with choking on food — airway and gastrointestinal system are crossed; and lack of adaptability to a new environment, as with insulin resistance, since we are eating more high-glycemic carbs than our ancestors did.

The drug companies would have you believe that every disease is a design error and needs to be fixed by a new chemical concoction or surgical operation. In reality, most modern diseases are caused by diet and stem from lack of adaptability. These

---

[*]I explain in chapter 4 of *The Live Food Factor* that bacteria do not "attack" us. It is their metabolic waste products that poison us.

diseases began with agriculture. We have clearly not adapted to diets rich in carbs and especially grains and legumes filled with antinutrients.

Dr. Lindeberg points out the limitations and contradictions found in scientific nutritional studies:

- Epidemiological research, which involves observing factors affecting the health and illness of populations, is unreliable because we cannot control all variable factors.

- Molecular biology is hard to rely on, since lab animals are not biologically the same as humans. Furthermore, there may be many as yet undiscovered nutrients and molecules that can impact the studies.

- An intervention study with a controlled trial has the flaw that people often simultaneously improve their lifestyles in other respects, such as giving up smoking or exercising more.

- Then there is publication bias, as studies with a positive outcome get published more often.

- There is funding bias, since scientists want to please those who finance their studies so they can get more work.

- Citation bias also occurs: drug studies get quoted much more than nutritional ones do.

- Then there is the influence of preconceived ideas: of course, every researcher hopes that his or her hypothesis will be confirmed.

Evolutionary nutrition provides an important complement to traditional scientific methods. The new field of *nutrigenomics* looks at the effects of foods and food constituents on gene expression. It considers the diets that people evolved eating. Traditional peoples on their traditional diets have been observed to be free of modern-day illnesses.

Those who were best suited to the food that was available were the ones who had the greatest chances of surviving. Adaptation is very slow, often taking about 40,000 years.[*]

---

[*]Physicist Guy-Claude Burger calculates that it would take 1 to 2 million years for complete biochemical adaptation. Adaptive tolerance is not the same as true adaptation.

For illustration, take the last 365 million years and convert them to a calendar year, making each million years one day. On January 1, we have our first amphibian ancestor. The earliest mammal is born on June 10. Our first primate ancestor arrives on October 28. *Homo sapiens* is born December 31 at 7:30 PM. Agriculture develops at 11:45 PM. At 11:59:50, just 15 minutes after agriculture and 10 seconds before the end of the year, cardiovascular disease begins.[2]

If agriculture begins 20,000 years ago as now thought, processed food begins appearing right about 11:59:59.8, less than one second before midnight on the last day of the year, assuming processing started about 400 years ago with sugar refining. The types and amounts of processed foods have steadily increased and accelerated throughout this past century to include microwaving; irradiation; insertion of chemical additives, artificial flavorings, and sweeteners; and marketing of nonfoods like soft drinks, margarine, Olestra, and many more.

Lindeberg also dispels the myth that Stone Age peoples had short life spans. He explains that it becomes difficult for osteologists to make estimates on a middle-aged skeleton other than simply saying "40 years or older." So whether a person reached 40 or 90 years cannot in many cases be determined.[3]

Furthermore, by studying the few remaining modern "Stone Age" people, he found that the health of traditional peoples remained quite good up to the end of their lives. The quality of life in the Trobriand Islands is quite high until they suddenly deteriorate rapidly shortly before dying.[4] This is how it should be and how it is with wild animals in pristine environments.

Man Evolved Eating Meat

Archeology tells the story of our ancient omnivorism in so many ways. Hunting spears were often found by the skeletons of our forebears. Excavations and cave art demonstrate that the Cro-Magnon of Europe and Asia hunted and ate large game: bears, lions, hyenas, wild horses, bison, reindeer, woolly mammoths, deer, and woolly rhinoceros.

In the Americas, the animals included over 100 species, including wolves, mammoths, giant beavers, camels, and more. Between 40,000 years ago and 10,000 years ago, many of these animals became extinct due to overhunting. Many researchers believe this lack of big game forced us to develop agriculture.

In addition, in cold places like Europe (and many more areas were very cold during ice ages), plant foods would have been scarce. The only way to survive winters would have been to eat meat.[5]

In fact, Professor Caleb Finch, PhD, of the University of Southern California believes that early man developed meat-adaptive genes that enabled him to survive the hazards of meat eating, such as cholesterol, phytanic acid, and infectious pathogens.

Brain evolution was crucial to the evolution of meat eating; we may consider as "meat-adaptive" the genes that enabled further brain developments.[6]

Finch also believes it was these genes that extended man's life span beyond that of the apes.

Let's look at a brief review of man's predecessors and their diets. Methods of figuring out the diets of skeletal remains include tooth morphology and microwear, carbon isotope analysis, trace element analysis, analysis of "food refuse" from archeological sites, and more.[7]

The first primates were very small and lived as early as 65 million years ago. They were primarily insectivores and only later ate fruit.[8]

This is interesting because it means mammals evolved eating animals (insects) right from the beginning. About 50 to 30 million years ago, their diets expanded to include meat from other mammals. Even a pro-vegetarian diet website warns us that man's dietary history was not vegetarian.

You sometimes hear the argument that humans are "naturally vegetarian" or that they evolved as vegetarians. This is somewhat dangerous to pursue, as the scientific evidence all indicates that we are omnivores; i.e., we can survive on a wide variety of plant and animal foods ...

What foods then has Nature programmed Man to eat in order to maintain health, growth, activity, and reproduction? Boyd and Konner state that "from about 24 to 5 million years ago, fruits appear to have been the main dietary constituent for hominids. ... Since 4.5 million years ago, our ancestral feeding pattern included increasing amounts of meat."[9]

From 7 to 5 million years ago, there was a divergence of chimpanzees into two separate lines,

one of which was proto-human.[10]

Ardipithecus ramidus was the first hominid that walked on two feet. He lived 5 to 4 million years ago. The skeleton of one, named "Ardi," was a biped whose feet, pelvis, legs, and hands suggest she was a biped on the ground but a quadruped when moving about in the trees.

The first upright hominid that walked on two feet lived 4 to 3 million years ago. The famous "Lucy" skeleton was from that era. Lucy and her family were called *Australopithecus afarensis*.

Next, between 3 and 2.6 million years ago, Australopithecus diverged into three lines of australopithecine species, one of which gave rise to humans.

They ate their food raw, but unlike other primates, they created crude stone tools to collect food more efficiently. They were bipeds, but restricted in agility. According to anthropologist Robert Foley, ScD, australopithecines were likely "occasionally carnivorous."[11]

The first of the genus *Homo* arose approximately 2.3 million to 1.4 million years ago: *Homo habilis*. They were hunter-gatherers, gathering wild plants and hunting and scavenging for dead animals. Unlike their australopithecine ancestors, they were runners. They were athletic and more active.[12] Often called "handy man," *Homo habilis* was the first species of this genus to make tools, as famed anthropologist Richard Leakey suggests.

It is reasonable to suppose that meat eating, either scavenged or obtained by hunting, was a factor, and possibly the major one, in the gradual emergence of the homo line from the basic hominid stock, leaving a predominantly vegetarian niche to be occupied by the australopithecines.[13]

But he adds that the rise of a hunting and gathering existence is more likely to have occurred as early as *five million* years ago when we broke off from the chimpanzees. Our ancestors may well have been eating meat for four to five million years, though big game hunting likely began no more than two million years ago.

Homo erectus thrived from 1.7 million to 400 thousand BC. Hunting increased. Hand axes 1.4 million years old were found in Africa that were so complex it took modern archeologists several months to acquire the skills to produce replicas of the quality they found.[14]

These guys had heavy jaws and large teeth — perhaps because they ate their meat raw — and also had low foreheads. They eventually gained control of fire about 1.4 million years ago, but it was not generally used for cooking until at least 50,000 to 40,000 years ago.[15]

The use of fire enabled *Homo erectus* to leave his ancestral home in Africa and move to colder climates. Around 400,000 BC, an archaic *Homo sapiens* appeared.

How Our Brains Developed

Around 150,000 BC, a subspecies of archaic *Homo sapiens* began to develop, *Homo sapiens neanderthalensis*, the Neanderthals, who thrived about 100,000 to 30,000 years ago in Europe and western Asia.

Another subspecies of archaic *Homo sapiens*, called *Homo sapiens sapiens*, our immediate ancestors, remained for some time in East Africa. Every single person alive today can trace his or her ancestry back to a single female skeleton found from that era. She is called Eve.

Even if you don't believe we descended from the same branch as apes, there is ample proof in the DNA that we all descended from this omnivorous woman. Here is what Wikipedia, an online encyclopedia of communal authorship, says about Eve.

Mitochondrial Eve refers to the matrilineal "MRCA" (most recent common ancestor). In other words, this was the woman from whom all living humans today descend, on their mother's side, and through the mothers of those mothers and so on, back until all lines converge on one person.

Because it is generally passed from mother to offspring without recombination, all mitochondrial DNA (mtDNA) in every living person is directly descended from hers by definition. Mitochondrial Eve is the female counterpart of Y-chromosomal Adam, the patrilineal most recent common ancestor, although they lived thousands of years apart.

Mitochondrial Eve is generally estimated to have lived around 200,000 years ago, most likely in East Africa, when *Homo sapiens sapiens* ("anatomically modern humans") were developing as a population distinct from other human sub-species.[16]

They (we) almost became extinct, but then something happened. Dr. Barry Sears, PhD, explains one theory about when we discovered brain food (shellfish, fish, and eggs).

Our immediate ancestors were perhaps only one or two generations from complete extinction, just like the other 97 percent of previous primate species. But something happened that gave them a second chance: they learned to scavenge a new food source that wouldn't have been found in the African savanna. This food was the shellfish found along the shores of the lakes in the East African Rift Valley. Shellfish consume algae and therefore can accumulate algae-derived fats in higher concentrations, in turn giving our immediate ancestors more of these algae-derived fats than have been consumed at any time in history.[17]

He explains that eating shellfish was alien to them, since they had hunted land animals. But desperate times call for desperate measures. This one move of eating large quantities of DHA increased the size of their brains. They stumbled upon brain food, and this gave them a cognitive leap that enabled them to conquer the world. The frontal cortex, where thinking and reasoning take place, gave them a huge evolutionary advantage.

The Neanderthals and 97 percent of the unsuccessful primate species before them died out. *Homo sapiens sapiens* remains. As we shall see, another theory (by Dr. Stephen Cunnane) puts the discovery of brain food much earlier, right at the beginning of when our brains started expanding.

At 40,000 years ago, the brains of our ancestral *Homo sapiens* peaked. There was a sudden explosion of new art, stone and bone toolmaking, culture, religion, and social organization. Humans migrated around the globe for the next 40,000 years.

There have been only a few significant genetic changes in the most recent 40,000 years, one being that some people, the Northern Europeans, have partially adapted to dairy with the retention of intestinal lactase to digest dairy into adulthood.

From 35,000 to 15,000 BC, the *Homo sapiens* Cro-Magnons thrived in Europe and added a lot more meat to their diets with big game hunting. If a Cro-Magnon man were alive today, he would be visibly indistinguishable from modern man.

The paleolithic period describes all the time from 2.6 million years ago, when the first homo line began with *Homo habilis*, until 10,000 years ago, when agriculture became prevalent and the neolithic period began. It has been proven that during that entire paleolithic time, man was a hunter and gatherer. It would be nonsense to say that we have not adapted to meat or that meat is toxic to us. How then did we thrive for 2.6 million years?

It has been proven by anthropologists that man was aggressive at obtaining, systematically transporting, and butchering animal carcasses, and that this increased meat consumption coincided with evolutionary changes resulting in larger brains, dental reduction, and gut modification.[18]

From the beginning of the homo lineage 2.6 million years ago until 40,000 years ago when brain size peaked, our brains were getting bigger and more sophisticated. Our guts shrank at the same time. We no longer have the big, protruding belly that chimps have. Such bellies are characteristic of vegetarian animals.

Drs. Leslie Aiello and Peter Wheeler came up with the Expensive Tissue Hypothesis. They noticed that the brain and digestive systems take up a lot of metabolic energy. In order for our brains to use up so much energy, we had to give up energy from somewhere else. That place was found to be the digestive tract, which actually got smaller. So as our guts shrank, our brains grew. We effectively traded the ability to digest cellulose for increased intelligence.

A considerable problem for the early hominids would have been to provide themselves, as a large-bodied species, with sufficient quantities of high-quality food to permit the necessary reduction of the gut. The obvious solution would have been to include increasingly large amounts of animal-derived food in the diet.[19]

A brain uses up a lot more calories — roughly 16 times as much as skeletal muscle tissue![20] — which is why man needs more calories per unit of

A brain uses up a lot more calories — roughly 16 times as much as skeletal muscle tissue! – which is why man needs more calories per unit of weight than do other primates. Fully 20 to 25 percent of our calories go to brain metabolism, compared to only 8 to 10 percent for other primates.

weight than do other primates. Fully 20 to 25 percent of our calories go to brain metabolism, compared to only 8 to 10 percent for other primates.[21] Brains are expensive to grow and maintain — using ten times more energy for maintenance than most other tissues.[22]

Have you ever eaten a big meal and noticed brain fog? This is because the digestive system suddenly needs a lot of energy, and it competes with your brain for that energy. But if you eat some very lightly cooked meat with raw or steamed vegetables or some fruit by itself, minimal energy goes to your digestive tract, and your brain continues to function well.

Dr. Loren Cordain, PhD, et al. showed that modern human foraging populations typically derive 45 to 65 percent of their daily calories from animal foods, since these are much more calorie and nutrient dense than plant foods.[23]

In all primates, the bigger the brain, the higher the diet quality must be. Also, large-bodied primates have expanded colons that are able to digest high fiber amounts, fermenting them to extract additional energy in the form of volatile fatty acids. Humans' short digestive tracts are midway between those of herbivores and those of carnivores, adapted to an easily digested, nutrient-rich diet.[24]

Large herbivorous mammals spend a lot more time foraging, feeding, and moving to feed than do those that eat meat.[25] Even chimpanzees spend 75 percent of their waking day in search of plant foods.[26] One would have to forage all day to get the nutrients found in just one small animal. Early man probably didn't like working long hours any more than modern man does.

Furthermore, to chew all the plant food needed to sustain oneself, early humans would have had to spend 42 percent of waking hours chewing, about five hours a day according to Harvard primatologist Richard Wrangham.[27] He claims that the amount of time spent chewing is related to body size in primates, and this is how he got that figure.

Humans had to expend a lot more calories than we do today, remember. Between foraging and chewing, a whole day would be spent in feeding. By hunting and eating meat, they found time for socializing with the tribe. Modern hunter-gatherers have generally been observed to put in four-hour days concludes Katharine Milton, an anthropologist at the University of California, Berkeley.

We would never have evolved as large, socially active hominids if we hadn't turned to meat. ... The vegetarian primates (orangutans and gorillas) are less social than the more omnivorous chimpanzees, possibly because collecting and consuming all that forage takes so darned much time.[28]

Hunting forced early men to collaborate to a degree not displayed by any of our primate cousins, says Richard Leakey.

Meat eating was important in propelling our ancestors along the road to humanity, but only as part of a package of socially oriented changes involving the gathering of plant foods and sharing the spoils. ...

A plant-eating existence tends to make the individual members of a troop very self-centered and uncooperative. In spite of the intense social interactions that take place, especially in our closest relative the chimpanzees, and even though there is group awareness of a sort in the search for food, to be a vegetarian is to be essentially solitary. Each individual tears the leaves from a branch, or plucks fruits from a tree and promptly eats them.[29]

Leakey explains that chimps experience no communal eating or even sharing of food with close relatives. Hunting, however, demands collaboration.

When early man eventually gained more energy from a diet high in meat, he no longer needed extra digestive room to process all the plant roughage. He therefore lost the chimp's or gorilla's ability to digest massive amounts of greens and vegetables, instead going for the nutrient- and calorie-rich animal foods and becoming more efficient at digesting them. Since our ancestors also had hands, unlike other animals, they could break open an animal's skull and eat its brains. This increased man's brain size, since brains are rich in DHA, needed by our own brains.

There are several different theories as to how early man got this extra energy to feed a larger

brain, though all agree it was from animal meat. These theories attempt to account for how we got larger brains and smaller digestive tracts, teeth, and jaws. Large teeth and jaws like those that other primates have are needed to grind fibrous plant food that has low energy density.

Richard Leakey says of the tooth size reduction that it was "probably an adaptation produced by a shift in diet from one made up exclusively of plant foods to one that included meat."[30]

The Savanna Theory holds that the climate in East Africa got so harsh and dry that the newly bipedal australopithecines were forced to rely less on fruit trees, which were disappearing. The savanna was abundant in grasses that supported plant-eating animals, but lacked fruit- and nut-bearing plants. Humans therefore had to hunt the abundant herbivores for food.

A brain's growth also depends on the fatty acids DHA and *arachidonic acid* (AA). Wild plant foods available on the African savanna (tubers and nuts) were found to have only trace amounts of DHA and AA, whereas the organs and muscle meat of wild African ruminants contained these important fatty acids.[31]

Later it was found that East Africa didn't get that dry, and there would have been more trees. So it transformed into the Woodlands Theory. The problem with this theory, as we shall see, is that the woodlands did not provide enough of the brain-specific nutrients.

Another theory is the Aquatic Ape Theory. It postulates that certain primates spent a lot of their time in the water, and these evolved to become humans. By eating seafood rich in DHA and EPA, their brains developed.

Then there is the Cooking Theory, that cooking made us human. You can imagine what I, as a raw fooder, think of this theory! The theory goes that we had to use fire for warmth and to keep predators away as we came down from the trees, so we discovered that cooking food makes it give us more energy.

Although no pots and pans over 20,000 years old have been found, Richard Wrangham points out that traditional peoples find ways to cook without pots. An example is to poke a hole in an egg and set it by the fire. Cooking food enables more of the calories to be absorbed, which is one reason people lose weight on raw food diets.

The issue I see here is that a few hundred calories a day isn't that big of a deal, certainly not enough for our brains to evolve so well. Also, most plant food — raw or cooked — is not high in DHA or its omega-3 precursors, so the brain would need a lot of in order to expand, as we will see in chapter 8.

Besides, I believe we ate at least 50 percent raw and likely much more until roughly 10,000 years ago when agriculture became well established. That is when we began eating so many foods (grains and legumes) that are too toxic to eat raw unless properly soaked and rinsed, as will be explained in chapter 15.

Without adequate intake of minerals found naturally in seafoods, we cannot reach full intellectual potential.

The theory I find most plausible is the Shore-Based Scenario, which theorizes that it was not the meat from land animals that made our brains grow. Rather it was eating brain food from the ocean, rivers, lakes, or seas. This differs from the Aquatic Ape Theory in that early man did not live in the water. Instead he discovered shellfish, eggs, and seaweeds washed up on the shore.

In his textbook *Survival of the Fattest: The Key to Human Brain Evolution*, Dr. Stephen Cunnane explains that the theories that eating land animals made our brains grow larger are flawed.

Our australopithecine ancestors may well have been able to hunt animals if they cooperated as a group, as chimpanzees have been observed to do, but chimps do not readily share their meat — except for male monkeys who trade meat for sex! It is therefore unlikely the australopithecine would have done so either.

Yet an abundance of meat-sharing would have been absolutely necessary because babies and children need a lot of brain food for their fast-growing brains. Young children could not easily have hunted land animals but could easily have gathered shellfish. They have been observed doing so in modern hunter-gatherer societies. Therefore, the development of children's brains would not have depended on the sharing of meat.

Furthermore, we now know that seafood, shellfish especially, is brain food due to its DHA and EPA content. Shellfish (and fish and eggs to a lesser degree) contain five brain-specific minerals that work together synergistically. When there is a deficit of even one of these minerals, a person's brain cannot function well, let alone evolve.

These are iron, iodine, selenium, copper, and zinc. Without adequate intake of these minerals, found naturally in shellfish and fish, we cannot reach full intellectual potential. Iodine is the most critical one. Stephen Cunnane attributes the 11 percent brain shrinkage that began 10,000 to 11,000 years ago to the shortage of iodine typically found in inland soils.

People inland, especially in the mountains, often are deficient in this critical brain nutrient. As a consequence, refiners in the US were required to add an inorganic form of it to table salt starting in 1924 in order to combat goiter. Many of those who are aware of how toxic table salt is have cut back on it without adding iodine from other sources, such as sea vegetables, part of the reason why there is an epidemic of hypothyroidism today.

Dr. Cunnane points out that getting our extra brain energy could not have happened on vegetarian or even insect diets. The energy expended in searching for nuts, digging up tubers, and raiding termite colonies would not have yielded extra energy for the brain to grow. If vegetation were all that was needed, why didn't the other primates, who shared our brain's genetic potential for expansion, also evolve in the same direction that ours did? Clearly there was a branch of australopithecines that discovered brain food, and this led to the evolution of their brains on the path to becoming human.

Cunnane explains that to evolve, man's brain needed to have a steady, easy supply of nutrient-dense food. The shores of lakes, rivers, and oceans provided that supply. It was thus environmental permissiveness rather than environmental pressure that led to our evolution.

Having the secure source of food, we had leisure time to play with sticks and stones, invent tools, and play in the sand to make art. Our time was freed up. Even today, Cunnane points out, "These traditional groups measure affluence not in material possessions, but in time available for story-telling, music, and dancing."[32]

Cunnane explains that another reason there had to be an abundant, relatively easy way to access food is that people (especially women and babies) had to be able to get a bit fat. By having surplus food stores, a woman could eat enough to have a baby with plenty of baby fat lasting three to five years. This baby fat, unlike adult fat, is rich in DHA stores. This assured proper brain nutrition in the human, who has a very vulnerable brain in early development.

In fact, if mother's milk with its DHA is not available, the infant's body fat DHA will last for two to three weeks. By age three, the toddler could relatively easily find shellfish or go egg hunting by himself, if need be. Thus there is a great disadvantage in a baby born prematurely or with a low weight.

Cunnane further asserts that we are still in the shore-based phase of human evolution and still need a shore-based food supply. The main brain food is shellfish with fish second. Eggs from chickens fed omega-3-rich feed are also brain foods, but they don't contain much copper. Copper is relatively easy to obtain from plant foods however.

One fifth of the world's population consumes diets that do not support brain development. In the mountainous regions of several continents, many people are mentally challenged because of iodine deficiency. Remember, Dr. Price found that coastal tribes exchanged seafood for plant food from mountainous tribes despite the fact that they were at war with each other! The mountain people found that they could get by only three months without seafood.

The Fat Debate

All anthropologists agree we evolved eating meat. They disagree on the ratio of plant food to animal food, and they also debate whether the meat was low or high in fat. Dr. Stanley Boyd Eaton, MD, one of the authors of *The Paleolithic Prescription*, argues that the cave man diet was low in fat,

but others cite evidence that we ate large quantities of animal fat.

Bison and camels had humps composed largely of tallow (fat). Organ meats are known to be treasured by traditional peoples for their rich nutrients, including healthful fats. People needed the fat-soluble vitamins, such as A and D found in animal fats.[33] There may also have been differences in dietary ratios of meat and fat among paleolithic peoples according to the foods available in each region.

Our Meat-Based Dietary Origins

Dr. Loren Cordain, PhD, professor at Colorado State University, is one of the world's leading experts on the paleolithic diet. He is author of the book *The Paleolithic Diet: Lose Weight and Get Healthy by Eating the Food You Were Designed to Eat.*

R.B. Lee, a Canadian anthropologist, had written a paper explaining that paleolithic man ate a diet consisting of a 65:35 ratio of plants to animal foods. Dr. Cordain ran a computerized nutritional analysis of the 65:35 plant to animal ratio. He found that for a human to get enough calories on a plant-based diet, he would have to gather 12 pounds of vegetation, which would have been unlikely. He also found that Lee was including shellfish under gathering, though it is clearly an animal product. Lee also included only 58 of the 181 hunter-gatherer societies.

When Cordain revised the analysis, he found the ratio to be flipped at 65 percent animal foods and 35 percent plants. This corresponds almost identically to the Zone Diet, which is 40 percent carbs (plants), 30 percent fat, and 30 percent protein. Consider also that before agriculture with its increased cooking, it would have been difficult to obtain much food from plants because of all the antinutrients found in grains, beans, and other foods. Antinutrients evolved in plants to prevent predators from eating too much of them.

Nowadays, it would be unsustainable for the planet and financially untenable for most individuals to eat that much animal food. Also, as man domesticated animals, they were given progressively inferior diets to consume, accelerated in the past century, which makes them less healthful to eat today. It may not be necessary to eat such a high ratio of animal foods for health if you consciously keep your insulin levels under control and also eat some seaweed and algae for brain food.

Our brains and nervous systems are about half composed of complicated, long-chain fatty acid molecules that do not occur in plants. These fats are found in human milk in order for a baby to grow a large brain, but not in cow's milk, since cow's brains are only a fifth to a third as big as ours despite their much larger body size. Bones of prehistoric people have been found with animals, and sometimes the animals' skulls were broken, indicating that people ate their brains.[34] By eating the animals' brains, they could feed their own brains.

Dr. Henry Bunn, PhD, professor of anthropology at the University of California at Berkley states it bluntly.

I contend that the procurement and consumption of meat by early *Homo erectus* is knowable from the Plio-Pleistocene archaeological record and created selective pressures for the evolution of human behavior.[35]

He notes that the pattern of bone damage of thousands of mammalian specimens shows this.

The fragmentation occurred predominantly when the bones were fresh, rather than during fossilization. A high degree of fragmentation is a common feature of humanly broken bones at more recent archaeological sites, in contrast to the relatively more complete bone elements characteristic of many bone accumulations generated by large carnivores.[36]

Man may have been a scavenger, or even a "power" scavenger initially, aggressively driving predators from their kills. But because 95 percent of the carcass fat is found in the brains, organs, and muscles, not just the bones, there was a need for man to hunt the animal directly.[37]

Gnawing bones left over from another animal's kill would simply not have provided enough nourishment, according to anthropologist Dr. Martha Tappen, PhD.

Scavenging opportunities are too unpredictable and rare to be a highly ranked food item for early hominids because deliberate search for them has a high rate of failure.[38]

Indeed, the evidence is strong that we were not just scavengers or hunters of small animals only. For example, in America there are 10,000-year-old fossil remains of 300 buffalo near the Arikaree River in Colorado. These animals were trapped by being driven down sloping banks of ice. Their bones were found arranged in an orderly fashion, indicating there may have been an assembly line for butchering.

A 120,000-year-old Cro-Magnon cave painting shows bison with spears piercing them. A rock painting in the Transkei of South Africa shows an eland herd being driven over a cliff by Late Stone Age hunters. There is evidence in the ancient Near East (Tel Abu Hureyra) that animals were driven into a corral to be killed, similar to the Native American practice of driving bison or antelope herds over cliffs.

Evidence of meat eating dates back to 2.6 million years ago, with the size of the brain steadily increasing since then, especially starting about 1.9 million years ago.[39]

Not only has man *adapted* to eating meat over the past 2.6 million years, man has actually developed — for peak health, at least — a *dependency* on meat! As we will later see, it is the high-carb diet that most people have not adapted to. It spikes the blood insulin, and this wreaks havoc on the body.

The caveman diet consisted of vegetables, fruits, nuts, greens, roots, and meat. Cereals, potatoes, bread, and milk were not eaten at all. His diet was not the cause of his shortened lifespan, according to Mark Thomas, professor of evolutionary genetics at University College London.

Paleolithic man may have died earlier than we do now, but he didn't die of bad nutrition.[40]

The Human Diet in Recent Pre-agricultural Societies

Dr. Weston Price was a practicing dentist active in the 1920s. He spent 10 years of his retirement traveling all over the world to examine the last of the traditional peoples, those who had not yet assimilated into modern diets and lifestyles. His *Nutrition and Physical Degeneration* is a classic, arguably the most extensive study of native nutrition we have. This book is an in-depth examination of extremely healthy people and their diets, including a number of different races and genetic variations, not just one.

He found that people everywhere ate animal products. Organ meats such as liver were considered the most nutritious. Some even regarded them as sacred. The people he examined who continued on the traditional diets had almost no cavities and were very happy, with robust health. If someone had health problems, it was common knowledge that the solution was to be found in nutrient-rich animal products.

Hygienic author Arnold De Vries researched the available literature extensively and wrote the book *Primitive Man and His Food*. By *primitive*, it is meant that technology had not yet developed. The people themselves were anything but primitive.

As I read about all the journeys and all the observations documented throughout the world, one thing stood out: All primitive peoples were not only healthy, but also intelligent and happy — *very* happy. There were no signs of mental illness or depression in any of them.

There is a belief among many spiritually inclined people nowadays that if you are ill, you must work deeply on your "spiritual issues" in order to heal. Yet, few of these guys had any spiritual (happiness) issues. So, which came first, the unhappiness and spiritual issues that led to disease, or the disease that led to unhappiness and spiritual issues?

I think the answer should be obvious.

Very few of these guys suffered from physical illness, let alone unhappiness or lack of intelligence. Yet nowadays we say, "Oh, it's just my cross to bear" if you're a Christian or, "Oh, it's just my karma" if you're into the Eastern thinking.

I think it's pretty clear in this chicken-and-egg matter that the modern high-sugar, high-grain diets lead to disease. The disease and nutrient deficiency permeating our entire civilization lead to the unhappiness. So to fix all of our mental woes, our depressions, our physical illnesses, we must return to our traditional ways of eating.

De Vries's research revealed that "primitive" people from all over the world ate a mostly raw diet consisting of a wide variety of whole, unrefined foods, sometimes including raw meat. The food that was cooked was exposed to heat only for a short time.

The percentage of animal products varied according to the tribe, ranging from high in complex raw carbs with some meat once every couple of weeks and daily raw milk and cheese (the Hunzas) to extremely low in carbs and 95 to 100 percent meat (the Eskimos).

Most people think that considerable pain and length of delivery time are necessary evils of childbirth. However, traditional women throughout the world gave birth with little or no discomfort and quickly — less than an hour. They were often expected to do so without any assistance. Many would go right back to work after giving birth, while modern women often take weeks to recover.

People on their traditional diets were able to withstand very extreme hot or cold temperatures. Though furs were available, they were often not used in bitterly cold weather.

For example, natives of Australia would sleep without clothes in the cold. In Chile, during the coldest winters, weather that would kill birds, women would wash their heads in cold water and not dry their hair. The Indians of Tierra del Fuego would survive the cold climate without clothing.

Weston Price noted of the Peruvians, "They can sleep comfortably through the freezing nights with their ponchos wrapped about their heads and their legs and feet bare." The torrid jungles of the Amazon region were also well tolerated without fans or air conditioners.

People's teeth very rarely had cavities. People kept their teeth into old age. The women were nearly always beautiful, another sign of health. Cancer and other degenerative diseases were nearly nonexistent. Many people did not have gray hair, even when old, and men were not bald. It was not uncommon to live to be 100.

It is often said in the vegetarian community that meat could not be man's original food because man could not possibly run as fast as his prey. Yet, the Native Americans of the Great Plains would run a hundred miles in a single stretch without stopping for rest.

The need for sleep would make itself apparent before physical exhaustion, and it was only this, and possibly hunger, that forced a halt to the run. A tribesman would start chasing a deer in the morning and continue the race until sundown if necessary, until the animal was worn out and caught. The Indian was a creature built for speed — a free, swift, graceful animal — and his physical power in running was always noted by the white explorers making first contact with the people.[41]

The explorer Dominguez found Indians from Brazil to be so "swift of foot and so long-winded that they tired out the deer and would catch them with their hands."[42]

De Vries attributes the following reasons for the superior diet leading to peak health in tribal peoples: proper soil care; proper feeding of domesticated animals; no stimulating, irritating, or intoxicating foods or beverages; no canned or processed foods; no pasteurization of dairy products; cooking kept to a minimum in temperature and time; all infants breastfed; foods eaten fresh soon after gathering; use of whole grains instead of refined; use of honey or natural sweeteners instead of sugar; liberal consumption of fruits, nuts, and other foods eaten in their raw state; maximal variety of healthful foods.[43]

The Biological Case for Omnivorism

If you go to vegetarian websites or books, you can see charts that compare the human digestive tract with those of herbivores. Other sites compare the human digestive system with those of carnivores. *The Stone Age Diet* has one that shows how similar we are to dogs, reprinted in *The Vegetarian Myth*. So which is right? Both are. We can digest both meat and plants.

Listen to Drs. Michael and Mary Eades, MDs.

Although in anthropological scientific circles, there's absolutely no debate about it — every respected authority will confirm that we were hunters — many people still believe in the dangers of meat eating in light of our supposed vegetarian past. We've had at least twenty people send us copies of the same tables published in an anti-meat book from the 1970s showing how sundry parts of our anatomy or physiology are more like those of herbivores than of carnivores, thus "proving" our vegetarian inclinations. We are, of course, neither. We're omnivores, able to subsist on meat and plants — hence the intermediate size of our intestinal tract.[44]

One such chart by vegan raw fooder John Coleman compares various body parts and attributes to conclude that humans are frugivores.[45] As we will see, it really depends on which parts are compared. Coleman omits parts that don't suit his agenda.

Dr. Walter Voegtlin argued that our digestive systems are similar to those of dogs. Sally Fallon and Mary Enig, PhD, summarize the observations of Dr. Walter Voegtlin's *The Stone Age Diet.*

Like the carnivorous dog, man has canine teeth, ridged molars, and incisors in both jaws. His jaw is designed for crushing and tearing, and moves in vertical motions. Mastication of his food is unnecessary [but improves human digestion], and he does not ruminate. His stomach holds two quarts, empties in three hours, rests between meals, lacks bacteria and protozoa, secretes large quantities of hydrochloric acid and does not digest cellulose.

His digestive tract is short relative to body length, the cecum is nonfunctional and his appendix vestigial [now it is thought to be involved in immunity]. His rectum is small, contains putrefactive bacterial flora [if the food is cooked], and does not contribute to the digestive process. The volume of feces is small [depending on fiber content], digestive efficiency borders on 100 percent; his gallbladder is active and well-developed. Both the dog and man feed intermittently and can survive without a stomach or colon.

The herbivorous sheep, by contrast, lacks canines, has flat molars, and incisors only in the lower jaw. His jaw is designed for grinding and rotary movements. Mastication and rumination are vital functions. His stomach holds eight and one-half gallons, contains bacteria and protozoa, never empties, and has but weak production of hydrochloric acid. His colon and cecum are long and capacious; the cecum performs a vital function; the bacterial flora of his rectum is fermentative rather than putrefactive: feces are voluminous; gallbladder function is weak or absent; and total digestive efficiency [if food is cooked] is 50 percent or less.

The sheep feeds continuously. He cannot live without his stomach or colon. His entire digestive tract is about five times longer, as a ratio of body length, than that of man and his dog.[46]

Unlike herbivores, human eyes focus forward like those of predators, and humans have ample hydrochloric acid for digesting meat when healthy. We have small incisors for cutting meat that we no longer need since we have tools. Our digestive tract is intermediate in length. It is neither as long as that of an herbivore nor as short as that of a carnivore. Meat does not putrefy in the intestines if eaten raw or rare. Unlike herbivores but like carnivores, we have gallbladders that help us digest fats.

We have only two stomach compartments, unlike cows, which have four. We also do not have much of the bacteria they have to help digest the cellulose of high-fiber plant food.

Herbivores would die without plant food. We can live without plants, as we have no biological need for carbohydrates in order to live. Without protein or fat, we would die. The Eskimos often ate only the plant food found in the stomachs of seals, yet they were the healthiest of traditional peoples. This is not ideal, just possible.

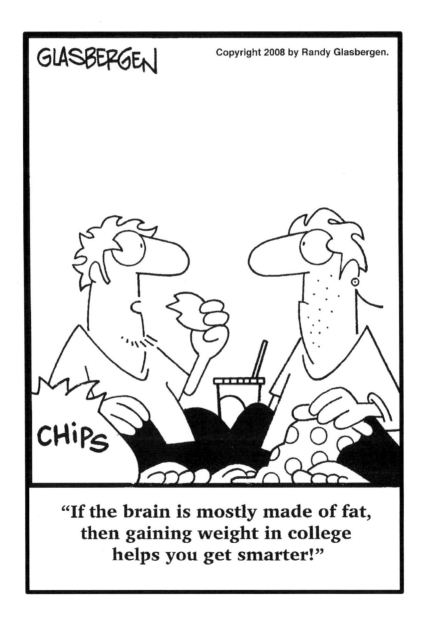

"If the brain is mostly made of fat, then gaining weight in college helps you get smarter!"

Chapter 7

Agriculture: Civilization, Hierarchy, Disease

Archaeologists studying the rise of farming have reconstructed a crucial stage at which we made the worst mistake in human history. Forced to choose between limiting population or trying to increase food production, we chose the latter and ended up with starvation, warfare, and tyranny.

Hunter-gatherers practiced the most successful and longest-lasting lifestyle in human history. In contrast, we're still struggling with the mess into which agriculture has tumbled us, and it's unclear whether we can solve it. —Jared Diamond, PhD, *Discover Magazine*, May, 1987

The beginning of agriculture arose 10,000 to 20,000 years ago, occurring at roughly the same time period all over the world. Some believe that the addictiveness of the opioids in wheat was a large incentive to settle down, grow these crops, and learn how to grind and cook them to make them more edible. Other opioids are found in milk, and milking also began with agriculture.[1]

Other factors include the recession of the last Ice Age glaciers, which created a warmer global climate. Another possible scenario was that humans overpopulated and were running out of wild game to sustain them.

But the *real* population explosion began with agriculture.

Whatever the reason, man has never been the same after having created civilization and a hierarchy of power. The diseases of civilization arose at the same time: cancer, heart disease, diabetes, arthritis, dental cavities, and infectious diseases.

Skeletons began to shrink because the phytates in grains and legumes bind up key minerals, making them unavailable to our digestive systems. Surviving skeletons show loss of bone density and signs of arthritis beginning in that time period.

Paleolithic people had had robust skeletons, due not to just a higher bone density, but also to a more favorable bone structure.[2] The bones of hunter-gatherers reveal that their diets had no deficiencies. They also were not subject to the perils of crop shortages and famines. The hunter-gatherers were found to be taller and free from modern degenerative diseases.

Once agriculture began, human bones were found to have symmetrical osteoporosis, known by several other names, such as porotic hyperostosis,

cribra cranii, and hyperostosis spongiosa. The cause was anemia due to insufficient meat. Infectious diseases arose due to bacteria and parasites in farm animals, which are definitely inferior to wild animals as a food source.

For millions of years, we relied on wild foods 99.8 percent of the time. We ate a variety of wild animals and had *thousands* of plants from which to select our food. Only 150 of these have been cultivated, and only about 20 are main crops.[3]

The aristocratic elite have always known the superiority of wild animals: in England they even made it illegal for the commoner to hunt wild game, reserving this for themselves.[4]

As shown in the previous chapter, our ancestors were hunter-gatherers long ago. The men mostly did the hunting (they still love "the chase" in courting women and job promotions), and women were mostly gatherers (we so love to shop). They were nomads, moving constantly and looking for wild game. They knew they had to keep the population down, even if it came to infanticide.

They had to work only a few hours a day. They had perfect health and no dental cavities. It was heaven in some ways (except for the infanticide), but they didn't have books, computers, shops, fancy clothes, cars, and houses. It was not our modern vision of paradise.

By settling down, we became able to form schools, hospitals, and all other modern institutions. We developed cool inventions like the printing press, machinery, light bulbs, computers, TVs, and all kinds of gadgets — many of which I haven't even kept up with, such as iPods and phones with text messaging.

You might say we traded health for technology

and increased knowledge, but this came at a price. We have also had to work more than 3 or 4 hours a day to accomplish all that, so we have sacrificed our leisure time. We have also given up a more egalitarian existence, for whoever could store and accumulate grains could dominate the field workers. Possessions didn't accumulate in a nomadic life, but hoarding became a habit in the civilized life.

Agriculture brought into play many social transformation forces. Since people could now hoard grains, some got power over others. Hierarchies with elites arose, as anthropologists Gregory Cochran and Henry Harpending note.

> Since the elites were in a very real sense raising peasants, just as peasants raised cows, there must have been a tendency for them to cull individuals who were more aggressive than average, which over time would have changed the frequencies of those alleles [alternative forms of genes] that induced such aggressiveness.[5]

The authors go on to discuss how the gene that is associated with ADHD (hyperactivity) is almost absent in East Asia.

> The Japanese say that the nail that sticks out is hammered down, but in China it may have been pulled out and thrown away.[6]

People's personalities gradually changed as well. The hunter-gatherer could be free to talk, gossip, and sing. Leisure time afforded a great social life and time for art. They could share, since there were no refrigerators to store extra food. They didn't have to deny immediate gratification for the same reason: eat the food now, or it will perish!

Those who succeeded as farmers, on the other hand, were hard working. They also accumulated more wealth by stinginess. They had to defer gratification for long periods of time to survive. If they ate the seed grain when they were hungriest, right before sowing time when food from the previous crops was exhausted, they wouldn't have any seeds to sow.

One of the biggest advantages of civilization was the accumulation of knowledge, since schools could educate people. We may have lost our health due to agriculture, but those of us who used that accumulated knowledge to study health decided we wanted our health back and figured out how to do it.

We learned that we had to go back to the old ways of eating because that was the way our ancestors ate for 2½ to 3 million years. The most recent 10,000 is just a blink in our evolutionary history. But where are the wild berries? Where is the wild game and heirloom, nonsugary fruit?

Thanks to grains and the depletion of our fossil fuels for fertilizers and farm machinery, we have cultivated nearly 7 billion people. The human population took about 200,000 years to reach a billion. Then, after the discovery of oil around the year 1800, the population went to 2 billion in 1930. Just 30 years later by 1960, it jumped to 3 billion. About 14 years later (1974), it added another billion, and 13 years after that (1987), another billion to make it 5 billion. In just 12 more years (1999), it was 6 billion. It is nearly 7 billion now.[7]

Is there enough wild game, nonhybrid fruit, wild berries, and fresh greens to feed 7 billion? No. The fact is that we can't at this point feed everyone on the planet a diet that will offer peak health, at least not until governments and corporations make that a priority over money, power, and war profiteering.

Meanwhile, is it any wonder that government officials put grains as the most important and frequently eaten food on the food pyramid? Traditionally, a government that cannot feed its people is subject to revolution. If the truth of what constitutes peak nutrition were to be announced, there would be revolutions worldwide as people realized they could not afford to feed their families the best diet. This may be the *main* reason the vegetarian diet is now touted as being politically correct.

Yet that doesn't change the ideal diet needed by our bodies to be at their healthiest. Our population is increasing by leaps and bounds, but that doesn't change our human nutritional needs.

You may choose for philosophical reasons to live on a deficient, toxic diet of grains and soybeans, but that won't put a dent in the population problem. Meantime, your health may suffer.

Chapter 8

Our Shrinking Brains

The precipitous drop in the intake of long-chain omega-3 fatty acid in America ... may represent the greatest public health disaster of the past century in our country. Without adequate levels of DHA in the diet, do we run the risk of regressing as a species? I'm afraid the answer may be yes.
— Dr. Barry Sears, *The Omega Rx Zone*

Most shockingly, our brains have shrunk 10 to 15 percent in the last 10,000 years.[1] Size is not everything. Also important is the density of the synapses, which is directly related to crucial nutrients, such as iodine and zinc. Nonetheless, brain size in proportion to body size is important to the evolution of our brainpower.

The best explanation for our brain shrinkage is the fact we are no longer eating as much brain food. In pre-agricultural times, our consumption of meat and fish was as high as 55 to 60 percent of our calories. Now it is much less.

We are no longer getting sufficient DHA to feed our brains, 60 percent of whose solids are composed of fat.[*] About half of that is DHA. DHA makes up 40 percent of the polyunsaturated fat (PUFA) of the brain and 60 percent of the PUFA in the retina.

Due to food processing, the average person eats a mere sixth of the omega-3 fats typically consumed in 1850.[2] Furthermore, many of us are no longer getting enough iodine, the most crucial of the five brain-dependent minerals.

You might question how our brains could have shrunk when we have so much more technology than we did 10,000 years ago. Obviously this shrinkage is an average. Some people, such as brilliant inventors and scientists, probably don't have smaller brains. Some may even have slightly larger ones. It largely depends on the diets of the mothers when pregnant with them, as well as on the diets they themselves have eaten. The dietary effect can even go back several generations.[†]

Even domesticated animals have lost around 30 percent of their brains![3] This is because they are no longer free to eat a wide variety of wild foods and because we feed them artificial, processed foods not biologically suitable to their species.

We Need Brain Food

As mentioned in the earlier chapter on our dietary legacy, we differ from other primates in that our brains are larger. We need food that nourishes those brains to develop and maintain them. Brain cells are said to turn over more slowly than other body cells, but that still leaves 40,000,000 new ones being born every day.[4]

As we saw earlier, the Shore-Based Scenario contended that our brains grew because of brain food: shellfish, fish, and eggs, which are all rich in DHA and five key minerals. Fish is also very rich in *dimethylaminoethanol* (DMAE), a phospholipid important for focusing, learning, and remembering. Most of us have been eating far less of these foods since the onset of agriculture.

It doesn't matter whether you believe in evolution or not. You can believe in the Shore-Based Theory, creationism, or even that we were genetically engineered by aliens! The fact of the matter is that studies prove our brains thrive on seafood and eggs.

In Jewish tradition, eating fish is thought to increase a certain type of intelligence, according to Rabbi Harav Yitzchak Ginsburgh, an authority on Jewish mysticism.

Although fish is not sacrificed in the Temple, it is a very important factor in our diets, particularly appro-

---

[*]See page 136.

[†]The Pottenger experiment on cats proved that on a cooked diet, each generation got worse. Dr. Gian-Cursio observed the same with three generations of his patients who were on a de-
(continued in the next column)

---

ficient raw diet. Instinctive eaters have observed that animals also get worse health or better health with each generation, depending on diet.

priate as part of the festive Shabbat meals. While the scholar who studies the revealed portion of the Torah is likened to a land animal, the fish that swim in the water represent the scholars that study the inner dimension of the Torah.

If a person desires to sharpen his mind to learn the revealed portion of the Torah, it is recommended that he eat meat. If he wishes to sharpen his mind for the study of the concealed part of the Torah, it is recommended that he eat fish.

In Kabbala, we are taught that the souls of great *tzaddikim* ("righteous ones") are present in fish more than in any other type of food. When we eat fish in holiness, we incorporate the holy spark of the *tzadik* ("righteous") within ourselves, transforming ourselves to holy fish.[5]

Survival of the fittest is part of the theory of evolution, the authors of *The Driving Force* argue.

If one asks that conventional question about the "fittest" today (one could use the quantitative measurement of the financial markets, exchange rates, trade surpluses, drive, and financial intelligence), the Japanese recommend themselves as being pretty fit. Based on the growing budget deficits of 1981–1989 in the US and the growing surplus cash in Japan, the US has collapsed into a position of such debt that the Japanese could just about buy up the US. ...

The Japanese can be said to be the one remaining successful hunter and gatherer culture, but they specifically hunt and gather the sea. They eat five times more fish than the British. To replace their seafood by agriculture, they would require seven times their present amount of land. No nation would have indulged itself to that extent had it not been led on by a superabundance. Is it possible that nutrition has played a role in shaping the success of nations?[6]

DHA and EPA: Crucial for Weight Loss, Brain Health, and General Well-Being

Omega-3s needed by the brain and the rest of the body are fatty acids that include alpha-linolenic acid (ALA), docosahexaenoic acid (DHA), and eicosapentaenoic acid (EPA). EPA is needed for creating hormones that defend against trauma and infection. It is also influential in behavior and mental health.

☞ Omega-6 fats are also crucial, but few people have problems getting these in a modern-day diet. In fact, a half tablespoon of soy or corn oil contains the maximum amount of omega-6 fat that we should consume in one day according to one expert.[7]

DHA is crucial for the nervous system and brain function, including intelligence. It is critical for the retina of the eye, for synapses that control the flow of neurotransmitters, and for the mitochondria in each brain nerve cell that makes ATP and provides the energy to keep those cells alive. One study even found that DHA can help prevent and treat breast cancer.[8]

These omega-3 fats are critical for optimal health. They lower the risk of heart attack, lower serum LDL ("bad" cholesterol) levels, inhibit cancer tumor growth, fight inflammation, help prevent diabetes, and help maintain muscle mass. They boost the brain in the areas of mood, increasing serotonin levels and attention span. They cause the "raw glow" radiance to the skin that every raw foodist is aware of. They are very important in energy production within the mitochondria. They decrease symptoms and severity of rheumatoid arthritis and skin conditions such as eczema. They improve the immune system. They are used in cell formation and maintenance.

Omega-3s are powerfully anti-inflammatory. Inflammation is linked to obesity, aging, and disease, playing a big role in getting and staying slim. They increase thermogenesis, which means they can get the body to waste calories in the form of increased body heat instead of storing them as fat. They switch on key genes involved in fat burning. They decrease the appetite, stabilize the blood sugar, and increase insulin sensitivity, lessening the roller-coaster ride of carbohydrate highs and lows.

They are used in the creation of hormone-like messenger chemicals which regulate key metabolic functions. They also stimulate the secretion of leptin, a hormone important in suppressing appetite.

The brains of people with Alzheimer's disease have 30 percent less DHA than those of healthy people. Dr. Barry Sears has worked with giving fish oil to Alzheimer's patients. Results included regaining memory of one's identity and loved ones, regaining the ability to walk, being able to play cards and tell jokes again, and even getting out of the nursing home![9]

In a study published in the *American Journal*

of Clinical Nutrition, researchers found that among nearly 15,000 older adults living in China, India, or one of five Latin American countries, the odds of having dementia generally declined by as much as 19 percent as fish consumption rose.[10] Such was the conclusion of the study's head, Emiliano Albanese, PhD.

The fact is, the more fish you eat, the less likely you are to get dementia.[11]

Note that this will not be true if you eat those fish polluted with neurotoxic mercury.

One study at Tufts University found that eating fatty fish slashed the odds of getting Alzheimer's by 41 percent, while eating lean fish made no difference.[12]

The omega-3s in fatty fish also improve leptin sensitivity and help prevent Alzheimer's.[13] Chapter 12 will go into more detail on leptin.

DHA and EPA are linked to increased intelligence, enhanced immune system, improved emotional well-being, and better attention span. Fish oil supplements rich in DHA and EPA have been used to treat mental disorders, such as attention deficit disorder, manic-depressive disorder, and schizophrenia.

Food Sources of Omega-3s

The main plant food sources of ALA are flaxseeds, hemp seeds, chia seeds, walnuts, and their oils. Smaller amounts are found in nuts, wheat germ, greens, sprouts, navy beans, kidney beans, and soybeans. Seaweeds, grasses, and other greens also have omega-3s, but since they are very low in fat content, they should not be considered a primary source. Plant foods rich in ALA can be converted to DHA and EPA, but as we will see, conversion is not always possible or efficient.

Direct sources of DHA and EPA so desperately needed to maintain the brain are found in high amounts in these sources: cod liver oil, oily fish (sardines, mackerel, herring, salmon), shellfish, organ meats, the fat of grass-fed animals, and egg yolks from chickens fed fish meal, flaxseeds, hemp seeds, or chia seeds.

Don't overdo shellfish, as they tend to have high toxin content from spending their lives in today's polluted coastal waters. Eating them raw can

be deathly toxic, and I don't recommend it. If you do, it must be done when they are very fresh, as it is easy to get food poisoning from them. Also make sure they are from a reputable source and don't have a foul smell. But even absence of a foul odor is no guarantee of safety. Oysters in particular are considered to be safe to eat raw only in the winter months.[14]

Some algae are also a direct source of DHA, though as will be discussed in the next chapter, they are usually not a good source of EPA and have other drawbacks.

Most healthy people can eat ALA from plant sources like chia and flaxseeds, and it will be transformed into EPA and DHA. However, only 7 to 15 percent of the dietary ALA may be converted to EPA. Much less is converted to DHA. And this is in a healthy *young* person!

[In] adult men conversion to EPA is limited (approximately 8 percent), and conversion to DHA is extremely low (less than 0.1 percent). In women fractional conversion to DHA appears to be greater (9 percent).[15]

The conversion rate is far less in the unhealthy or elderly. Some people have an impaired enzyme, Δ6-desaturase (D6D), and are unable to convert ALA into DHA and EPA.

People with cancer, diabetes, advancing age, viral infections, allergy-related eczema, or high stress levels may have impaired their ability to make D6D enzymes. Furthermore, toxic lifestyles, such as overeating saturated or trans fatty acids, over-consuming alcohol, smoking, taking prescription drugs, or eating processed foods with additives may impair production of these enzymes. A premature baby will not make the enzyme until six months old.

Certain people termed *obligate carnivores* have no ability to manufacture DHA and EPA from plant food. These are people whose ancestors lived in coastal regions and habitually ate seafood, so they got plenty of direct DHA and EPA without having to convert it.[16]

These people must eat some meat or fish to get elongated fatty acids (DHA and EPA), as they lack sufficient enzymes to synthesize them from essential fatty acids.[17]

Fish and Fish Oil

The case can be made for those who are poor converters and who don't eat fish every day, or who need a temporary boost for healing, to take purified fish oil to directly obtain the purified EPA and DHA instead, since fish oil EFAs do not require the D6D enzyme to produce EPA and DHA. Just make sure the fish oil is pharmaceutical grade and says so on the label, which means the mercury has been sufficiently removed. Otherwise, you will be consuming mercury and other toxins which concentrate in the animal fat. Even fish oil with a "mercury free" label could contain trace amounts.

Pharmaceutical-grade fish oil is a great source for quickly rebuilding one's DHA stores. Dr. Sears recommends you experiment until you find the right amount for you. He suggests starting out with 2.5 grams of long-chain omega-3 fatty acids from fish oil a day. This would be 1 teaspoon or four capsules of pharmaceutical grade fish oil. Then get a triglyceride/HDL test as well as an AA/EPA test to see if you need to adjust it upward or downward.[18]

Give it a month to kick in, though you should feel more energy, a sharper brain, and other benefits faster. Krill oil is five times more bioavailable than fish oil, so one gram a day should be plenty for healthy people.

According to Dr. Barry Sears, a person who uses fish oil to bring back his brain function will find improvement within weeks in the following areas: greater concentration, improved memory, better management of stress, increased calmness, and increased creativity.[19] This was certainly my experience.

You don't want to take a dose that would be too much, because, according to Sears, too much of the "good" hormones created from these fats can cause flatulence and diarrhea. It can also depress your immune system, increase the incidence of stroke, increase the "bad" LDL cholesterol, increase the time for blood clotting, and/or increase blood sugar in diabetics. He suggests getting a blood test after a month on his program to see if you are at the right level.[20]

The problem with many fish oil supplements is that they often have rancid fats called *lipid peroxides,* which are toxic. Up to 50 percent of capsules may contain rancid oil.[21] The fact that these supplements have toxic lipid peroxides does not make them a suitable long-term solution.

In my experience, taking 8 to 9 grams a day for about three weeks brought my memory back. I later tapered down to 3 grams. I lowered this to about a gram a day after learning about the toxic lipid peroxides, and after I realized it was unsustainable for my health not to eat fish, meat, and eggs.

I now take cod liver oil in liquid form. Fish oil in gel caps may already be rancid before you buy it. It spoils rapidly. It is best to keep it in the freezer. Even with these precautions, liquid fish oil should be used within six months of opening the bottle.

Dr. Nicholas Perricone starts his patients who want fast weight loss on a megadose of 9 grams of purified fish oil per day! This is only temporary and is much too high for the maintenance diet of a healthy person. Studies show that over 3 grams a day is at best a waste of money and at worst a way of increasing your bleeding time, your insulin resistance, and your LDL cholesterol. More of a good thing is not always better.

If you are a vegetarian, you might want to consider becoming at least a *piscetarian*: one who eats fish but no other animals. Fish is easier for most people to digest than land animals. Some anthropologists suggest this is because we ate seafood long before eating a great deal of land animals. Fish also has a lot less connective tissue, making it easier for gastric enzymes to break apart its proteins.

Seafood is what our brains evolved on. Seafood, especially shellfish, contains DHA, EPA, DMAE, and the five key minerals needed by our brains: iodine, iron, selenium, copper, and zinc. The B_{12} from fish is also more bioavailable than from many other animal foods.[22]

Dr. Barry Sears claims that food is druglike in its effects. If so, oily fish can be thought of as the

> *Studies consistently show that the happiest people on earth eat lots of fish, particularly wild-caught salmon.*

Prozac of foods, resulting in increased serotonin. Here is what Dr. Earl Henslin writes in his book *This is Your Brain on Joy*.

> Probably the number one supplement we recommend for brain health and for happiness is high-grade fish oil. Studies consistently show that the happiest people on our planet eat a lot of fish, particularly wild-caught salmon.[23]

This is interesting to me because I always wondered why my father was so happy all the time. He was very cheerful even on his deathbed. At nearly 85, his mind was still sharp, able to crack jokes, do crossword puzzles, and hold intellectual discussions. His favorite food his whole life was seafood. He didn't let living in inland Indiana stop him: he would often crack open a can of sardines or eat frozen fish.

Fish should be eaten wild, because farmed fish is often fed grain, fed chemical dyes to render its flesh orange, not exercised, and contained in small, crowded confinement. In other words, factory-farmed fish is like factory-farmed mammals: they won't provide the omega-3 fat profile, don't taste good, are full of antibiotics, and are unethical to eat.

> Ocean fish that contain mercury also contain substances called alkylglycerols that remove mercury from the body, but organically bound mercury in fish from industrially polluted waters is toxic and has caused deformities and mental deficiencies in the children of Japanese women who ate mercury-contaminated fish from Minamata Bay. A similar contamination poisoned natives near the Hudson Bay in Canada.[24]

Avoid lake fish at all costs, as they are very toxic from all the inland water pollution.

Ocean fish should be of the smaller varieties. Avoid large fish like tuna, swordfish, and shark. If you absolutely must have some on occasion, take a handful of chlorella (the "metal magnet") before your meal to hopefully absorb some of the mercury. Cilantro is also a good mercury-chelating agent. Small, oily fish such as sardines, herring, and mackerel are the best brain food and contain relatively little mercury.

Mackerel and herring, especially the hearts, are rich in the energy-production co-enzyme *ubiquinone* (CoQ_{10}). In fact, hearts from *all* animals are high in CoQ_{10}. Cooking reduces its content by 14 to 32 percent. CoQ_{10} has beneficial effects on the heart, blood pressure, and migraine headaches. Its consumption is also thought to increase life span.

It's not just the size of the fish that counts, but also where they swim. Anchovies are even smaller, but they are coastal and therefore more polluted.

One study found that the benefits of eating fish outweighed the harm resulting from its toxins. Finnish fishermen and their wives are a population with high fish consumption and high serum concentrations of dioxins and PCBs. In this study, they were shown to have lower mortality from all causes, from ischemic heart diseases, and from respiratory diseases than the respective general male and female populations. The fishermen (but not their wives) also had decreased Alzheimer's disease and suicide.

The high intakes of environmental contaminants in fish were not seen to result in excess mortality. It is possible that exposure to environmental contaminants was not high enough to cause excess mortality, or the beneficial health effects of fish consumption (or some other factor) outweighed the potentially hazardous health effects.[25]

A big concern with taking these oils is that overfishing threatens the ocean ecosystem. Fishing grounds are becoming rapidly depleted. Large fish are quickly disappearing.

Large marine animals like whales and seals depend on krill for food. Although krill has been called a "renewable resource," it remains to be seen how renewable it will be when its popularity as human food catches on! Global warming may also be reducing the krill population. If we have more incidents like British Petroleum's 2010 Gulf of Mexico oil spill, will only the wealthy be able to afford fish or fish oil?

Deliberate Dumbing Down in Education?

Allow me to digress a bit in order to prove a point: we may be intentionally being dumbed down by more than one method.

Throughout history those with power have conspired to control their serfs. Why? Because when you have all the money, sex, food, and possessions that you want, power is the only thing left for the ego to pursue.

I read *The Deliberate Dumbing Down of America* by Charlotte Thomson Iserbyt, who worked her way up to the job of Senior Policy Advisor in the US Department of Education and then became a whistleblower. Her book is filled with Congressional reports that prove that there is in fact a conspiracy to dumb Americans down through the school system. The ulterior motive was to create a mainstream people that would be docile and accept without question whatever government policies were created.

Americans were once one of the best educated people on the planet. About 3 percent couldn't read due to learning disabilities, but educational bureaucrats came up with "solutions" which ended up, over the course of many decades, creating a much higher percentage of illiterates. Now we have a society that ranks very low in education compared to other developed populations. In 2008, the Organization for Economic Cooperation and Development placed the US at number 18 out of 36 industrialized nations in educational attainment.

This may appear to have been blubbering accidental stupidity on the part of the country's leaders, but Iserbyt proves through countless Congressional records that it was intentional.

Only about 3 percent of us continue reading once we get out of school. You can't tell me that we can learn as much by watching movies, documentaries, or even brilliantly composed YouTube videos. When we watch stuff like that, no matter how informative the material, our brains are not very active. If we do this more than an hour or so a day, we get bored on some level because we are not using our full brain potential. Most of us can devour information much faster through reading. In the time it takes to watch a 2-hour documentary, we could have read several times as much information. Furthermore, when we read, we are able to access footnotes and bibliographies to further investigate matters. I therefore save those shows for when I am exercising or when I need to unwind.

Watching TV also puts a person into a hypnotized state of mind. It is much more difficult for a reader, as opposed to a passive viewer, to be brainwashed, deceived, manipulated, or controlled.

In fact, studies show that even the Internet is altering our brains. We are doing more scanning and skimming at the expense of the deep reading that leads to deep and creative thinking. Hyperlinks create distraction and lead to a restless mind. More information results in less knowledge, says Nicholas Carr in *Shallows: What the Internet Is Doing to Our Brains*.

> When we go online, we enter an environment that promotes cursory reading, hurried and distracted thinking, and superficial learning.[26]

As a teacher in the school system in California for many years, I noticed there was a subtle "deliberate dumbing down" going on. For example, I was actually reprimanded for teaching grammar at an inner city high school!

I thought, "Well, these kids do not know grammar, the foundation for writing. So I will transfer to elementary school to make sure they learn grammar."

When teaching second grade, my jaw dropped when I was told, "Grammar? We don't need to teach grammar! You know grammar without having been taught directly. *Everybody* knows grammar!"

When I cautiously mentioned my observations to veteran teachers, they concurred that this dumbing down was happening slowly, though less so in the areas where rich kids went to school. The parents would never tolerate it there.

I knew that kids weren't getting the best educations, especially in the 1980s when universities came out with an absurd "whole language" notion that kids could somehow "absorb" phonics without being taught directly. All they had to do was read the book with the teacher over and over, and they would somehow get the correlations between letters and sounds. Actually the kids were just memorizing the text.

There ended up being an entire generation of kids that barely became literate. I have a friend who teaches college English, and she says most of her students come to her without having read even one adult-level, full-length book.

This doesn't even go into the behavioral aspect of kids at school, which also has gotten progressively worse, to the point that some teachers even fear for their lives. Teaching in most public schools is about as stressful as it gets, right up there with air traffic control.

In all human and animal studies, processed, highly cooked diets deficient in nutrients have led to behavioral degeneration, including violence and antisocial behavior. American diets have grown progressively worse over the decades, and this is reflected in the negative behavior and learning difficulties of the children.

I saw school districts waste millions of dollars on worthless programs and unnecessary curriculum changes. If government officials were serious about children's success, they could have spent a fraction of that money on fish oil and other nutrients for the kids. In one study, simply adding a vitamin and mineral supplement increased IQ scores of children by as much as 20 points in three months.[27]

> *Dr. Barry Sears calls the alarmingly low levels of DHA in breast milk "the greatest public health disaster of the past century" and claims we "run the risk of regressing as a species."*

Dietary Dumbing Down

I uncovered so much research pointing to the dumbing down of America that I felt no surprise when I noticed that much of the media creates a bias in favor of low-fat, vegetarian diets when it is now so obvious to me that our brains need the critical saturated fats and DHA found in animal products.

As will be shown later, much of this misinformation and disinformation was due to the corporate quest for the higher profits found in vegetable oils and carbohydrates. I began to wonder whether there could be a further motive, a deliberate *dietary dumbing down*.

A population that is in a brain stupor from grains, especially wheat, the most common one; that is lacking in both DHA and cholesterol, another nutrient needed by the brain; that is fatigued by all the blood sugar swings; would surely not object to all the money spent on wars. They would not object to high taxes, outrageous inflation, policies that benefit corporate chieftains but not the public, and rigged elections. Even if they did, they would not have the energy or intelligence to do much about it.

I argue that the most extreme dumbing down is

not happening in the schools. It is happening in the diet. According to Dr. Barry Sears, the intake of long-chain omega-3s in America has decreased by 80 percent. The consequent decrease in DHA has been proven by testing the amount in breast milk. The breast milk of American mothers is one of the lowest in the world.

The milk of vegan mothers is *alarmingly low* in DHA, since DHA is rare in the plant world. Low DHA levels in breast milk mean the brains of these babies are not getting the nutrients they need to develop properly. Dr. Barry Sears calls this "the greatest public health disaster of the past century" and claims we "run the risk of regressing as a species."[28]

The modern diet, with its high omega-6 fatty acid content (which competes with omega-3s) and high carb content (which stimulates insulin), leads to obesity. One study in 2009 showed that obesity is linked to brain degeneration.

A team headed by Paul Thompson, University of California at Los Angeles professor, and Cyrus Raji, a medical student at the University of Pittsburgh School of Medicine, compared the brains of people who were normal weight, overweight, and obese.[29]

Overweight people were found to have brains that had 4 percent less brain tissue and looked eight years older than brains of those with a healthy weight. For the obese, it only gets worse: Obese people were found to have brains that had lost 8 percent of their brain tissue and looked 16 years older!

Obese people lost brain tissue in the frontal and temporal lobes critical for planning and memory, in the anterior cingulate gyrus (attention and executive functions), hippocampus (long-term memory), and basal ganglia (movement).

Overweight people lost brain tissue in the basal ganglia, the corona radiata, white matter comprised of axons, and the parietal lobe (sensory lobe).

Raji said in a statement to the press, "It seems that along with increased risk of health problems such as Type 2 diabetes and heart disease, obesity is bad for your brain: we have linked it to shrinkage of brain areas that are also targeted by Alzheimer's." The good news is that if you avoid being overweight, you lower your risk of dementia.

Another study conducted by French scientists revealed that the greater one's weight, the lower one's IQ. People with a Body Mass Index of 20 or less could recall 56 percent of the words on a vocabulary test, whereas those with a BMI of 30 or more (considered obese) could recall only 44 percent. Dr. Maxime Cournot, Assistant Professor at Toulouse University Hospital, headed the study.

Since obesity is a widely known cardiovascular risk factor, due to the thickening and hardening of the blood vessels, the same happens with the arteries in the brain.[30]

Trans fats, hydrogenated oils found in processed and deep fried foods, also dumb us down. Cooking fats causes them to become hydrogenated, which is why it is best to eat them raw. Hydrogenated fats are dangerous, according to nutritionist Patrick Holford, Director of the Food for Brain Foundation in London.

[These fats] can be taken directly into the brain and appear in the same position as DHA in brain cells, where they mess up thinking processes. They also block the conversion of essential fats into vital brain fats, such as GLA, DHA, and prostaglandins.[31]

Alcohol also dumbs us down by blocking the conversion of fats into DHA and dissolving fatty acids within the brain's membranes, replacing DHA with a poor substitute.[32]

Other dietary dumbing down includes mercury in fish, fluoride in water, pesticides in produce, bromine in grains and sprayed on strawberries, and excitotoxin[*] additives, such as monosodium glutamate (MSG), sucralose, saccharin, aspartame, and refined sugar, found in processed foods.

---

[*]*Excitotoxins* are neurotoxins, exposure to which stimulates a metabolic process by which nerve cells are damaged and killed by glutamate and similar substances.

Chapter 9

Your Brain on a Plant-Only Diet

Scientists have discovered that going veggie could be bad for your brain — with those on a meat-free diet six times more likely to suffer brain shrinkage. ... The link was discovered by Oxford University scientists who used memory tests, physical checks, and brain scans to examine 107 people between the ages of 61 and 87.
   —Anonymous, "Eating veggies shrinks the brain," *Times of India*, 14 September 2008

Former vegan Chet Day makes the following claim on his website.

> A famous writer and ex-vegan by the name of Upton Sinclair, the activist who forced the meat-packing industry to clean up its act many decades ago when he wrote *The Jungle*, found he couldn't maintain his work levels on a vegan diet.
>
> Writing sadly that he hated to give up veganism, Sinclair did so nonetheless because he found his brain just wouldn't function at an optimal level on fruits, vegetables, juice, nuts, and seeds. He turned to Salisbury steak as his answer.
>
> Although Upton Sinclair was nearly crucified by his vegan friends for changing his diet and writing about the positive results from the change, he maintained that he went where the truth led him.[1]

A myth in the vegetarian community is that if we just eat like our primate cousins, we'll do fine. But what they don't take into account is that we now know that most primates are not strict vegetarians. More important, our brains are much more developed than those of primates — and if we want to keep our brains, we must feed them.

This requires significant amounts of DHA in our diet, or at least plants high in omega-3 fats that can convert to DHA if we are young and healthy. But studies have shown that eating plant omega-3s is not enough for most people to get sufficient DHA.[2]

According to nutritionist Patrick Holford, "Relying solely on nuts and seeds to make complex brain fats such as DHA is close to useless." He explains that India, which has the world's largest vegetarian population, has one of the highest rates of blindness, since both the eye and the brain are built from DHA.[3]

Your brain's solids are 60 percent fat, and a big portion of that fat is DHA. On a plant-based diet, DHA is scarce. It is known to be prevalent only in marine algae and purslane, a weed. Since weeds are very low in fat, you would need enormous amounts to get enough DHA.

The body of a young, healthy person can convert omega-3s into DHA and EPA needed by the nervous system, but the conversion is inefficient. Also, this cannot happen if the person is eating an abundance of nuts other than walnuts, and seeds other than chia, flax, and hemp, because of their high ratio of omega-6 to omega-3 fats. It also can't happen if the person is sick or toxic, and may be harder if the person switched to a vegan diet later in life.

> *"Relying solely on nuts and seeds to make complex brain fats such as DHA is close to useless."*
> —*nutritionist Patrick Holford*

As previously stated, some people are even obligate carnivores because they lack the enzymes to convert plant omega-3s to the DHA and EPA needed by the brain. Often these are people whose ancestors lived in coastal regions and habitually ate seafood, so they got plenty of direct DHA and EPA without having to convert it.

For these reasons, it is always best to get the DHA directly from oily fish, the fats of wild meat, or eggs from omega-3-fed chickens. These eggs are usually labeled on the carton as high omega-3 or DHA eggs.

A ratio of 1:1 or 2:1 omega-6 fatty acids to omega-3 fatty acids in the diet is thought to have been what caused *Homo sapiens* to develop a more evolved brain than other mammals. In fact, carnivores are more intelligent than herbivores precisely because they eat meat and get more omega-3s.[4]

Some raw fooders might think this ratio doesn't matter if the food is eaten raw. There are two arguments against that. First, the paleodiet, which was almost all raw, is believed to have had a 1:1 ratio of these fats — at most 2 parts omega-6 to 1 part omega-3.

Second, dolphins — the only creature thought to be as intelligent as man, having an even bigger brain-to-body ratio — have also been found to have this 1:1 ratio of fats in their brains, and dolphins do not cook their food.[5]

Dolphins evolved by managing to balance the abundance of omega-3s in ocean food with omega-6s. The amount of omega-3s in the ocean is plentiful, so dolphins seek out omega-6s by consuming squid and certain sea plants.

Man, a land creature, managed to balance his ratios as well. Plants are plentiful in omega-6s, so he turned to ocean food to find omega-3s.

Vegans often take algae supplements. According to Brian Clement, author of *Supplements Exposed*, the processing of algae supplements creates toxic by-products that make them nonideal sources.

Dr. Barry Sears warns that algae contain "strange fats that can lead to significant gastric side effects."[6] Furthermore:

> All vegetable oils are extracted with hexane, whereas fish oils are not. The algae oils rich in DHA must also be extracted with hexane to pull the oil out of the algae cells.[7]

Hexane is toxic to the nervous system, and not all of it is removed in processing.

Most algae oils, with certain exceptions, contain about 30 percent DHA and no EPA. The body can convert some of its DHA into EPA, but not much. There is only about a 15 percent conversion of DHA to EPA. Depending on the capsule size and concentration, some would need to supplement with about 10 capsules to get 150 mg. of EPA.

Unfortunately, the metabolic conversion of ALA to EPA and DHA, and DHA to EPA from algae oils is very limited. The best way to obtain EPA and DHA is from direct consumption via fish rich in DHA and EPA. They can also be obtained in concentrated form from ultra-refined pharmaceutical-grade fish oils. Since it is better to stay away from ultra-refined foods when possible, cod liver oil may be a better option. (Carlson is a good brand.)

Krill is another option. Although *neither* of these choices is as sustainable as algae, both are more natural and healthful options, considering that our ancestors' brains evolved through eating fish, not algae.

There is perhaps a more healthful vegan alternative, and that is to supplement with blue-green algae, which contains DHA. It is very expensive, but could be used as a supplement by vegans. Note that some people believe algae contain neurotoxins, yet another reason to make fish or krill an exception to an otherwise vegan diet.

Of course, man evolved eating fish and shellfish, not algae. So it can be argued that a strict vegan runs the risk that another nutrient in fish or other animal foods will be discovered later down the road, something not found in plant food.

> At this point in time, the concentration of EPA or DHA [in algae] is low and expensive but, as the technology develops, marine algae-derived EPA and DHA will become a viable source for strict vegans.[8]

Your Brain on Soy

As mentioned earlier, most processed soy is bad for the brain, at least according to many studies. Soy reduces brain-derived neurotrophic factor (BDNF), which is needed for the survival and genesis of brain cells.[9]

It was formerly believed that adults did not regenerate brain cells, but psychiatrist Dr. David Amaral explains otherwise.

> A decade ago, we still had the notion that you acquired all the neurons you would ever have by the sixth month of pregnancy. ... It turns out that nothing could be further from the truth.[10]

Genistein, a phytochemical in soy, reduc-

> *Genistein, a phytochemical in soy, reduces DNA synthesis in the brain and inhibits the proliferation of brain cells, manifesting as brain atrophy.*

es DNA synthesis in the brain and inhibits the proliferation of brain cells, manifesting as brain atrophy. Soy is thought to be good to reduce cancer because of this initiation of *apoptosis* (programmed cell death), which enables it to kill cancer cells. Unfortunately, healthy cells in certain parts of the body are also destroyed, including brain and testicular cells![11]

Effects of Vegan/Vegetarian Diets on Mood

The insufficient amounts of good saturated fats and dietary cholesterol found in plant-only diets (except for coconut, palm nut fat, and white cacao butter) have also created mood and mental health problems for many people. Adequate cholesterol in the diet is needed for neurons to form the new synaptic connections that are needed for learning new information. The cholesterol issue will be explained in more detail in chapter 11.

Good dietary fat is also needed for emotion and mood stability. Fish oil is often used for depression, hyperactivity in children, and manic-depression, or bipolar disorder. People who eat seafood are the happiest people in the world.

I must emphasize that many of the following issues also apply to omnivores who lack sufficient brain foods in their diet.[*]

Vegans are known to be kind and compassionate, but for some, this compassion is reserved only for animals, not for people who disagree with their idealistic views. People who are into animal rights sometimes become violent, even if only verbally, but occasionally they rise to the extreme of becoming homicidal in defense of animals.

Long-term vegans are often susceptible to getting depressed, sometimes even suicidal, as will be discussed later. Yet ironically the only thing that can soothe this mental state is to do exactly what they feel is wrong: eat animal products.

It is very honorable and enlightened on their part not to wish any harm to animals, yet they are in denial of nature and the way their bodies have evolved. Their consciousness has in some ways evolved beyond their bodies' evolution. The only solution for them is to give in to the way things are instead of resisting nature — either that or forgo optimal mental health.

Aajonus Vonderplanitz once told me that he was giving a lecture about the raw animal food diet. Some vegetarians and vegans were getting very, very angry with him. He remained calm throughout. Then he said, "Look, guys. Look at who is getting irritated and upset. Whose diet is better for the nervous system?"

Lierre Keith, who had been vegan for 20 years, wrote in a similar vein.

> Even vegans talk about "the vegan police." Admit you know what I'm talking about: aggressive, rigid, on a hair trigger, and in a semi-constant state of rage. That's what happens to a human with a brain deprived of protein and fat.[12]

She explains that she had a full-blown anxiety disorder and lost most of her youth to the "dull, gray nothing of depression." She felt a lot of rage. She said the tiniest task became inexplicably overwhelming.

> No amount of will can melt it, because it's a biological reality. Hence the fat binges, the cravings. It will only change when the brain is allowed to consume what it needs.[13]

Lierre even lost a vegan friend to suicide.

Lierre explains that she and her vegan friends all craved sweets. This was because of hypoglycemia, typical on high-carb diets, and a lack of quality proteins to build serotonin and endorphins in the brain.[14] A sugar hit will give a quick-fix adrenaline rush for temporary endorphins, but quality protein gives the brain that steady flow it needs for optimal brain health.

In an online article entitled "The Naïve Vegetarian," Dr. Barry Groves, PhD, agrees.

> *Many of these issues also apply to omnivores who lack adequate brain foods in their diet.*

---

[*]See chapter 8.

As we know, when it needs food, our body indicates this to us with the feeling of hunger. But there are also other signals if specific nutrients are deficient. Meat is the best source of several nutrients. When our bodies are deficient in these, we become irritable and aggressive. This is a perfectly natural signal built into our genetic make-up over our evolution: our bodies are telling us to go out and kill something to eat. This is why strict vegetarians tend to be so vociferous.[15]

Food expert Steve Gagne, author of *Food Energetics*, agrees.

These days, followers of exclusively plant diets often preach about the association of eating the flesh of animals with anger, irritability, and elevated sensual passions. However, among traditional peoples, meat has been associated with strength, courage, bravery, and a psychological sense of earthly realism.

Followers of meatless diets also unjustly claim superiority above meat eaters in their cleanliness, devotion, compassion, and spiritual idealism. But realistically, while a diet heavy in meat has its share of drawbacks, so too can a meatless diet. For many, a meatless diet can result in various forms of malnourishment as well as feelings of instability, fanaticism, and unrealistic idealism.[16]

As explained later in chapter 11, studies show that low cholesterol levels increase the likelihood of violence. Usually the violence is only verbal, or a threat.

Tom Billings has been a vegetarian for 30 years and experimented with all sorts of vegan variations until he settled on a lacto-ovo-vegetarian diet, avoiding meat for spiritual reasons. He set up a website that shows the pitfalls of veganism and even provides plenty of proof that we evolved eating meat.[17] He claims to have received death threats for doing this, despite the fact that he is a vegetarian himself.

The blogger Natasha was a vegan activist, but gave it up after 3½ years for health reasons. When she blogged about it, she actually received death threats! Some people even accused her of being an "anti-vegan troll who has been plotting this for years, or in the employ of the meat industry."[18]

I have also had people say spiteful, false, and absurd things about me on blog posts after learning that I am no longer vegan. If I dared mention fish oil in my newsletter, they would unsubscribe. If people wrote asking for my thoughts on their health issues who I felt could benefit from adding some raw egg yolks to their diet, they would get angry or upset.

In order to write this book, I had to get to the place within myself where I wouldn't care if people unsubscribed, wrote ridiculous things about me on blogs, or even wrote me angry hate mail. I just decided this was an issue that needed to be more openly discussed. I know that I am not alone.

Not everyone becomes ungrounded or fanatical on a vegan diet. My colleague Tonya Zavasta is neither judgmental nor "vegangelical."

I do not take any B_{12} supplements at present. So far, I've not eaten raw eggs either. Some raw foods people do; some don't. I am not going to throw stones. ...

One thing for sure: I will not think twice about losing the status of "TRULY vegan" if my health depends on it.[19]

Then there is the friend and former housemate in San Diego who first told me about the raw vegan diet 23 years ago. When I met her for lunch to tell her that I'd had a hard time with veganism and was now eating raw meat, she encouraged me to write about it.

She was amazed at how much *better* I looked than I had on a *vegan* diet. She agreed that there must be different metabolic types. Although *she* does well with a high-carb diet, it is obvious to her that *I* don't. She also added this.

When I see a 20-something person has just turned vegan, I know he has no clue how hard it is going to be. I have seen so many give up. It doesn't work for everyone.

I also received many e-mails from people who failed at vegan diets thanking me for tackling this subject in a book. Here's one example.

> *"Vegetarianism is harmless enough, though it is apt to fill a man with wind and self-righteousness."*
> *—Robert Hutchison, address to the British Medical Association in 1930*

Thank you for your new book. Many of us faced health consequences on a vegan diet because our metabolisms needed the DHA, B_{12}, D, AA, CLA, etc. available from animal-based foods. Many of us moved to nonvegan raw diets out of necessity and found great health returned. Yet we were disbelieved and even vilified by the vegan and raw vegan communities. Either we were "detoxing" still, or we were "eating too much _____ (fill in the blank)," or we were just traitors.

Moral Superiority of Vegetarians

Food is a funny thing; it can bring us together, but it can divide us as well — vegetarian, carnivore, vegan. —Tara Weaver, author of *The Butcher and the Vegetarian.*

For some, the attitude of nonmeat eaters borders on cultish. They exude the moral superiority, a "holier-than-thou" attitude, found in many religions. Many refuse to have friends who eat meat.

I myself once posted a bumper sticker on my car that proclaimed "Friends don't let friends eat meat." I too was guilty of feeling morally superior to those "crude meat eaters with dense consciousnesses."

Here's more from Tara Weaver.

I'll let you in on a little vegetarian secret: Not eating meat is like a guilt-free pass. I can sleep easy knowing that I'm not contributing to the ethical and environmental issues brought on by meat production.

The world's wild fish supply may disappear in the next few years, but it's not my fault; I don't even like fish. Whatever ills there may be in modern animal husbandry, none of them are being done in my name. Being a vegetarian earns you a healthy serving of virtuosity. This can also creep into a distressingly common case of vegetarian self-righteousness, it must be said.[20]

Later on, when she explored the world of meat, she found herself a victim of this moral superiority.

What I didn't expect is that the fringe might begin to loathe me. Don't I get credit for all those years of alfalfa sprouts and brown rice?[21]

Some vegans feel morally superior even to vegetarians, claiming "milk is meat" because the male calves of dairy cows are sold as veal. Such smugness is more prevalent among young, zealous vegans, because for them it is almost a religion. One former vegan told me that his decades of dealing with vegans convinced him they think they "sit at the right hand of God."

Former vegan Tom Billings, who remains a vegetarian but has not eaten meat in 30 years, says, "Such attitudes are really self-righteous, egotistical, and the dietary equivalent of racism."[22]

I also had a vegan friend that I fought with verbal violence over certain issues, even over petty things. Sometimes the phone would be slammed down. After I started taking fish oil, I never had any fights with her at all. She told me one time that she noticed she could never get a rise out of me anymore. I said it was because my brain was now being fed what it needed: good cholesterol, DHA, EPA, B_{12}, and saturated fats!

When I told her about writing this book, she condescendingly remarked, "I had such *high hopes* for you!"

Some vegans go to such an extreme with their cause that they think people should sacrifice their health instead of eating animal products. I have seen bloggers proudly say things such as, "Even if I learned that my body and brain needed fish, I would *die* before eating it!"

Some people even suggested that those of us who couldn't remain healthy as vegans should willingly sacrifice our health for the cause. As a feminist, [I found] this body-hating rhetoric infuriated me.[23]

Forgetful Vegans

I have a friend who eats mainly raw but due to blood sugar issues was never able to become vegan. Being active in the raw food community, she has a number of vegan friends. She complains about how erratic they can be. Many are "flaky" and unreliable. Again, this also applies to omnivores who lack sufficient brain food in their diets.

I explained to her that such behavior is caused by years of depriving their brains of essential fats. The brain needs saturated fats, DHA, EPA, and B_{12}, which are often lacking in vegan diets unless they are very carefully planned. Furthermore, a zinc deficiency can cause one to become spacey and ungrounded.

The memory is also affected from inadequate DHA and B_{12}. Once I gave a small talk on my book. A woman definitely no older than 50, possibly younger, approached me and said she would like to get together with me because she was having memory problems. She said she was a vegan.

I replied that she needed more DHA than a vegan diet provided. I discovered she lived in my neighborhood and suggested we get together, giving her my phone number (which I rarely do). She never called. I ran into her at the Raw Spirit Festival about a month later, and she didn't even recognize me!

At the same festival, I encountered another vegan friend. We talked for five minutes and hugged before parting ways. Later, a mutual friend said that he commented that he didn't run into me at the festival!

I have yet another friend who wasn't even a strict vegan but a vegetarian for spiritual reasons. After over a decade of eating this way, she became overwhelmed and could barely function. Her mood swings made her dysfunctional and erratic. When she followed my advice to take fish oil and eat seafood, she amazed herself by growing better, calmer, and more functional by the day.

Many vegans consume soy products, which can lead to Alzheimer's disease.[24] Even vegans and vegetarians who shun soy are susceptible to dementia due to B_{12} deficiency.[25] In a German study on vegetarians, they were found to have a somewhat higher rate of deaths by nervous system diseases, mental disorders, and accidents (which could have been caused by these disorders).[26]

Part 3

Finding Balance in Fats, Carbohydrates, and Protein

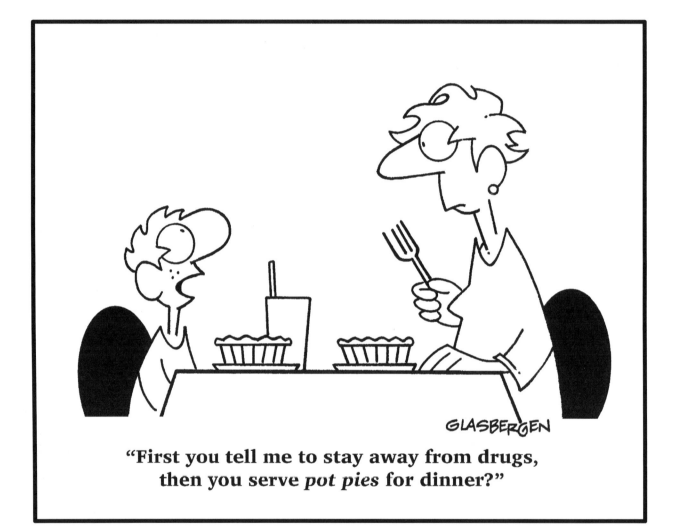

"First you tell me to stay away from drugs,
then you serve *pot pies* for dinner?"

Chapter 10

Metabolic Types: Why We Can't All "Go Veg"

Although there are some foods that are not good for anyone (processed, refined, altered, etc), arbitrary rules of what is good or bad for people cannot possibly apply to everyone. For every food that exists, there has been some 'expert' who claims it will irreparably harm health and another 'expert' who claims it will miraculously heal. Humans are not like car engines with a general instructional manual that works for everyone.
   –Judith A. DeCava, CCN, LLC, *Price-Pottenger Journal of Health and Healing*, 2001, v. 25, #4

In the world of nutrition, nothing will drive you nuttier than all the controversy over the correct percentages of macronutrients (fats, carbohydrates, and proteins). Some studies indicate that a diet high in *protein* is toxic, or at least not conducive to longevity. Some indicate that high *fat* is a recipe for poor health. Others indicate that a diet high in *carbs*, leading to high insulin levels, is at the root of all health evils.

If you were to examine a number of studies on weight loss, you would find some that "prove" a low-fat diet is best and others that "conclusively demonstrate" the superiority of low carb. Is it any wonder Dr. Barry Sears of the Zone Diet concluded that we should balance ourselves by eating about a third of our diet from each category?

Another thing to consider is this: What kinds of carbs, proteins, and fats were used in many of the controlled studies? We know there are "good carbs" (whole food, high fiber) and "bad carbs" (refined, fiberless, and/or high sugar). There are also "good fats" (fish oil, coconut oil, oils rich in omega-3s) and "bad fats" (heated, rancid seed oils high in omega-6s, fats in meat of animals fed grains, heated animal fats, and trans fats). There are also "bad proteins." Many of the studies on protein will use casein, a protein from dairy that has been implicated in cancer.[1]

In fact, in one study, the protein used was casein, the fat was corn oil (rancid and heavy on the omega-6), and the carb was sucrose (refined sugar)![2]

Even using healthful foods, it's not always clear which ratios are best. Much of this confusion is cleared up when you realize that people come in different metabolic types. This may explain why some people do much better on high-carb vegan or vegetarian diets than do others.

It has long been observed by health practitioners that people vary widely in their ability to metabolize nutrients. There are individual differences in ability to digest, absorb, assimilate, transport, utilize, and excrete nutrients. Give everyone the same diet, and one will show up with deficiencies while another will thrive.

The late Roger J. Williams, PhD, former professor of chemistry at the University of Texas at Austin, who wrote the seminal classic *Biochemical Individuality*, is considered the "father of biological individuality." He found that this manifests even in rabbits, rats, and cows.[3] He documented the huge anatomical variations in human organ sizes and shapes, such as some stomachs that could hold six to eight times the volume of others.[4]

Most relevant to the issue of meat eating is the length of the intestines. In 1885, English surgeon Frederick Treves found that human intestinal lengths from fresh male cadavers ranged from 15.5 to 31.1 feet.[5]

Dr. Melvin Page, DDS, later observed that coastal Nordic meat and fish eaters had short guts, while inland mid-Europeans who ate grains as well as animal foods had long guts.[6]

Jay Cooper, MS, author and wellness director of the Green Valley Spa in St. George, Utah, noted in his study of metabolic types that those of our

> *Dr. Roger J. Williams, PhD, found that biological individuality manifests even in rabbits, rats, and cows.*

predecessors who lived in warm climates had longer digestive tracts and were able to live on plant foods, whereas those living in colder climates had shorter guts and could process more animal foods.[7]

One of the pioneers in metabolic typing was Dr. George Watson of the University of Southern California who found in the 1950s that patients differed in how they metabolized fats and carbohydrates into energy. He labeled those who burned carbs quickly *fast oxidizers* and those who burned carbs slowly *slow oxidizers*. Fast oxidizers do well on low-carb diets, while slow oxidizers do well on low-fat, higher-carb diets.

Metabolic experts William Wolcott and Trish Fahey, authors of *The Metabolic Typing Diet*, found that there appear to be three metabolic types: carb, protein, and "mixed." So some people can do well with a high-carb diet, some need a high-protein diet, and others do best on mixed.

Family physician and Internet health guru Joseph Mercola observed the same with thousands of patients in his practice. For some patients, juicing worked wonders, but a diet high in meat was a disaster. For others, it was the opposite, validating the saying that one man's meat is another man's poison.

Dr. Mercola doesn't believe these types correspond to the blood type theory proposed by Dr. Peter J. D'Adamo, ND, who has written popular books based on his theory. Mercola is a blood type A, which should be vegetarian (actually piscetarian, since type As are told to eat fish), yet he classifies himself as a protein type.

> Now that there's so much heterogeneity of the population and mixing of the genes, it's difficult to make broad, culture-based recommendations. So we basically use a Nutritional Typing profile to help people learn if they need to eat lots of protein and fat (i.e., a protein type) or virtually very little of that, and mostly vegetables (a carb type). There is also a mixed type, which is very common.[8]

I took Dr. Mercola's test and that of Wolcott and Fahey. I was found to be a mixed type in both tests. It makes sense that I am not a carb type because I have been diagnosed with hypoglycemia and definitely hold the *Syndrome X* pattern in my genes, the tendency to become insulin resistant when carbs are overindulged. I wish I were a carb

type. Then I could enjoy my carb culinary preferences with impunity.

There are many, many more who have theories on various metabolic types, including Ann Louise Gittleman, William Donald Kelley, DDS, and John Lawder, MD. Even Dr. Barry Sears, inventor of the Zone Diet, acknowledges that people vary in the level of carbs tolerated.[9] The book *Metabolic Man* by Dr. Charles Wharton, PhD, is a fairly comprehensive guide on the topic.

Dr. Eric Berg, DC, author of *The 7 Principles of Fat Burning*, theorizes that there are four metabolic types, and I seemed to fit his *adrenal type* most. The developing bags under my eyes were one clue. People of this type need more protein than the others.

Nonetheless, I find that I don't need quite as much protein as Mercola and Wolcott claim is needed for a mixed type — so long as I eat most of it raw. I can get by fine with around 20 percent (or less) of my calories in protein. I just add more good, healthful, raw fats to make up the difference, since I am sensitive to excess carbs.

When Dr. T. Colin Campbell, PhD, retired Cornell University nutrition professor and author of *The China Study*, writes that protein causes fatigue, I am caught thinking, "What planet is he from? In my body it is *carbs* that cause fatigue." When he says that people can eat a diet high in carbs, and the calories are "lost as body heat" rather than stored as fat, I know he has never lived in *my* body.[10]

Carbs make me fat, but I can eat a few hundred calories extra on a low-carb diet, and they don't stick. I am definitely not a carb type. When not on the correct diet, I become insulin resistant, storing fat easily, and get fatigued.

When the low-fat craze gained popularity, high-carb diets began to be prescribed universally. By the end of the 1980s, one in four Americans was overweight. Now it is one in three, with half of the overweight being obese. Type 2 diabetes can no longer be called *adult onset* diabetes, since it is now so prevalent in children.

Many people, if not the majority, do not do well on high-carb diets, especially with highly processed, refined carbs. Practicing Arizona physician Scott Rigden, MD, describes what is called *carb sensitivity*.

"Carb-sensitive" people, after consuming simple carbohydrates and sugars, experience a rapid spike of blood sugar that triggers, in turn, a spike in insulin and associated metabolic cellular messengers and leads to negative consequences: the body receives the signal to store, not burn, fat; and the spike in insulin causes a rapid drop in blood sugar; this in turn creates uncomfortable symptoms like fatigue, irritability, headaches, and brain fog. These symptoms stimulate the individual to seek even more carbohydrates and sugars to remedy the uncomfortable feelings associated with the rapid drop in blood sugar.[11]

Many of us have this sensitivity because modern diets incorporate so much cooked, refined grain; oversweet, hybridized fruit; refined sugars; and other processed carbs that our paleolithic ancestors never ate.

> *Dr. Williams found that people's internal anatomical characteristics varied as much as their outward appearances.*

I am not alone as someone who does poorly on low-fat, high-carb diets, as Dr. Eleftheria Maratos-Flier, MD, director of obesity research at Harvard's Joslin Diabetes Center, confirms.

For a large percentage of the population, perhaps 30–40 percent, low-fat diets are counterproductive. They have the paradoxical effect of making people gain weight.

☞ Low-fat diets tend to be high in carbs because protein in nature usually comes bound with fats. Since you go low on fats and proteins, you eat high carb by default.

Raw diet advocate Gabriel Cousens, MD, also sees different metabolic types.

A person with a slow oxidative metabolism processes glucose too slowly in the glycolysis cycle. ... The result ... is a slow-down of the production of energy in the cells. Adverse psychological effects of this include documented cases of anxiety, depression, and obsessive-compulsive disorders. ... Slow oxidizers do best on a diet that is high in complex carbohydrates, moderately low in protein, and low in fat. ...

Fast oxidizers are people whose metabolism burns glucose quickly and have too much activity in the glycolysis cycle. ... Fast oxidizers do best on variations of the "Zone" diet.[12]

Dr. Roger Williams realized that the internal anatomical characteristics of people varied as much as their external characteristics. He found that individual bodies also vary greatly in their physiological and chemical composition. The metabolic differences include organ and glandular function, bodily fluid composition, detoxification ability, blood cholesterol control, and more. Because of this, people exhibit highly individualized nutritional needs for optimal functioning.[13]

Metabolic types probably depend upon genetic origins. In 1988, some still-surviving hunters and gatherers were found to differ quite widely in their macronutrient ratios. The ratio of plant (carbs) to animal (protein and fat) foods varied considerably:

- The Eskimo ate 10:90 plant/animal.
- The Filipino Agta ate 40:60 plant/animal.
- The Paraguayan Ache ate 50:50 plant/animal.
- The Botswanan !Kung San ate 65:35 plant/animal.
- The Tanzanian Hadza ate 80:20 plant/animal.
- The Australian Aborigine ate 90:10 plant/animal.[14]

Regardless of their macronutrient ratios, these groups of people were all disease free.

At last there is scientific proof of the different metabolic types! A striking piece of evidence is shown by the Apo gene test and its relationship to differing optimal ratios of the macronutrients. Pamela McDonald, NP, author of *The Perfect Gene Diet*, found in her practice that those with the ApoE e2/e2 and e2/e3 genes do better with diets rich in fats (35 or 30 percent respectively), moderate in carbs (50 or 55 percent respectively), and low in protein (15 percent).

Those with ApoE e4/e3 and e4/e4 genes do better with low-fat (20 percent), high-carb (55 percent), moderate-protein (25 percent) diets. Those who consume over 2,800 calories/day should eat 20 percent fat, 20 percent protein, and 60 percent carbs.

The e4/e4 gene indicates susceptibility to heart disease and Alzheimer's. Those with it are advised to eat a diet high in plant food and low in animal foods.

Note that if you turn out to have the ApoE e4/e4 gene, known for its high risk in Alzheimer's and heart disease (unless you adhere to a diet that keeps the gene switched off), you may be in danger of losing your job or health insurance. About half the states don't protect people from this. So you should do the test anonymously, with a number, not a name.[15]

Those with the ApoE e3/e3 and e4/e2 genes are mixed types and do better with diets of 25 percent fats, 20 percent protein, and 55 percent carbs.[*] Note that every diet is limited to 60 percent carbs, and no diet exceeds 25 percent protein. None of the diets go below 20 percent fat.

Of course, most of us can just listen to our instincts without all the associated caloric calculations. This is especially true if you eat a whole-food, raw diet. Did the cave man have diet books and calculators to make sure he was on track?

If I get too low in fat, I start craving it. Even on a raw vegan diet, when I got too low in protein, I craved large amounts of nuts, which made me gain weight.[†] But it is good to check ourselves once in a while with the calculations to make sure we aren't getting gradually out of balance.

Endocrinologist Gerald Reaven, MD, of Stanford University tested the ability of healthy nondiabetic adults to metabolize sugar and carbohydrates. He found that 25 percent had no trouble metabolizing carbs, and another 25 percent handled them very poorly. The latter were labeled "impaired glucose metabolism" or "insulin resistant." The other 50 percent fell somewhere between.

He figured that perhaps one person in four is a carb type, one in four is a protein type, and the rest are mixed. These were all *young* people too. Young people handle carbs better as a rule. We become more insulin resistant as we age, at least if we eat diets high in carbs. So maybe the percentage of *adults* who do well with carbs is much smaller than 25 percent.

According to the American Association of Clinical Endocrinologists, one in three Americans is insulin resistant.[16] That means 67 percent don't handle carbs well, particularly refined or cooked carbs, which have higher glycemic levels, because they enter the bloodstream faster.

To find out your metabolic type, you can order Dr. Mercola's test at www.mercola.com or take the test in William Wolcott's book *The Metabolic Typing Diet*.

Or you can just experiment. Go a week or so on a high-carb diet and later on a low-carb diet. Keep a journal and note how you feel: How are your energy, mental focus, and mood? Do you experience hunger or cravings? Especially take note of how you feel throughout the day after a carb-based breakfast vs. a protein-based one.

Some people can change types sometimes, at least temporarily under certain conditions. For example, if you are suddenly very active in physical labor or athletics, you can increase your percentage of carbs. If you develop diabetes or hypoglycemia, you will need to decrease carbs and increase healthful raw fats. If you are trying to build muscle with weightlifting, you may need to increase your protein to some degree.

According to British sports authority Janet Pidcock, living in high altitudes also enables one to tolerate high-carb diets.

Wherever you are, as an active athlete, you boost your capacity for endurance by eating a high-carb diet.[‡] But this becomes even more critical if you soar to high altitude. During both short and long-term altitude exposure, there is a decrease in the use of fat as an energy source, together with an increased reliance on carbohydrate. It's thought that this shift makes it easier for oxygen to dissolve into the blood.

Thus, there's a need for an even higher carbohydrate intake than usual. At altitudes over 5,000 meters [about 16,000 feet], experts have recommended that carbohydrate foods should be increased to as much

---

[*]McDonald describes each metabolic type and its corresponding optimal macronutrient ratios in pages 10–34 and 123–28 of her book.

[†]See chapter 15 to understand why.

[‡]Paleo diet proponents would of course argue her on this point.

as 70 per cent of total energy intake. A number of researchers have found that people spontaneously increase their carbohydrate consumption when at high elevations.[17]

Also, the healthier you get, the more flexible your body is to adaptation, says nutritionist Judith DeCava.

As people become increasingly well, they tend to shift towards a middle ground, able to eat a little of everything. Healing bodies have very different requirements from healed bodies.[18]

Carb Excess Is Poison for Some

If you are vegan, everything you put into your mouth has carbs. Think about it. Every morsel of food is adding to your glycemic load.

Now if you are a raw vegan, at least you are not eating many grains, hopefully. At least you are not eating processed, highly refined carbs. But even that fruit and agave spike your insulin unless you are on a very low-fat diet or buffering the fruit with greens, as in green smoothies. If you are successful on a Nathan Pritikin or Dean Ornish 80 percent carb/10 percent protein/10 percent fat-type diet or the Doug Graham raw version, and if you still feel great a few years into it, then congratulations! You are a carb type.

But if you feel fatigue and experience dry skin and depression, you are not getting enough fats. If you are losing muscle mass, you are not getting enough protein.

Syndrome X

Syndrome X is also known as metabolic syndrome or insulin resistance syndrome. It includes insulin resistance with hyperinsulinemia (excessive blood insulin). The National Cholesterol Education Program Adult Treatment Panel III currently includes five features of metabolic syndrome, three of which a person must have in order to be diagnosed with it. These include the following:

- elevated waist circumference: greater than 40 inches for men, 35 inches for women
- triglyceride levels above 150 mg/dl
- decreased HDL: less than 40 mg/dl for men and below 50 mg/dl for women

- blood pressure over 130/85
- fasting blood sugar above 100 mg/dl.

Syndrome X is highly correlated with coronary heart disease, hypertension, strokes, Type 2 diabetes, and obesity.

The cause is partly genetic, as evidenced in the populations of the Pima Indians and Australian Aborigines, both of whom developed severe insulin resistance after eating modern diets. But even genes can largely be controlled by lifestyle: diet, exercise, fasting. These people had no problems when eating their traditional diets.[19]

People who are apple shaped are more likely to have this issue than the pear shaped. The waist-to-hip ratio is a common test: Standing upright with feet apart, measure the smallest part of your waist, just above the belly button, and the widest part of the hips. Divide the waist measurement by the hip measurement to get the ratio. If the ratio is over 0.95 in men or 0.90 in women, it is an indicator of syndrome X. A ratio of 1.0 or higher indicates a risk of diabetes, insulin resistance, cardiovascular disease, stroke, and various cancers.

If you are overweight, this is an indicator that you have developed insulin resistance to some degree.

My Battle with Hypoglycemia and Carb Addiction

I recall that when we were children, my brother and sister both had their appendices and tonsils removed. After my sister had her tonsils removed, I stood staring at her, envious that she was being doted upon by my parents.

She received the gift of a Casper-the-Ghost puppet for no other reason than that she was sick. She got to eat Jell-O and ice cream for dinner. Not I. I had to be the healthy one who was forced to keep all my internal organs.

I soon discovered my weak link: the pancreas. As soon as I turned 16, I couldn't wait to get my first job. I worked as a waitress, where I was overjoyed to get a quarter for a tip. (This was 1972.) One day I was walking to clean the tables when I suddenly blacked out and collapsed on the floor. As a pom-pom girl, I again fainted in the midst of practice.

My blood sugar sometimes got too low, with symptoms that include weakness, dizziness, fatigue, sleepiness, shakiness, and more.

Finally my parents took me to the doctor, who hospitalized me for a battery of tests. I was in the hospital for one week. That has been my only hospital stay, by the way, except for visiting other people.

The upshot of all these tests was that I had *hypoglycemia*. The doctors almost apologized for the diagnosis. It was a new diagnosis at the time. There were even some doctors who called it a "fad disease" and weren't even sure it was real.

After that, I dutifully counted my carbs and limited them to, if memory serves, 100 grams a day. Not much when you consider that a potato — one potato alone — has 63 grams of carbs! I was miserable. I tired of not being able to consume my staples of potatoes, dry popcorn, and graham crackers. Before counting my carbs, I had often eaten an entire package of graham crackers daily, having discovered they were only 30 calories each.

Soon I sided with the doctors who said it was merely a fad disease. I decided it was a quack diagnosis. I knew sweets were bad, but I really, really loved my potatoes, graham crackers, and popcorn! After all, these were low in fat and calories. How bad could they really be? I figured since I didn't faint anymore, I must have been okay.

Throughout all of this, I had slipped into *anorexia nervosa*, the obsession with thinness. Three years later, this anorexia flipped into bulimia, which it commonly does, since the body becomes starved of critical nutrients.

While at the university, I grew so desperate that I went to see a counselor. He said something that I will always remember, though it took me years to fully understand, and has since become my credo: "Always rule out physical causes of illness before assuming there is a psychological or emotional one."

He ordered an extensive blood sugar test.

"Always rule out physical causes of illness before assuming there is a psychological or emotional one."

Again I got the drawn-out test that takes hours as they test your blood sugar every couple of hours. I was pronounced hypoglycemic again. The diagnosis couldn't escape me. The counselor explained that my body's over-reactive, high-insulin response to carbs made me hungry, craving still more carbs, especially sweets.

By this time, 1976, I sensed that the disorder had gained more credibility in the medical establishment. Again, I tried to monitor my diet for a while, and I again forgot the diagnosis and went on to eat whatever I wanted.

In the late '80s, I became a cooked-food vegetarian for a couple of years — it was the cool, hip thing to do. Besides, it allowed me more carbs than ever, so it was really an easy thing to do. I took naps after every meal. The oatmeal, the pasta, the beans — they made my blood sugar plummet! I got chubby, fatigued, depressed. But at least I wasn't in danger of heart disease, I thought.

Then I discovered the Zone Diet and learned to stabilize my blood sugar. But once again, this was no fun! Eating a sparse 40 percent of my calories in carbs was pathetic, but my blood sugar became stable and my waist slim.

I discovered the raw diet years later. Even as a raw fooder, I sometimes had bouts with hypoglycemia. This occurred if I overindulged in dates, honey, dried fruit, kombucha, agave, or raw desserts.

Where did this carb conflict come from? When I was a child, my father dubbed me the Potato Queen.

I was frequently told the story of my great-great-grandmother (not sure how many greats), who fled the potato famine in Ireland in the 1840s. She was quite young and one of the very few survivors when the ship hit the dock in Montreal, Canada. Most died from some sort of plague from the rats on board.

My ancestor roamed the streets of Montreal, devastatingly broke, until she ran into a man who was a friend of her family's. Though he was 20 years older, she married him. It was *she*, I was told, from whom I inherited my lust for potatoes.

Years later, it dawned on me: Ireland is not a big country, and it's part of an island. Why hadn't she simply relocated to the Irish shore where she could have fished for food? But my taste buds immediately answered that question: because carbs taste better than meat, especially fish!*

This is the lengths we will go to feed our carb addictions: eat junk food, eat a macrobiotic diet (better), eat a raw vegan diet (better yet). And we pat ourselves on the back for contributing to sustainability and morality because we aren't killing animals. My ancestor even risked her life by crossing the great ocean in order to feed her carb addiction.

Prehistoric man went to great lengths, climbing trees and risking bee stings to get honey. It was a seasonal rare treat, but the lust for sugar overrode the fear of all those bees.

People don't get addicted to protein. You don't see many people bingeing on meat and eggs not loaded with addictive substances like MSG, salt, or sugar. You don't see people going to great lengths to get a meat-only fix. Unless starving, children don't cry for, and cannot be easily bribed with, protein products.

On the other hand, carbs are definitely addictive, so much so that I used to go to the movies and eat popcorn even after being an otherwise raw fooder for several years and even if the movie was pathetically boring. My friend who shared it with me would exclaim, "This stuff is like crack cocaine! I just can't stop eating it!"

A seemingly innocent, low-calorie baked potato has the same effect on your blood sugar as a lump of sugar. That's why I just had to laugh when I read a comment to my book review of praise for Lierre Keith's *The Vegetarian Myth*.

Susan sounds like someone who has been waiting a long time to have someone else okay her decision to stop being vegetarian.

Nothing could be further from the truth! On the contrary, it's carb addiction I struggle with. I used to use anything as an excuse to indulge in carbs.

---

*A friend of mine who studied the history of the Irish potato famine insists that the Irish (serfs of the English) couldn't fish because they couldn't afford fishing boats. At first glance, it does seem odd that they could afford what must have been an outrageous fee to take a ship ride across the Atlantic, but Wikipedia states that "they could get passage cheaply (or free in the case of tenant evictions) in returning empty lumber holds."[20] Also, the reason so many died on my ancestor's ship could be because it may have been a *coffin ship*, an overly insured boat in which deaths were rigged to occur for insurance purposes.

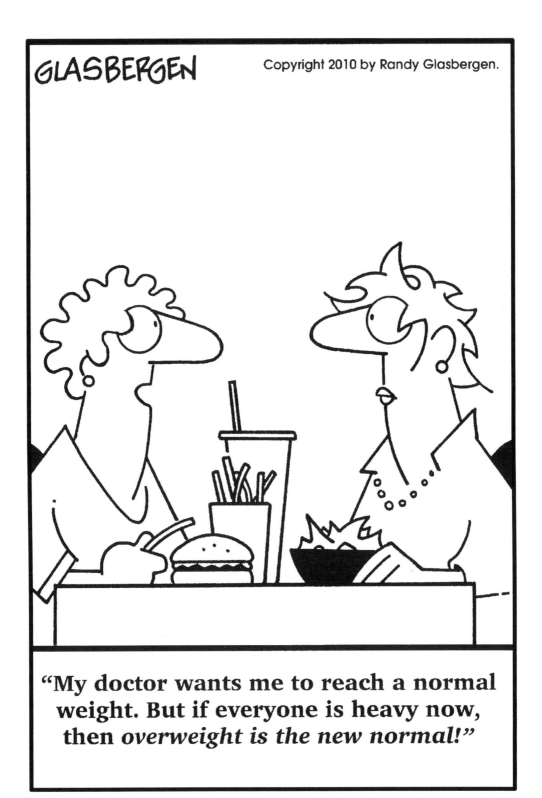

Chapter 11

Falling for the Big Fat Lie

For years, "heart-attack food" was synonymous with red meat, eggs, and butter. The evidence is in. That is utterly and completely wrong. Fast-acting, concentrated carbohydrate is the ultimate heart-attack food, particularly for those with a sedentary lifestyle.

—Richard K. Bernstein, MD, *The Diabetes Diet*

As early as the 1800s, long before the Atkins and Zone diets, doctors told people who wanted to lose weight that they had to reduce starches and sugary foods and replace them with protein foods, such as meat, dairy, and eggs instead. Conventional wisdom had it that bread, doughnuts, cakes, grains, and potatoes would fatten you up, as well as keep you hungry, while proteins and good fats (there weren't as many bad fats around until the 20th century) kept you full and satisfied.

So how did the fat-as-villain myth begin? How did this deadly lie go mainstream, now proven to be so blatantly false, not to mention contrary to the way man has eaten for millions of years? Investigative journalist Gary Taubes spent five years researching that question, and the extensive results are in his book *Good Calories, Bad Calories*, which reads like a political science text on the politics of nutrition.

It began with Ancel Keys, PhD, a University of Minnesota physiologist, who came up with the theory that dietary fat raises cholesterol levels and gives you heart disease. We now know that dietary fat influences only 15 to 20 percent of the cholesterol levels, and high blood cholesterol is not really a cause of heart disease.[1]

Furthermore, if you go on a low-cholesterol diet, your liver, which makes about 80 percent of your cholesterol, will simply compensate by making more. In other words, if you don't eat much cholesterol, your liver makes up for much of the difference. If you eat a lot of cholesterol, your liver backs off.

Dr. Keys made the cover of *Time* magazine in 1961 with his hypothesis and prompted the American Heart Association to publish its first official endorsement of a low-fat, low-cholesterol diet as a means to prevent heart disease. Saturated fat is higher in cholesterol, and most saturated fat comes from animal products: meat, dairy, and eggs.

Thus began the myth that animal fats, which our ancestors lived on for 2.6 million years, are bad for you. This was merely a hypothesis, mind you, not a proven fact.

Whenever an epidemiological study contradicted this theory, it was called a "paradox." For example, when the French had a low rate of heart disease yet indulged in diets rich in saturated fats, it was the "French paradox." When the Italians of Rosetto ate copious amounts of animal fats and even cooked with lard, yet had a strikingly low percentage of deaths from heart disease, this was thought to be another exception.

The Masai of Africa lived on very little besides milk, blood, and beef yet were free of heart disease and had low cholesterol levels. Eskimos eating their traditional diets, which often consisted of 100 percent animal meat for long stretches of time, were so healthy that they had no medicine men.

There is even a study that demonstrates an American paradox.

These effects include the paradox that a high-fat, highly saturated-fat diet is associated with diminished coronary artery disease progression in women with the metabolic syndrome, a condition that is epidemic in the United States.[2]

There were so many more paradoxes — the Greek Paradox, the East African Paradox, the Swiss Paradox, the Pacific Island Paradox, the Japanese Paradox — that Dr. Malcolm Kendrick, MD, author of *The Great Cholesterol Con*, queried, "How many paradoxes do you need before the only paradox left is the diet-heart hypothesis itself?"

Yet Dr. Keys's theory received a tremendous amount of publicity because there were *profits to be made* from it. Interestingly, Keys himself recanted the theory decades later, stating, "There's no connection whatsoever between cholesterol in food and cholesterol in the blood. None. And we've known that all along" (*Eating Well*, March/April 1997).

He also admitted that his lipid hypothesis, originally based on rabbits, herbivores by nature, applied *only* to rabbits. His retraction came after a man who ate 20 to 30 eggs a day for 15 years was found to have healthy plasma cholesterol![3]

Still, the lipid hypothesis grew because it was such a cash cow for the vegetable-oil and other food-processing companies, as well as for the pharmaceutical industry, the main beneficiaries.

This theory became instilled into mainstream consciousness in 1977 after Senator George McGovern announced the publication of the first *Dietary Goals for the United States*. Investigator Gary Taubes takes us behind the scenes, to show us that this dubious theory was decided by academic and corporate *politics*, not real *science*. Yes, you read that right. Government health guidelines — a dietary disaster for so many of us! — were basically the result of some closed-door wheeling and dealing from behind the scenes.

It turns out that this established "wisdom" was determined by a handful of men in a good ol' boys' club of academia, *none* of whom even worked with obese patients! These men included Jean Mayer, Fred Stare, Jules Hirsch, George Bray, Theodore Van Itallie, Albert Stunkard, George Cahill, and Philip White.

Meanwhile, Dr. Robert Atkins, MD, was writing about his tremendous results with patients who were able to shed the shackles of obesity without getting hungry, feeling deprived, or even "going low calorie." One of the good ol' boys, Van Itallie, had a personal grudge against Atkins and wrote that his work "lacked scientific merit" — despite the endocrinological science behind the fact that insulin, stimulated on high-carb diets, causes the body to store fat.

☞ Don't get me wrong. I am *not* an Atkins Diet fan! That diet is usually too high in protein and mostly cooked, but Atkins was a modern-day popularizer of the need to lower insulin levels.

Other MDs — William Banting, Alfred Pennington, and Herman Taller, author of *Calories Don't Count* — had likewise been getting astounding results in weight loss with their obese patients by using carbohydrate-restricted diets.

The late Dr. Frederick Stare, PhD, former head of Harvard University's nutrition department, began his career with articles warning about the nutritional deficiencies created by diets that included white flour. He even wrote about a study that found that diets high in vegetable oils correlated with heart disease.

But after becoming the department head, he sold out to the food industries in exchange for grants. His articles soon assured the public that white flour and processed foods were harmless. He even advocated eating *refined sugar*!

Stare and his colleagues at Harvard ensured that anyone who claimed that carbohydrates were uniquely fattening would be labeled a quack. Stare and colleagues White and Mayer publicly condemned Taller's low-carb book.

When did they denounce it? They badmouthed the low-carb diet one year after Harvard University's nutrition department broke ground on a new $5 million building, a lot of money back in the 1970s. Where did most of the donations for the building come from? As you might guess, the lead "gift" came from a corporation vested in carbs, General Food Corporation, maker of very carb-rich cereals.

Over the next decade, Harvard's nutrition department continued to receive funding from the sugar industry. Stare "coincidentally" became a staunch advocate of sugar and carbs.

So there you have it folks. Our health was placed on the sacrificial altar of corporate profits. Our health was *sold* when the lie was *told*. Harvard University professors profited from the lie.

The food companies were delighted with the lie because calorie for calorie, starches and sugars are the cheapest nutrients for them to produce. They yield the highest profit.

Grains can be stored, so having longer shelf lives makes them cheap and abundant. This is why grains have been called "the staff of life" — because they can be stored and used during times of famine.

Finally, the public was happy with the lie because carbs taste sweet and are like narcotics to the brain. Most people prefer pizza, crackers, doughnuts, cakes, pretzels, chips, and cookies (even fat-free ones) to yogurt, eggs, and meat. People get addicted to carbs, *not* protein.

Grain Merchants behind the Scenes

Who else may have been behind this great low-fat conspiracy to lead the public to purchase more grains and vegetable oils? According to researcher Dan Morgan, author of *Merchants of Grain: The Power and Profits of the Five Giant Companies at the Center of the World's Food Supply*, there are seven secretive families that monopolize the world's grain supplies.

According to Morgan, since these grain companies had been privately owned for centuries and mostly still are, there were no public stockholders and therefore no financial statements that had to be openly published, despite the fact that they received billions of dollars in government subsidies — at least those operating in the US.

These grain companies make money whether grain prices rise or fall. Farmers and commodities speculators alone shoulder the risks of bad weather, changes in governmental policies, and falling prices. (Since Morgan's book was written, at least one of these companies has gone public.)

These seven reclusive families own or control the five big grain companies: the Fribourgs at Continental Grain Company (New York City, US); the Hirsches and Borns at Bunge (no nationality); the Cargills and MacMillans at Cargill, Inc. (Minneapolis, US); and the Louis-Dreyfuses (Paris, France) and Andres (Switzerland) at the companies with those names.

Few people even know the names of most of these companies and fewer still have ever heard of the oligopolists who own them. Their families like to keep it that way.

They are likely behind the entire low-fat craze, since they are the ones who profit most. They are likely behind the soy craze, since soybeans are one of the farm crops they monopolize.

No doubt they are behind the "eat grains for fiber" propaganda (now proven bogus), as well as the food pyramid, which suggests we eat 6 to 11 servings of grain a day! Grains — generally the worst food for humans — are at the *base* of the food pyramid.

The Great Cholesterol Con

Heart attacks and heart disease used to be very rare, even though people indulged in pork lard, beef tallow, eggs, and steaks. When Dr. Paul Dudley White, personal physician to President Eisenhower and lead author of a text on coronary disease, decided to specialize in coronary heart disease, he was recommended to find a more profitable specialty, because heart problems were so rare.

By the 1950s and 1960s, heart disease became the leading killer. What had changed in just a few decades? Factory farming practices had begun in the 1920s, degrading the quality of our meats and resulting in damaged arteries a few decades later. Animals were fed grains to fatten them up, for example, which skewed their omega-6:3 ratios. Also to blame was the widespread dietary replacement of animal fats with toxic, rancid vegetable oils high in omega-6 fats. Worthy of note as well was the increase in carb consumption, especially refined sugar and other highly processed foods.

Yet the simplistic dietary fat theory was promoted as the chief culprit.

Despite a huge brainwashing of the masses to eat less saturated fat and lower their cholesterol levels, heart disease only increased. A reduced death rate has resulted from improved emergency care, but progression of the disease itself is relentless.

Despite masses of people giving up smoking and taking up exercise, heart disease continues. The ulterior motive here from corporations? To sell the food companies' vegetable oils, to sell the high-carb foods, and especially to sell the drugs that lower cholesterol.

Dr. George V. Mann, MD, a Johns Hopkins-educated biochemist and physician who was the associate director in the Framingham study of cholesterol, later studied and wrote about the Masai cattle-herding people in Africa. Their unique diet was nearly all meat, blood, and fatty milk. During some periods of their lives, that was *all* they ate. He found these people to be completely free of heart disease.

Although there was significant atherosclerosis, raised plaques were rare, and cholesterol levels were very low, as his study states.

The intake of animal fat exceeds that of American men. Measurements of the aorta showed extensive atherosclerosis with lipid infiltration and fibrous changes but very few complicated lesions.[4]

He also found that the Pygmies living in the African rain forest had low levels of cholesterol despite eating large amounts of meat.[5]

Dr. Mann called the lipid hypothesis the greatest scam in the history of medicine.

When we find the real cause and prevention of the cholesterol problem, it will seem to many that there was an unwholesome conspiracy.[*]

A world-renowned heart surgeon from Houston, Dr. Michael DeBakey, MD, devoted extensive research to the cholesterol theory of heart disease. He found that out of every ten people in the US who have atherosclerotic heart disease, only three or four (30 to 40 percent) had high cholesterol levels. That 30 to 40 percent is the same percentage of the general population that has elevated cholesterol!

In other words, 30 to 40 percent of people with heart disease have high cholesterol levels, but so do 30 to 40 percent of healthy people with no risk of heart attack. A study he undertook proved that there was no correlation between heart disease and high cholesterol.[6]

> *"When we find the real cause and prevention of the cholesterol problem, it will seem to many that there was an unwholesome conspiracy."*

Other studies have found such correlations, but not a simplistic cause-effect one. There are other more important factors.

Author Michael Murray, ND, calls the fixation on cholesterol by the drug companies and doctors "one of the greatest medical injustices of all time."

Half the people who die of a heart attack or a stroke have low to normal cholesterol levels. How do the drug companies and the government respond to this fact? They simply recommend making the suggested target cholesterol levels even lower, thereby effectively casting an even wider net for potential customers. ...

Six of the nine expert members of the government panel that drafted the new cholesterol guidelines had either received grants from, or were paid consulting or speakers' fees by, the companies that make some of the most popular statin drugs. ...

These new guidelines should dramatically increase the number of patients on statin drugs. Keep in mind that statins are already the biggest moneymakers in the drug industry.[7]

Cholesterol Is Absolutely Necessary!

Cholesterol is one of the most important substances in our bodies. Without it you would die. Cholesterol gives our cell membranes their necessary stiffness and stability. Without it, you would "melt down like the Wicked Witch in *The Wizard of Oz*," as Drs. Michael and Mary Eades say.

Cholesterol is used to make our hormones, including estrogen, testosterone, progesterone, cortisol, aldosterone, and DHEA. Cholesterol is a precursor to corticosteroids, hormones used to deal with stress.

It is a precursor to vitamin D, which is needed for healthy bones. Sunlight on the skin interacts with cholesterol to produce vitamin D. If your cholesterol levels are too low, you risk the degenerative diseases that come with vitamin D deficiencies.

Cholesterol is needed in maintaining the health of the intestinal wall, which is replaced every four or five days. It prevents leaky gut syndrome and other intestinal disorders.

Cholesterol is needed to repair wear and tear on the skeleton and muscles, repair injured tissues, and renew hair, skin, and nails.

The brain is rich in cholesterol and needs cholesterol for serotonin receptors to function. Without sufficient cholesterol, people and animals become depressed. Low levels of cholesterol are linked to depression, suicide, homicide, and violence, because a serotonin deficiency is often behind all these conditions. Low cholesterol levels over time cause the brain to shrink and may eventually result

---

[*]In an editorial published in the *New England Journal of Medicine* in 1977, Dr. Mann called the cholesterol theory of heart disease "the greatest scam in the history of medicine."

in Alzheimer's disease.

Depression, Suicide, Violence, and Homicide Worse with Low Cholesterol

Lowering serum cholesterol levels by diet or drugs has been shown in numerous studies to increase the rate of death by suicide or violence.[8]

Nutritionist Nathan Pritikin was among those who popularized low-fat diets. After many years on his diet, while still relatively young in his early 60s, he was diagnosed with cancer and depression. This led to his committing suicide. Cancer, depression, and suicide are all now well-researched and proven consequences of insufficient cholesterol.

My own life has been a continuous experiment in diets. When I look back at my deepest, darkest night of the soul, the period during which I was severely depressed, it coincides with the late '80s and early '90s when I was on a low-fat diet! (Two of those years I was also a cooked food vegetarian.) I was dysfunctional in both relationships and my professional life.

I had been duped like everyone else into eating a lot of grains and fat-free products, such as no-fat salad dressings and fat-free cheeses. Like everyone else, I threw out the egg yolks and ate the whites only. So depressed was I that I took Prozac, which made me gain 40 pounds within six months!

I snapped out of this depression only when I moved on to the Atkins Diet and later the Zone Diet. Even then, I was not eating healthful raw fats, but at least I could dump the Prozac. I became happier on a raw diet full of good plant fats, but I am now happier than ever since I added fish oils, raw egg yolks, and cod liver oil with its DHA and EPA.

Saturated Fats Are Critical for Health

We know that overdoing saturated fats can lead to strokes, Alzheimer's disease, and even diabetes, but completely eliminating saturated fats from the diet can lead to other problems in those people who are unable to synthesize enough in their bodies.

Saturated fats have also been maligned by the entire low-fat industry. They have been blamed for clogging arteries when in reality only 26 percent of

the fat clogging the arteries is saturated. Most, 74 percent, is unsaturated, of which 41 percent is polyunsaturated, the kind found in vegetable oils that were supposed to make our arteries healthy.[9] In fact in one study, the progression of atherosclerosis was shown to be greater in those who took the least saturated fat.[10]

Saturated fats constitute at least 50 percent of our cell membranes, giving them stiffness and integrity. Sally Fallon and Mary Enig, PhD, cite a study showing that 50 percent of our dietary fats need to be saturated in order for calcium to be effectively incorporated into the skeletal structure.[11]

"Half the people who die of a heart attack or a stroke have low to normal cholesterol levels. How do the drug companies and the government respond to this fact? They simply recommend making the suggested target cholesterol levels even lower, thereby effectively casting an even wider net for potential customers."

Vitamins A and D, found only in animal fats, help with protein and mineral absorption. Animal products are the richest sources of dietary saturated fats, with the exceptions of coconut, cacao butter, and palm oil. Protein cannot be utilized without dietary fats. In nature, protein and fats usually come together, as in eggs, milk, fish, and meat from land animals.

Other fat-soluble vitamins found in some animal fats include vitamins E and K. Dr. Price referred to these fat-soluble vitamins as "activators" or "catalysts" and observed that without them we cannot absorb the water-soluble vitamins and cannot utilize the minerals, no matter how much of them we ingest. This is why the whole "low-fat milk" and "low or zero animal fat" craze is crazy!

People who promote that have clearly not studied Dr. Price's research.

I recall that when I grew up, everyone suddenly switched from butter to margarine, believing the propaganda that it was "better for the heart." Now we know the opposite is true: margarine is often made from soy, which is toxic to humans, and contains trans fats — even worse, as nutritionist Mary Enig, PhD, and collaborator Sally Fallon explain.

Saturated fats maintain cellular integrity everywhere in the body. Why? Because *every* cell membrane is ideally made up of about 50 percent saturated fat. When we eat too much polyunsaturated oil and not enough saturated fat (or carbohydrates that the body turns into saturated fat), our cells don't function correctly. Those cell membrane fatty acids need to be saturated for the cell to have the necessary "stiffness," or integrity, and to work properly. When the cell walls do not contain enough saturated fat, they actually become "floppy" and cannot work properly.[12]

Sally Fallon discusses the benefits of butter and other animal fats in her classic book *Nourishing Traditions*. These fats contain the "Wulzen factor," named after researcher Dr. Rosalind Wulzen, which gets rid of stiffness in the body: arthritis, hardening of the arteries, cataracts, and calcification of the pineal gland.

Butter also contains conjugated linoleic acids, but only if the cows were completely grass fed. Animal fats (from animals fed their proper diets, not grains) are rich in omega-3 fats and have the right ratio to omega-6 fats, unlike the vegetable oils that are too high in omega-6s. Even lard, which we used when I was a kid, is better than the rancid omega-6 vegetable oils that replaced it! Lard is an excellent source of vitamin D.

Though it is best to eat everything raw, if you must cook, animal fats are more stable when heated than vegetable oils are. Saturated fats are more stable and safe to use at high temperatures in cooking. So when we used to fry things in lard, it was actually much less harmful than using vegetable oils, which are unstable, toxic, and rancid when heated.

Even coconut oil was badmouthed by the food industries eager to sell us their vegetable oils. Coconut oil, though it doesn't contain the crucial vitamins found in animal fats, is stable when used for cooking and helps in weight loss.

One study found that a reduction in dietary saturated fat resulted in lower levels of the "good" HDL cholesterol.[13] Even more powerful, researchers Ronald P. Mensink and Martijn B. Katan reviewed 27 studies and found that *saturated fat elevated HDL* whenever it was used instead of carbohydrates! This effect diminished with increasing use of unsaturated fats.[14]

Saturated fats also protect the liver from foreign substances, assist in bone growth, protect against infection, influence hormone function, and protect against heart disease.[15]

Nutritionist and weight-loss coach Dr. Jonny Bowden, PhD, CNS, outlines the reasons saturated fats were blamed for heart disease:

- A diet high in saturated fats can be a problem when they are eaten as part of a high-carb diet.

- Saturated fats were demonized because much of the research on diet and disease lumped saturated fats in with dangerous trans fats.

- Modern saturated fats usually come from poor sources: corn fed, hormone-treated cows, with their unhealthful dairy products, deli meats, etc.[16]

So What Causes Heart Disease?

Studies show that the percentage of dietary cholesterol has little effect on the risk for cardiovascular disease.[17] There is great controversy in the idea that eating a high-cholesterol diet increases blood cholesterol levels. Even if it did, there is no proof that high cholesterol levels alone result in heart disease. Neither is there proof that lowering cholesterol levels will eliminate heart disease, unless they get so low one's mental or emotional well-being might be endangered.

The only concern for cholesterol is that HDL should be high relative to LDL, and the ratio of triglycerides to HDL should be low.[18] As far as LDL, the "bad" cholesterol, goes, there are two types, A and B, indicating whether the LDL particles are light and cottony (A) or small and dense (B). Having a type A LDL pattern is healthier.[19]

According to Robb Wolf, author of *The Paleo Solution*, the type B LDL pattern is "born from the

VLDL [very low-density lipoprotein] that is the product of *high-carbohydrate intake*" [emphasis his].[20] Gary Taubes concurs.

Carbohydrate-rich diets not only lower HDL and raise triglycerides, they also make LDL small and dense.[21]

Furthermore, cholesterol abnormalities are considered *symptoms*, not *causes*, of heart disease. As Taubes explains, "The cholesterol seems to be an innocent bystander."[22]

So now that we have found that animal fats, dietary cholesterol and saturated fats are not as lethal as previously thought, what has been shown to be the real cause of heart disease?

One theory is a high blood level of the amino acid *homocysteine*, a metabolite of the amino acid methionine, is to blame. *Methionine* is a sulfur-containing amino acid found chiefly in flesh foods, nuts, and seeds. Consumption of vitamin B_{12}, as well as vitamins B_6 and folate (found abundantly in organ meats and chicken liver, but also in green, leafy vegetables), helps lower excess serum homocysteine levels. A high homocysteine level is also considered to be a risk factor for dementia.

The less B_{12} one has, the higher blood homocysteine levels rise. The richest source of B_{12} is meat. Studies show that vegans and vegetarians tend to have higher levels of homocysteine than do nonvegetarians because of consuming less B_{12}.[23] On the other hand, too much methionine-containing protein (common in meat) can increase homocysteine beyond acceptable levels, so balance is key. Eat enough animal foods to get adequate B_{12}, but not enough to overdose on methionine.

Another factor in heart disease is high blood levels of insulin. To get one's insulin levels down, one must eat a diet low in carbs. In such a diet, it is usually necessary to include meat, fish, or eggs, since they are the only foods that contain no carbs. The American Heart Association agrees that high-glycemic diets rich in low-fiber carbs are related to heart disease.[24]

Another factor in heart disease is a blood level high in triglycerides, which increase when insulin levels are high.[25] The ratio of triglycerides to HDL should be low. In one study, those people with the highest triglyceride ratio had a 16 times greater risk of heart attack than those with the lowest ratio.[26]

HDL should be high, the higher the better. An article published in the *New England Journal of Medicine* explained that HDL is "a biomarker for dietary carbohydrate." In other words, a healthfully high level of HDL indicates that one is eating few carbs. If it's low, it is likely you are eating a lot of carbs.[27]

Consider what Dr. Bowden has to say.

Triglyceride levels always come down on a low-carb diet. Always. Not "sometimes": *all* the time. (Which makes sense – the body takes all that excess sugar and packages it into triglycerides; so the less sugar in the diet, the fewer triglycerides in the blood.)[28]

Yet another factor in heart disease is inflammation, the C-reactive protein (CRP) theory. Inflammation is made worse by vegetable oils that replaced animal fats, because these oils are very high in omega-6 fats. Many of these fats, such as margarine, are hydrogenated trans fats, which increase the risk of heart disease and many other diseases.[29]

A high-carb diet, which is the norm with many vegetarians, also increases inflammation unless the carbs are mostly raw fruits and vegetables.[30]

All of those factors are exacerbated when one ceases to eat healthful meat from free-range farmed animals that were fed their proper, species-specific diets.

The total amount of meat consumed by Americans has risen dramatically in the past century. This increase, from toxic, factory-farmed animals no less, also plays a huge role in heart disease. It gets even worse when one overindulges carbs, so typical on vegetarian and vegan diets.

Ironically, getting rid of healthful animal fats has led to an increased risk of heart disease.

Factors in Heart Disease

- high homocysteine levels
- high insulin levels
- high triglyceride levels
- high CRP levels (inflammation)[*]
- high LDL cholesterol levels with type B
- high VLDL levels

---

[*]*worsened by a diet high in omega-6 fats*

Chapter 12

Benefits of Curbing Your Carbs

Low-carb is not even close to being a fad diet.
—Dr. James E. Carlson, low-carb nutritional and wellness expert

The price of food relative to income is probably lower in the US than anywhere else in the world. Two-thirds of Americans are overweight, and one-third are obese. Yet obesity is *worse* among the poor, which indicates that being overweight is not simply overindulgence, since the poor have limited funds.

I concluded after much research that it is the overabundance of cheap carbs and the excess of omega-6 fats found in vegetable oils and the meat of grain-fed animals that have created the obesity epidemic.

The terms *carbohydrate* and *saccharide* are used in biochemistry to refer to sugars. Carbohydrates include both simple sugars as well as starches, as in potatoes and grains. Some people think that starches are "good" carbs, although they break down into simple sugars in the digestive system nevertheless.

If you eat foods that are *low glycemic*, it simply means the sugar gets into your bloodstream more gradually than those that are *high glycemic*. Low glycemic is better.

Examples of high-glycemic foods would be sugary desserts, baked potatoes, popcorn, rice cakes, and white bread. Low-glycemic carbs would be broccoli, lentils, sprouted whole grains, and other foods having lots of fiber that make them slower to break down into sugars by diluting the body's digestive juices.

The *glycemic index* is an arbitrary rating scale that rates foods according to their effects on blood sugar levels one hour after consumption. The number is not always reliable because different individuals respond differently to various foods. Cooking also increases and may even *double* a food's glycemic index. Also, foods grown in different soils may vary in their GIs.

The *glycemic load* (GL) is the impact of the entire meal. It's a measure of the insulin response over the whole digestive process of a given food or meal.

Here's the good news: fiber will reduce the glycemic load. So if you combine something sweet with a lot of fiber, such as some psyllium husk or bran, the glycemic load would be lowered by the fiber.[1] Therefore, when you are counting the carb content, you can subtract the dietary fiber to get the effective carbohydrate content.[2] You don't count the fiber as carb because it doesn't act metabolically like a carb.

For example, if you eat a packaged snack that has on the label 13 grams of carbs and 10 grams of fiber, you subtract 10 from 13 to get only 3 *effective* grams of carbs. This calculation applies to the US and may not be applicable to other countries, which may use different labeling systems. In some countries, the subtraction has already been done for you, and the snack's label would list "3 grams of carbohydrates" and not bother with listing the fiber.

Now let's define what we mean by *low-carb diet*. Americans eat about 50 to 70 percent of their calories in carbs, around 300 grams per day. A low-carb diet is usually considered to be less than 40 percent of total calories in carbs and sometimes down to 10 percent or 20 percent. Some authorities consider even 50 percent to be on the low side.

Low carb is thought to be how our paleolithic ancestors ate, or at least those tribes who didn't have access to abundant fruit, such as those who lived in cold climates.

If you lower your carb quota to 20 to 40 percent, you may experience many benefits, *unless you are a carb type*. Your insulin sensitivity will improve. You will have less likelihood of diabetes. You will lose weight or find your ideal weight easier to maintain.

Your dental health will also improve. Nutritional anthropologist Dr. H. Leon Abrams, Jr., points out that "Archaeological and ethnological studies show that as humans increase their reliance upon carbohydrates, there is a corresponding rise in the incidence of caries."[3]

The debate over the relative merits of carbs vs. fats has been a hot one since the 1970s. Even in the raw food community, the camps vary widely. On one extreme, you have Dr. Doug Graham who insists that 80/10/10 (80 percent carb calories with 10 percent each of fats and protein) is optimal for nearly everyone. He is big on being 100 percent raw but states emphatically, "*If high-fat raw or low-fat cooked seem your only options, choose the low-fat option, every time.*"[4] He is claiming that *low fat* is even more important than *raw*!

On the other hand, you have Dr. Stanley S. Bass with all of his degrees and over 50 years of clinical experience. He and his hygienic mentor, Dr. Christopher Gian-Cursio, PhD, broke away from the prevailing vegan hygiene camp, adding raw eggs and dairy to their patients' diets. In 2003, hygienist Anna Nelson, along with Dr. Bass and some of his nonvegan hygienic professional colleagues, founded the International Natural Hygiene Society.

Dr. Bass has recently become firmly convinced that high insulin and leptin levels are responsible for most diseases. He advises people to go low carb, and it is nearly impossible to do this unless you eat very few calories or unless you include animal products, which tend to be very low carb, almost zero. He says if his patients can't eat their meat, dairy, and eggs raw, then it is better to eat a low-carb diet *cooked* than even a high-carb diet *raw*. So in marked contrast to Dr. Graham, Dr. Bass is stating that *low carb* is even more important than *raw*.

Low-carb diets are not all alike. Dr. Sears of the Zone Diet advocates what he calls balance in the macronutrients. The Atkins Diet advocated eating as much meat as you felt like. I believe many of the failures of the Atkins Diet came from eating too much meat. Excess protein is toxic. Dr. Ron Rosedale, MD, later wrote *The Rosedale Diet* and warned that even protein can stimulate insulin production.

If you are a carb type, much of the info in this chapter will not apply to you as strongly as to mixed or protein types. Nonetheless, it is good to keep insulin levels down with low-GL meals.

A Low-Carb Diet Increases Nitric Oxide

Nitric oxide (NO) is a gas. It should not be confused with nitrous oxide (N_2O), the "laughing gas" administered by dentists. A molecule of NO is made from one atom of nitrogen and one atom of oxygen. It is released from the lining of your blood vessels when you feel pleasure, and it then turns on neurotransmitters that carry messages between the brain and nervous system. One of the neurotransmitters increased by pleasure is beta-endorphin, which dulls pain and creates euphoria.

Nitric oxide facilitates healthy immune, nerve, gastrointestinal, and kidney functions. It enables blood vessels of the penis to dilate and for the blood to enter and form an erection. In fact, Viagra "works" by interfering with the body's breakdown of NO.

Nitric oxide aids cardiovascular function. Low levels of NO predict cardiovascular heart risk. NO also helps relax the uterus in childbirth.

An article published in *The Iranian Journal of Diabetes & Lipid Disorders* concluded from a study that calorie restriction reduces blood pressure and increases nitric oxide.[5] Still, most of the benefits that come from a CR diet occur because the people or animals are restricting their *carbs*. According to Dr. Rosedale, you will get nearly the same effect without the hunger and emaciated look if you just eat low carb.

Studies show that glucose neutralizes NO when it is exposed to human endothelial cells at levels close to those of diabetics. Furthermore, glycation, the binding of sugars to proteins, arising from elevated blood sugar causes red blood cells to bind tightly with NO. This prevents the NO from exerting its beneficial anti-clotting and artery-relaxing effects.[6]

Dr. Christiane Northrup, MD, praises NO in her book *The Secret Pleasures of Menopause*.

Nitric oxide is special because, quite simply, it resets your power grid and reboots your body the same way you reboot your computer in order to make it work better. The more nitric oxide your body makes on a regular basis, the healthier and happier you are on many levels. Nitric oxide is the mother of all "feel good" molecules; and it isn't illegal, immoral, or the least bit fattening![7]

[NO is] quite literally the spark of life — the physical equivalent of life energy, chi, or prana. It's what breathes life into us in the first place.[8]

She claims it is the molecule that determines physical, emotional, spiritual, and sexual wellness.

She lists ways to elevate levels of NO: think positively, eat healthfully, exercise, get enough sleep, take pride in yourself, have a healthy sex life. Now we can add to her list: eat a low-calorie, or at least a low-carb diet! In addition, give up smoking and eat more foods high in antioxidants.

Low-Carb Weight Loss

Studies show that lowering your carb intake is nearly as important as lowering your caloric intake for weight loss. In fact, it may be every bit as important if you want to be sure you are losing fat and not muscle fibers. It also prevents hunger, since you are not spiking your blood insulin levels, so it is much easier to reduce your calories.

Again, if you are a carb type, these caveats may not apply to you. Such people experience less hunger and can lose weight on a high-carb diet.

Numerous studies have confirmed that at least in certain metabolic types, weight loss is much easier on a low-carb diet. A large number of books have been written about it, starting with one as early as 1864 by William Banting. In fact, very often one can eat a high-calorie or maintenance-calorie diet and still lose weight if it is very low in carbs.[9]

In one study done in England, obese people were put on a low-calorie diet of 1000 calories a day. Some ate 90 percent protein, some 90 percent fat, and some 90 percent carbs. The high-protein dieters lost 0.6 pounds a day; the high-fat dieters lost 0.9 pounds a day, and the high-carb dieters actually *gained* weight![10]

One study showed that on a low-carb diet rather than a high-carb diet, a person also loses more body fat instead of lean muscle tissue. The higher protein group that ate low carb also had lower triglycerides, lower insulin levels, and greater satiety after eating.[11]

There appears to be a metabolic advantage on a low-carb diet for most people: more calories are burned, 100 to 400 extra per day. Dr. Jonny Bowden insists that if two people were to go on diets of the same number of calories, one low carb and the other low fat, the low-carb person would generally lose more weight.[12]

The reason for this is that the body doesn't behave like a checkbook or bank, simply adding or subtracting calories. Hormones are involved, not just calories. But low carb, high carb — either way, *calories still count*. Some people have the idea that they can eat endless calories on a very low-carb diet and still lose weight. This has been proven false.

The Importance of Controlling Insulin Levels

Many doctors argue that the most crucial indicator of a long, healthy life is insulin sensitivity, or low insulin levels. Dr. Rosedale sums it up.

Insulin sensitivity is going to determine, for the most part, how long you are going to live and how healthy you are going to be. It determines the rate of aging more so than anything else we know right now.[13]

Keeping your insulin levels down will keep you not only healthy, but also slimmer and younger looking. Even if you are a carb type, you need to and can keep insulin levels down with low glycemic loads. Also, as Dr. Doug Graham and others point out, do not mix carbs with fat.

Insulin sends a message to the body to lower blood sugar, but perhaps its main function is to store fat. For our paleo ancestors, finding sweet fruit or honey was a rare treat. Fruit back then was not hybridized to be oversweet, and it wasn't every day you were able to raid a beehive. So the main evolutionary purpose of insulin was to store fat for times of food scarcity.

In today's diet, we consume too many fiberless carbs and too much sugar, creating an overload of insulin and hence stored fat. As children, our insulin blood sugar regulation mechanism worked perfectly. We could handle eating a lot of carbs. The carb load nowadays is even too high for many children, and they develop "adult" onset diabetes!

Because of high-carb diets, which promote a lot of insulin secretion from the pancreas, our cells eventually become insulin *resistant* rather than insulin *sensitive*, refusing to listen to insulin's messages. This is why we get and remain fat. Will young, slim vegans who eat lots of carbs, especially cooked ones that are higher glycemic, become fat? Will the bestselling vegan authors of *Skinny Bitches* become Chubby Crones?

Eventually insulin resistance can lead to Type 2 diabetes. Dr. Rosedale says *we all have diabetes* to some extent — it's just a matter of to what *degree* you are insulin resistant.

One of insulin's messages goes to the kidneys, telling them to retain sodium and hence water weight. This leads to bloating, high blood pressure, and congestive heart failure in some cases. According to Dr. Rosedale, the insulin — not dietary fat, as we have been falsely led to believe — causes plaque to build up in arteries. In an article on Dr. Rosedale's site, he says that heart attacks are two to three times more likely to happen after a high-carb meal than a high-fat one.[14]

There is also a strong correlation between a diet that incites high insulin levels and the development of breast, colon, prostate, and pancreatic cancers.[15] My father was diabetic, for example, and suffered from both prostate cancer and colon cancer, eventually dying from the latter.

High insulin levels also contribute to osteoporosis. By keeping levels of insulin and leptin down, which happens on a low-carb diet that is also not too high in protein, you don't just prevent bone loss, but you can actually build bone density. According to Dr. Rosedale, no drug, over the counter medication, supplement, or exercise will build new bone mass as dramatically as simply lowering your leptin levels. We'll discuss more on leptin later.

As we age, we lose muscle mass and bone mass. Some MDs believe this is accelerated if we are running on sugar as fuel instead of fat. By lowering our insulin and leptin levels, we burn fat and prevent muscle and bone loss.

Having high insulin levels also causes us to lose muscle in another way. When insulin, a "building up" hormone, is too high, the body tries to restore balance by bringing in the hormones adrenaline and cortisol, which break things down. Unfortunately, cortisol breaks down the muscle.[16]

High insulin levels age your skin, according to rehabilitation specialist Dr. Adrienne Denese, MD, PhD.

Insulin takes an active role in thickening and hardening your arterial walls, a condition that is the precursor for heart disease and poor circulation. Poor peripheral circulation is one of the fastest ways to a decline of the elasticity, resilience, and radiance of your skin.

It also increases your blood cholesterol levels.

You may think that a six-ounce porterhouse steak will send your cholesterol soaring, but in fact, the consumption of red meat has a minuscule effect on your cholesterol levels compared to what an even moderately elevated insulin level can do.[17]

High insulin levels lead to fatigue. Think of how you feel after a plate of pasta or pancakes, and compare this to how you feel after eating some moderately cooked meat and vegetables.

Insulin resistance can also cause or contribute to polycystic ovary syndrome, infertility, impotence, and chronic kidney failure.[18]

Dr. Richard Bernstein, MD, explains that a high insulin level is toxic to the body, reduces longevity, and increases both blood pressure and damage to the lining of the *endothelium* (blood vessel walls).[19] He says our fasting blood sugar level should measure no more than 83 mg/dl, which is what he sees in slim, young, healthy adults.[20]

Reduced Water Retention

Edema (water retention) is also reduced on a low-carb diet. This is because when some people go low fat and low protein (high carb), they experience acute deficiencies of albumin — blood proteins that are synthesized from dietary proteins. This drop in albumin affects plasma osmotic pressure. Excess electrolytes then cause edema as they move into the intercellular space. When adequate protein is resumed, the edema is reduced.[21]

Some people think weight loss on a low-carb diet is due to water loss. Actually the low-carb diet just makes water weight more balanced and normal. In other words, it's not that low-carb diets get rid of excess water weight, but rather that *high-carb diets may cause too much water retention*.

A diet high in carbs can be bloating for another reason, which Robb Wolf points out.

When blood insulin levels increase, we make more of a hormone called aldosterone. Aldosterone causes our kidneys to retain sodium.

The body dilutes this otherwise toxic sodium with water, which can even lead to high blood pressure.[22]

Furthermore, a high-carbohydrate diet can eventually result in reduction of the hydrochloric acid needed to properly digest many foods.

Finally, high-carb diets tend to be high in fiber if whole grains, fruit, and starchy vegetables are consumed, which causes increased fermentation in the gut. This fermentation produces gases, and the acidity of the fermentation process causes intestinal inflammation. The combined impact of fermentation and acidity causes the intestines to swell like a balloon.[23]

One Cause of Dementia: High Insulin Levels

A diet high in carbs will often lead to spiked insulin levels, and this damages the brain, according to author and lecturer Dr. Mark Hyman, MD.

> [Excess insulin] increases inflammation and oxidative stress and ages your brain, leading to what is being called Type 3 diabetes (also known as Alzheimer's disease).[24]

Insulin resistance leads to a cascade of damage that produces inflammation in the brain and dementia.[25]

The process of mental decline due to insulin resistance begins in childhood and adolescence. Dr. Hyman provokes us with this startling concern.

> Given the epidemic of childhood obesity and the fact that we are seeing heart disease in twenty-year-olds, will we soon see an epidemic of Alzheimer's when (or if) these kids turn forty?[26]

☞ Those who are savvy about the dangers of cell phone radiation emissions already expect an epidemic of Alzheimer's to occur in today's youth when they hit their forties.

Will this generation survive the brain trauma of DHA deficit, insulin surplus, phone radiation excess, excitotoxins in processed foods, and the ever-increasing number of childhood vaccinations?

Other Advantages of Low-Carb Diets

Low-carb diets with adequate protein will also help preserve muscle mass and slow down the aging process.[27]

Leptin: The Master Hormone

Body fat was once thought to be simply a storehouse of extra calories, but now we know it is part of an active endocrine system that produces its own hormones. When we gain weight, our fat cells produce *leptin*, a hormone discovered as recently as 1994. A healthy body responds to excess weight by increasing leptin production, which suppresses the appetite and speeds up metabolism so that one loses those extra, unneeded pounds.

Leptin controls metabolism, oversees energy reserves, decides whether to induce hunger, and decides whether to store fat or burn it. It regulates the other hormones and impacts our emotions, cravings, and behavior.

When leptin was discovered, drug companies could hear the cash registers ringing. They thought of all the leptin pills they could sell for weight loss. However, it was discovered that obese people already had an abundance of leptin. Their bodies just weren't listening to it. Just as they were insulin resistant, they were also leptin resistant.

Because leptin is the master hormone, you have to bring it under control if you want to lose weight and attain peak health. The only way you can control leptin levels is through diet. As with insulin control, leptin control requires a *low-glycemic diet*, or at least the avoidance of mixing carbs with fats, as Dr. Doug Graham teaches.

Having optimal leptin resistance also requires eating healthful fats. Fats should be a balance of saturated, monounsaturated, and polyunsaturated fats. The polyunsaturated fats should include a ratio of 2:1 or 1:1 omega-6 fatty acids to omega-3 fatty acids. The American diet contains the outrageous ratio of 25 to 50 omega-6s to 1 omega-3!

You need the correct ratio because omega-6s compete with omega-3s for transport into cells and can crowd out the omega-3s, keeping the body from making use of them. You need the omega-3s for weight loss and making DHA and EPA for the brain. If you have too much omega-6, you will get an excess of eicosanoids, hormones that create inflammation, leading to pain and disease.

Furthermore, the trans fats and hydrogenated oils found in most processed foods should be avoided completely. They are man-made, toxic fats.

Studies which incited the fat phobia of the 1980s by showing fat to be dangerous were often including these fats. We now know that all these vegetable oils that became much more prevalent after the cholesterol hypothesis became popularized have led to cancer, heart disease, and diabetes — the very illnesses they were supposed to protect us from!

Chapter 13

Burning Fat Instead of Sugar

If I were to summarize in a single sentence what practice would best promote health, it would be this: Health and life span are determined by the proportion of fat versus sugar people burn throughout their lifetime; and so the more fat that one burns as fuel, the healthier a person will be, and the more likely he or she will live a long time; and the more sugar a person burns, the more disease ridden and the shorter a life span a person is likely to have.

—Dr. Ron Rosedale, *The Rosedale Diet*

Our cells normally burn two kinds of fuel: sugar and fat. When we are young, we burn sugar (carbs) more efficiently than when we are older. We can switch back and forth from burning carbs to burning stored fat and vice versa. So if we haven't eaten in a while or go on a calorie-reduced diet, we can switch from burning sugar to burning our stored fats as energy.

Things change as we age unless we keep our bodies in youthful condition by eating a high-raw diet, exercising, and fasting periodically. Otherwise, we lose the ability to switch gears quite so easily. Since agriculture began, most people have been on much higher carb diets than what we evolved on. They are used to burning more sugar than fat.

You normally burn the sugar in the food you have just eaten, but if you haven't eaten in a while and are no longer able to easily switch gears to burning fat, you'll get hungry.

Some doctors and researchers theorize that you will even cannibalize your own muscles and bones if you are in the sugar-burning mode and don't eat for some time, as Dr. Rosedale explains.

> Most people are good sugar burners because they've had a lot of experience doing so, due to our typically high sugar and starch diet. Even when you are not eating, your body's cells are still burning fuel to do their work. When you are a sugar burner, your body continues to burn sugar as its primary fuel and to sock away fat. I call this phenomenon "metabolic momentum." The body continues to burn the fuel it is accustomed to burning.
>
> Being essentially a 24/7 sugar burner can be very damaging. Your body can't store very much sugar. To continue to feed its sugar habit when you don't

eat, your body will break down the protein in its lean tissues — including muscle and bone — into sugar. Your body would prefer not to destroy itself in this way, so it will make you hungry and make you crave sugar. This makes you more and more leptin resistant. And instead of burning off excess fat, you make more of it, and you store more of it away. Over time you end up turning your muscle and bone into sugar and fat, and you get fatter, weaker, frailer, and flabbier. And you will always be hungry.[1]

Body fat cannot be burned so long as insulin remains in the bloodstream.

Body fat cannot be metabolized when insulin is present in the bloodstream.

This is because the hormone *glucagon* is needed to mobilize the burning of stored body fat, and glucagon can't operate when insulin is present. If you eat enough carbs to secrete insulin, glucagon can't do its fat burning, so you burn sugar.

What drives us to store rather than burn fat is the dominance of insulin over glucagon. Nutritionist Ann Louise Gittleman explains the process.

> High insulin levels promote fat storage and the inability to access stored fat because they activate the enzyme adipose tissue lipoprotein-lipase (AT-LPL). This enzyme acts like a master key to fat storage. Individuals who consistently eat foods that generate a high-insulin response, therefore, are promoting fat storage.[2]

Dr. Barry Sears, author of numerous Zone Diet books, says that people who are genetically sensitive to insulin, whose insulin secretion is stimulated on diets high in carbs, or too high in protein, fall into a "fat trap." Insulin causes fat storage, and it is harder in these people to access that stored fat for energy. If they use the common prescription of eating less and exercising more to lose weight, he claims that much of the weight loss comes from muscles, not just stored fat.[3]

Dr. Diana Schwarzbein, MD, also addresses the burning of muscle when you are running on carbs instead of fat for fuel.

A low-fat, high-carbohydrate diet burns muscle mass, especially if you are exercising.[4]

On the other hand, Hereward Carrington, author of books on fasting, such as *Fasting for Health and Long Life,* explained that muscle *fibers* are not lost: the body, in its wisdom, uses the fat, toxins, and junk proteins marbled within muscles and other tissues as fuel. Muscle mass shrinks, but the actual muscle fibers are preserved. In such a case, a person will have less bulk but retain his strength.

In the last few decades, we have witnessed an obesity epidemic. Genes cannot evolve that fast. What *has* changed is diet.[*] Our diets are now richer in carbs and in omega-6 fats from using vegetable and seed oils due to the fear of saturated fats and cholesterol (as well from eating meat from animals that were fattened on grain).

Though you can't change your genes, you can keep those genes which would cause you to get fat "switched off" with a diet low in carbohydrates and vegetable oils. You can also fight fat with fish or krill oil, which is very rich in omega-3 fats.

If you're relying on carbohydrates as your primary source of fuel, you need to eat more often. As soon as the fuel from the food you just ate runs out, you will crave more carbs or stimulants. This is why so many diets tell you to eat numerous snacks throughout the day, so you will keep up your blood sugar and not overeat later.

When you are burning fat, frequent eating is not necessary because you have a steady source of fuel, *your body's fat*! You might get a quick burst of energy from eating carbs. That is what they are great for — a turbocharger for running from the ti-

ger. Yet most of us don't need that sudden burst of energy unless we are constantly exercising, which allows us to safely indulge in more carbs.

For sustainable, long-term energy, burning fat is the way to go. Nature never intended for us to rely heavily on burning sugar for fuel and to be hungry throughout the day. It would have been very impractical in the wild or when food was scarce. Our hunter-gatherer ancestors never would have survived if they had depended on frequent meals; they sometimes went days without eating.

The average body stores about only 2,000 calories of glycogen (stored sugar) in the liver and muscles, and yet it can store hundreds of pounds of fat. If the body were meant to run on sugar, don't you think it would be the other way around?

Longevity through Burning Fat Instead of Sugar

Dr. Rosedale reviewed many calorie restriction experiments on animals and found some common biomarkers that nearly all the longest-lived animals had. These traits were low fasting leptin levels, low fasting insulin levels, reduction in fasting glucose, low body temperature, low percentage of body fat, reduced thyroid hormone levels, and low triglycerides. These were found in animals fed 30 to 40 percent fewer calories (with high nutrient density) than they would normally eat.

When Rosedale put his patients on his diet of low carbs, adequate protein, and what some would consider high fat (50 to 60 percent), his patients, even the sickest ones, obtained the same longevity profile after two weeks, *without restricting calories* and *without constant hunger.*

A low-carb, or at least low-glycemic, diet (something carb types can do too) is one of the best things you can do to ensure a long, healthful life. In a 1992 Italian study, researchers examined people who were at least 100 and mentally and physically fit to see what biomarkers they had in common. They found three factors these centenarians shared: low triglycerides, high HDL cholesterol, and *a low blood level of fasting insulin.*

Centenarians generally present a low concentration of insulin, with a mean insulin level of 7.1 ± 4.0 (normal values [n.v.] 3–35 IU/ml); and a normal lipid-

---

[*]Toxins in our external and internal environments have increased in the past few decades. They can increase our fat stores since the body tends to protect its organs from toxins by storing those toxins in fat cells. Some of the most "fattening" toxins include pharmaceutical drugs and pesticides.

ic equilibrium, with a cholesterol value of 182.3 ± 34.9 mg/dl (n.v. 120–200) and triglyceride level of 99.8 ± 33.7 mg/dl (n.v. 30–190) and intermediate values of HDL 46.7 ± 11.8.[5]

Dr. Ron Rosedale explains that longevity is not natural because it is not needed to continue the species. However, we can trick nature into thinking we are starving in the midst of some sort of famine by going on a calorie-restricted diet, which will turn on our longevity genes, those genes that enable scientists to predict one's ability to live a long life.

These genes slow the aging process so that your body can survive the "famine" and be able to reproduce when it's over. Instead of spending what little energy you have available on making babies, the body now directs its energy toward body maintenance and repair.

Low-glycemic, fat-burning diets are clearly the healthful norm.

Leptin is the master hormone that controls all the other biomarkers of the longevity profile. It is produced by, and stored in, white fat tissues. High levels of the hormone leptin are mammals' evolutionary signal that they have enough food to reproduce. Thus there is no need to turn on the longevity genes that instruct the body to focus on maintenance and repair activity to keep you around after the famine.

Just as excessively high insulin levels lead to insulin resistance, excessively high leptin levels in the fat tissues lead to leptin resistance. This keeps you from having the longevity profile that expands your health and extends your life.

Ketosis

Ketosis is a term that describes what happens when the body switches from burning sugar to burning fat as its main fuel source.[6] There is an increase in *ketone bodies*, biochemical by-products of fat metabolism when the body uses fat as an energy source.

Ketosis is often confused with diabetic *ketoacidosis*, a life-threatening condition, as Wikipedia explains.

Ketoacidosis is a pathological metabolic state marked by extreme and uncontrolled ketosis. Normal ketosis, by contrast, is a functional aspect of fat-based energy metabolism, induced by prolonged fasting or a low-carbohydrate diet. In ketoacidosis, the body fails to adequately regulate ketone production causing such a severe accumulation of keto acids that the pH of the blood is substantially decreased. In extreme cases ketoacidosis can be fatal.[7]

Some in the alternative health movement suspect that these terms have been deliberately confused to the public in order to discredit fasting, which enables the body to heal itself of almost anything without drugs.

People confusing these two terms therefore think ketosis is unsafe. Nothing could be further from the truth. When you switch to burning fat, your brain becomes sharper, your energy soars and stabilizes regardless of whether you eat regularly or not, your hunger diminishes, and your blood sugar stabilizes.

☞ Conventional wisdom holds that pregnant women, people with uncontrolled Type 1 diabetes, and people with kidney disease should all avoid ketosis. This is because the cooked protein they consume contains toxic by-products.

Being in a ketotic state doesn't mean you will lose weight: it just means you are eating a diet low in carbs. You could eat 10,000 calories of fat and actually gain weight in ketosis. Likewise, you can lose weight without being in ketosis if you are eating fewer calories than you use. Staying in ketosis simply assures that the weight lost will come from fat stores.

It can be argued that stored body fat was partly what we evolved to use for fuel, since food was rarely as plentiful as it is today. If food had been plentiful, how could we have thrived under the devastating effects of the high insulin levels that come from overeating? We are clearly not meant to have high levels of insulin, which indicates that a low-glycemic, fat-burning diet is the healthful norm. Think about it.

During the Ice Age prior to the arrival of agriculture, people often spent long winters with few if any plants, so they had to eat meat. People may have had to go days without successfully hunting an animal to eat. Ketosis would have enabled them to stay calm, not experience hunger cravings with the associated anxiety, and to burn their fat stores efficiently.

A ketogenic diet improves childhood epilepsy, Alzheimer's, Parkinson's, and (unless calories are high) obesity.[8] It improves the biomarkers insulin, triglycerides, HDL, and LDL.[9] Other conditions that possibly benefit from ketosis include migraine headaches, diabetes, adult epilepsy, hyperactivity, behavior disorders, leukemia, brain tumors, and other cancers.[10]

Ketosis is used in many popular weight-loss diets, most notably the popular Atkins and South Beach diets. Someone who is overweight and insulin resistant might have to go very low carb for a week or so to switch gears. We're talking below 20 to 40 grams in one day, just enough for some greens and nonstarchy vegetables.

A person also ends up burning 100 to 400 more calories on these diets, but that is generally not thought to be the reason for the weight loss. The reason you lose weight is that the body is burning much more of its fat stores, provided you don't eat an excess of protein and fat calories. There are many studies that prove this.

State-of-the-art body composition technology was used in one study. People put on a fast lost an average of 21 pounds, but most was lean body tissue; only 7.5 pounds was from body fat. But on a ketogenic, very low-carb diet — 1000 calories and only 10 grams of carbs — an average of 14.5 pounds was lost, and 14 of those were from fat! So fat stores were burned at twice the rate, muscles were spared, and the person got to eat.[11]

A ketogenic diet is great for protein-sparing, fat-burning weight loss, but you won't lose weight on it or any diet unless you eat fewer calories than what you burn. Since ketosis is a natural appetite suppressant, you can lower your calories rather painlessly once you're in it. Much like when you are fasting, you can go to a party or even prepare a buffet and not be tempted to indulge.

One of the best-known authorities on ketogenic diet, Lyle McDonald, explains, "Ketosis is the end result of a shift in the insulin/glucagon ratio and indicates an overall shift from a glucose- (sugar-) based metabolism to a fat-based metabolism."[12]

The amazing thing about ketosis is you don't have to eat a lot of protein to get there — that was just something people often did on the Atkins Diet, and it is dangerous. You just have to go very low carb or even do a water-only fast. You can eat protein adequate for most people, 10 to 30 percent of calories. In fact, more than 100 grams of protein is believed by some scientists to be toxic for most people.[13]

Just get the rest of your calories from quality fats. If you don't need to lose weight but want the benefits of ketosis, that would mean eating as much as 50 to 80 percent of your maintenance calories in quality fat: fat in clean meat from animals fed species-appropriate diets, avocados, olives, low-carb seeds and nuts, coconuts, coconut butter or oil, and oils (hemp, olive, avocado, walnut, flax) for your green salads.

It is not advised to stay on a ketogenic diet for a long time unless you need to for health reasons, since your body thrives better with more plant food than just plant fats. You can get some beneficial minerals and antioxidants on a ketogenic diet if your carbs consist of nutrient-rich produce, such as berries and sea vegetables. Also, some toxic by-products may result from ketosis.[14] This is especially true with cooked protein.

Other considerations: You need to maintain a good potassium and sodium balance, so you need to eat plenty of greens for potassium and a little seaweed such as kelp for both potassium and trace minerals. I also boil some potatoes and drink only the broth.

You may also find that it takes two to four weeks for you to get the same level of physical performance that you had before.[15] After that, you should find that you have more energy than ever.

> *On a ketogenic diet, you may find that it takes two to four weeks to achieve the same level of physical performance as before.*

You're no longer diverting fuel into your fat tissue, where you can't use it, and so you literally have more energy to burn.[16]

Your Brain on Ketones Instead of Glucose

On a very low-carb ketogenic diet, you have nearly the same blood concentration of ketones as when fasting for one week.[17] Fasting is known to make the brain very clear and sharp.

Gary Taubes writes this in his famous article "What If It's All Been a Big Fat Lie?" (*New York Times*, 2002).

> Rather than being poison, which is how the press often refers to ketones, they make the body run more efficiently and provide a backup fuel source for the brain. [Ketosis expert] Veech calls ketones "magic" and has shown that both the heart and brain run 25 percent more efficiently on ketones than on blood sugar.

National Institutes of Health researcher Dr. Richard Veech, MD, conducted many studies on ketones, finding that ketogenic diets have many therapeutic effects for the brain that could be used in treating Alzheimer's, Parkinson's, and epilepsy.[18]

Your mood improves in ketosis too, as Dr. Atkins noted.

> It's as delightful as sex and sunshine, and it has fewer drawbacks than either of them![19]

One study found that in ketosis there is an enhanced synthesis of *glutamine* and *gamma-aminobutyric acid* (GABA).[20] Glutamine is an amino acid that suppresses appetite, helps build and maintain muscle, enhances the ability to burn fat, and enhances growth hormone release. GABA is a neurotransmitter that reduces stress and anxiety.

The ketogenic diet may also have mood stabilizing benefits in the brains of depressed or manic individuals, or those with bipolar disorder.[21]

I wrote most of this book either in ketosis or hovering nearby on a very low-carb diet. I was amazed at how easy it was to remain focused for hours at a time. I often recalled which page number things were on. Though I have the habit of reading up to a dozen books at a time, I could remember which book contained a certain piece of information. Every day I awoke with joy and anticipation for learning, reading, and writing.

Chapter 14

Carbs and Fats Don't Mix

Sugar + Fat = High Blood Sugar   —Dr. Douglas N. Graham, *The 80/10/10 Diet*

Most people are ignorant about the fact that carbs don't assimilate well with fats in the bloodstream. This combo is nearly unavoidable in the usual modern diet: pizza, spaghetti, sandwiches, lasagna, doughnuts, cookies, cakes, bread with butter, etc. It is also a popular combination in raw food desserts: sweets with nuts. And this is why we are fat and tired. This is why we have high blood insulin levels leading to fatigue, overweight, diabetes, and all the other diseases of civilization, as nutritionist Robert Crayhon calls out.

Large amounts of fats and carbohydrates should not be eaten together. This was never done by Stone Age man. Diets that have high amounts of fat, as in the case with the traditional Eskimo diet, are also low in carbohydrates, while the diets of equatorial peoples that are higher in carbohydrates are usually lower in fats.[1]

He warns that disease results because the combination of high-carbohydrate and high-fat intake is new to mankind. Food as it comes from nature is typically not found in this combination. High-fat diets don't cause disease unless they are combined with a high intake of carbohydrates.

Drs. Michael and Mary Eades explain that if you add fat to your diet, your cholesterol may increase; but if you eat the fat *without carbs*, it *won't*. They also explain that diet affects only 20 percent of your total cholesterol. If insulin levels are reduced, the cells do not convert the dietary fat to cholesterol, no matter how much fat is eaten.[2]

Paleo diet author Robb Wolf gets more specific in blaming *saturated* fats.

A high intake of saturated fats, in conjunction with a high intake of dietary carbohydrate, is a hell of a combo for an early grave.[3]

Dr. Doug Graham also explains the damage resulting from combining fats with sugars in his book *The 80/10/10 Diet*. When we eat a high-fat diet, which he defines as being over 10 to 12 percent of our calories, the fat lingers in the bloodstream. It coats the sugars and slows down their assimilation by interfering with insulin's ability to latch onto them.

The resulting accumulation of sugar causes several things to happen. The pancreas sends more insulin to attach to the sugar, which also gets coated by fat. The microbe *Candida albicans*, beneficial at normal levels by consuming excess sugars and helping our bodies detox mercury from fish, air pollution, and dental fillings, then proliferates to unhealthful levels. The symptoms of candida overgrowth include fatigue, brain fog, irritability, itching, obsessive thinking, craving of sweets, headaches, skin problems, digestive problems, vaginal yeast infections, ADD, and more.

Furthermore, the receptor sites where insulin would leave the blood get clogged up with fat too, so that as more sugar accumulates, still more insulin is secreted, causing *Syndrome X*, insulin resistance syndrome. The increase of fat in the bloodstream reduces the oxygen-carrying capacity of the red blood cells. The resulting oxygen deficit from too much fat in the blood causes fatigue, as do the insulin and candida. For raw fooders like Dr. Doug Graham, the solution is to eat a very low-fat diet in which the fats must be eaten separately from all the carbs in fruit and starchy vegetables.

Insulin receptor sites get clogged up with fat. Still more insulin is secreted as more sugar accumulates in the blood, resulting in insulin resistance.

The problem with eating a diet low in fat is that when you lower the fat, you have to replace it with something else. It is not usually replaced with protein, because in whole foods that protein usually comes with more fat, in addition to the fact that overeating protein is also not healthful. So a low-fat diet almost always ends up being high in carbs, which is not healthful unless you are metabolically a carb type.

Eating carbs raw is not nearly as bad as eating a high-carb cooked diet since the carbs are not absorbed as quickly. It is nonetheless not ideal unless you are a carb type.[*]

> *Fruits picked unripe do eventually ripen after a fashion but never really achieve their full nutrient potential.*

A high-carb raw diet often contains a great deal of fruits, which are nowadays hybridized to be too sugary for their mineral content. One bit of evidence of this is that so many people eating high-fruit diets get cavities or outright lose their teeth! I have met at least a dozen people who experienced these tooth problems. In addition, commercial fruit is nearly always picked unripe so that it can be transported long distances without bursting or spoiling en route. It therefore contains less mineral content and is less alkaline. These minerals also aid in properly metabolizing the sugar.

Fruit picked before ripening will not have time to absorb all the minerals it should have that would contribute to its alkalinity. Unripe fruit has a high acid content that warns us against eating it in that condition. While most fruits picked unripe do eventually ripen after a fashion, they never acquire the mineral content and concentration they should have.

Add to that the sorry state of our depleted soils, extensive hybridization, and the fact that temperate fruits are less nutritious to begin with than tropical fruits, and a real problem exists for would-be fruitarians.

Besides all that, fruit sugar remains problematical, according to nutritionist Nora Gedgaudas.

There is no such thing as a "safe" low level of glucose. Glucose and other sugars, such as fructose, always glycate us [load us with crosslinked sugars and proteins] and attract free radical activity, to some on-going degree, no matter what.[4]

She explains that even though fructose doesn't have much impact on insulin, it is extremely glycating and does immeasurable damage to the arteries and tissues. She claims it is *20 to 30 times* more glycating than glucose! One study puts it at "only" 7 to 10 times as much.[5]

Glycation leads to premature aging and brain degeneration. It leads to wrinkling of the skin, cataracts, age spots, and even failure of major organs, such as the kidneys and heart.[6]

Another problem with a low-fat diet is that 10 to 12 percent of its calories in dietary fat is simply not enough fat for most people. Unlike carbs, dietary fat is essential. Carbs play a very minimal role in any sort of structural component of the body. Less than 2 percent of our body structure is composed of carbohydrate, and all of this can be manufactured without dietary carbs.[7]

Drs. Michael and Mary Eades claim that most of the problems that come with dieting simply result from a too-low fat content. These include dry skin, dull hair, hair loss, brittle nails, gallstones, menstrual irregularities, and a weak immune system that leads to colds or infections.[8]

Why We Need Fat

Meta analysis of worldwide studies implicates high fat consumption in breast cancer, but the association is very small or even nonexistent in Western populations.[9] It has been found that reducing *body* fat is more important than reducing *dietary* fat.[10]

Ann Louise Gittleman used to work at Pritikin's center where people ate a mere 5 to 10 percent of their calories as fat. She saw people develop all sorts of health problems after being on the diet a-while, including low energy, difficulty concentrating, depression, weight gain, and mineral deficiencies. People were hungry all the time.

Those who had been on the diet two years developed vertical ridges on the fingernails, a symptom of nutritional deficiency. "Pritikin said fat was the problem," she wrote. "I was seeing fat as the solution."[11]

Gittleman discovered that a main problem with fat was that people were overeating omega-6s rela-

---

[*]See chapter 10.

tive to omega-3s. Also, the fats were not eaten in their natural state. They were heated, hydrogenated, oxidized, and homogenized, which created all sorts of health concerns.

Dietary fat is needed for all kinds of reasons. Some fatty acids are essential nutrients, meaning that they can't be produced in the body from other compounds, and need to be consumed at least in small amounts. Fully 60 percent of brain tissue is composed of fat. Fat is used to stabilize the nervous system, which is why low-fat diets are associated with depression.

Further, low levels of blood fat (cholesterol) have been found to correlate with violence, suicide, homicide, and low self-control.[12]

Fat is used for building, rebuilding, and maintaining cellular membranes and nerve tissue. Fat is used to make hormones and neurotransmitters. Fat is needed to support the immune and lymphatic systems. Fat is used to create pro- and anti-inflammatory compounds.

Fat feeds the heart, other muscles, and the brain. Fat supports the proper utilization of proteins. Fat stores vitamins A, D, E, and K, nutrients we get from foods that contain fat.

Aajonus Vonderplanitz consumes raw fats liberally, especially from animal products.

Raw fats, especially unsalted raw butter, are the primary substances that dissolve and bind with toxicity, protect our cells, reverse the greatest number and most severe cases of diseases, and deliver the greatest strength and energy. In an ideal, healthy world, we would not need such an abundance of fat. In our civilized, polluted, disease-ridden world, we need an abundance of fat.[13]

When you go low carb, you have to replace the reduced carbs with another macronutrient, either protein or fat. Nutritionists agree that we shouldn't overeat protein but rather ingest *adequate* protein, 15 to 25 percent of one's calories, depending on the individual and his activity level. Overconsumption of protein stimulates insulin production and also increases acidity since protein is acidic. According to Dr. Rosedale, fat has no effect on insulin secretion whatsoever.

Fats from meat and cheese are acidic, while plant fats are neutral or alkaline. Cream and raw or lightly cooked egg yolks are neutral.[14]

We can control our leptin levels if we eat an abundance of good fats (not hydrogenated oils or trans fats) and if we eat them in the absence of carbohydrates.[15]

In Japan where low-fat diets were traditional, the official Japanese nutritional recommendations included increased consumption of fat and protein and decreased consumption of sodium to prevent strokes. Studies showed that these three factors would decrease the risk of stroke. Stroke rates went down when this advice was heeded.[16]

Increased saturated fats decreased strokes in Japan, but this was because the Japanese tend to have hemorrhagic strokes due to their high intake of salted fish. Western populations suffer primarily from ischemic strokes, which are caused by ingesting excessive amounts of saturated fats.

☞ Balance and moderation are the keys: don't overdo or underdo saturated fats or eat salted foods to avoid both kinds of strokes.

Nutritional anthropologist H. Leon Abrams, Jr., has came to these conclusions.

Cross-cultural data clearly demonstrate that all human cultures include some types of animal proteins and animal fats in their diets and esteem them highly. Consumption of these foods is determined, or limited, by ecological and economic factors. No exclusively vegetarian society has ever been discovered. ... The preference for and use of animal protein and fat appears to have been a dominant human dietary trait from the earliest times. ... Animal protein and animal fat, as preferred foods, are universally present in human diets.[17]

Doesn't Fat Make You Fat?

That eating fat makes you fat was a misconception popularized by the low-fat diets. The logic is that fat contains 9 calories per gram, whereas carbs contain only 4 calories per gram. Fats are thus more "fattening" because they are calorically denser. The thinking behind this is that hunger is appeased more with a high volume of food in the stomach. *But fat stays in the stomach much longer, keeping hunger at bay.*

However, some experts, such as diabetes specialist Richard Bernstein, MD, think that fat in the absence of sugars is actually only about 5 calories per gram after you factor in the energy used to metabolize fat versus carbs. This is true only when one is in (or perhaps near) ketosis.

Recent evidence has shown that while fat may gross 9 calories per gram, the net available for metabolism is closer to something like 5 calories a gram.[18]

Moreover, fat has no effect at all on insulin release, while carbohydrates have a strong effect! Most fruits (with the notable exceptions of olives, avocados, and durians) contain nearly zero fat. Eaten alone, they have an effect on insulin secretion, but the effect goes away quickly. Vegetables (except brassicas) are also very low in fat.

Drs. Mary and Michael Eades reviewed some experiments that varied the macronutrient percentages to see the effects on insulin levels. The diets that impacted insulin the least were those with substantial protein and fat, those with protein only, and those with high protein and low carbs. The diets that impacted insulin the most were those with carbs only, those with carbs and fats, and *worst of all* those with high carbs and low protein.[19]

> *"The reason nutritionists like to think (and like to tell us) that carbohydrates are somehow the preferred fuel for the body, which is simply wrong, is that your cells will burn carbohydrates before they'll burn fat. They do so because that's how the body keeps blood sugar in check after a meal."*
>
> *—Gary Taubes, Why We Get Fat*

Carbs versus Fat: Which Is More Important?

Let's look at the facts in this fat vs. carb controversy, probably one of the biggest controversies in nutrition!

How much carbohydrate does your body need? Zero. The brain needs glucose, but it can produce it without dietary carbs. Shocking as it might seem, *your body can be at peak health with zero carbs.* We know this because the Eskimos would go sometimes 6 months on zero-carb diets yet experience perfect health. They also ate their animals raw.

As for fats, your body needs a variety of dietary fats. It needs the essential omega-3 and omega-6 fatty acids that it cannot produce. Your body needs fat for energy production in the mitochondria, hormone production, skin moisturizing, brain maintenance, happiness, mental stability, and good memory.

Dr. Bowden explains how the liver transforms excess sugar into triglycerides, a type of fat. He then asks which is worse, sugar or fat? He answers. *Sugar is far more damaging to the body than fat.* In a very real sense, what the liver is doing is detoxifying sugar into triglycerides.[20]

Dr. Rosedale theorizes that the body — unless on a low-carb diet — probably burns sugar first *as a defense mechanism* to protect us from the potentially lethal effects of sugar and the ensuing insulin production.

Dr. Rosedale further claims that fats have no impact on stimulating insulin release, yet studies cited in the textbook *Food and Western Disease* indicate otherwise. Nonetheless, the author of that textbook rationalizes this.

The lack of standardization with respect to other dietary factors (e.g., grains and milk proteins) make it premature to state that a high-fat diet is sufficient to cause insulin resistance.[21]

In other words, it may have been the grains or carbs used in combination with the fat that stimulated the insulin.

I place my bet on fats as the better fuel. How many carbs do we need? Zero, none. Your body will die from lack of fats, but studies show we can live without carbs. It is not ideal, of course, but possible. Your body would certainly benefit from the fiber, alkaline minerals, and antioxidants by including an abundance of nonstarchy plant food.

Interestingly, uric acid, a by-product of metabolizing meat, is also a potent antioxidant. However, high blood levels of uric acid are toxic to the kidneys. Raw meat has more than sufficient ammonia (a base) to neutralize the acid, according to Dr. Rosedale, which explains why Eskimos didn't die of uric acid poisoning.

The brain requires a minimum of 120 grams of glucose a day in order to function, but it has no problem making it from certain amino acids found in protein and from the glycerol backbone of triglycerides.[22]

Dr. Eric C. Westman of the Department of Medicine at Duke University Medical Center elaborates.

> Although there is certainly no evidence from which to conclude that extreme restriction of dietary carbohydrate is harmless, I was surprised to find that there is similarly little evidence to conclude that extreme restriction of carbohydrate is harmful. In fact, the consequential breakdown of fat as a result of carbohydrate restriction may be beneficial in the treatment of obesity. Perhaps it is time to carefully examine the issue of whether carbohydrate is an essential component of human nutrition.[23]

We know of several traditional cultures that lived on very low (or even zero) carb diets, yet exhibited perfect health. These include the Masai of Africa, the Eskimos, the Plains Indians, and the Lapps.

One may think this ability is related to genetics, but Vilhjalmur Stefansson, a European explorer, went to live with the Eskimos and thrived on their diet: He was found to be very healthy after eating this way, according to the medical standards of the day.[24]

The Eskimo diet was sometimes 70 percent animal fat. Stefansson and Karsten Anderson participated in a study done at the Russell Sage Institute of Pathology at Bellevue Hospital, an affiliate of the Medical College of Cornell University. For a whole year, they ate *only raw meat* in the ratio of two pounds of fresh lean meat to one-half pound of fat each day, and were found to be in good health at the end of the experiment.[25] But they experienced blood pressure levels that would be considered much too high by modern standards, so their health was likely not perfect on this diet.

On the other hand, metabolizing protein to make energy produces toxic by-products. Since most people consume proteins and fats in cooked form, these deranged nutrients contribute an additional toxic burden. Simple carbs like fruit and raw fat are the only "smokeless" fuels.[26]

Carbs are also needed to get more tryptophan into the brain. This amino acid is used to produce serotonin, the feel-good neurotransmitter. Because tryptophan competes with other amino acids to get into the brain, little of it gets in. When carbohydrate is eaten, insulin is released, carrying tryptophan into the brain that results in a rise in serotonin levels. This explains why depressed people crave carbs.[27]

Chapter 15

A Closer Look at Plants as Protein Sources

Those who think they have no time for healthy eating will sooner or later have to find time for illness.

—Edward Stanley, 18th century British prime minister

When they first hear about the raw vegan diet, people's first question is nearly always, "But how do you get enough protein?" The standard answer is nuts, seeds, greens, and vegetables. There is even a scant amount of protein in fruit.

A study allegedly proved that if you eat the food raw, up to twice as much of the protein is absorbed. Don't forget, the meat industries have also brainwashed us into thinking that we need about twice as much protein as we really do.

For me, the raw vegan diet was an excuse to enter Carbohydrate Heaven! I just threw protein out of my consciousness. No more need to be concerned, I willingly gave up bland meat and fattening beans and grains (save the occasional popcorn cheat).

Now I could focus on what I truly loved — carbs — which I had restricted on previous low-carb diets like the Zone. I could also indulge in good, healthy fats like avocados, nuts, and olives that are off-limits on low-calorie diets.

So here is how I calculated my protein requirements: If the standard way of thinking is that I need 100 grams of protein a day, I should reduce that to about 50 because we don't need as much protein as they say. Then, I thought, if I eat it raw, I can cut that in half again and eat 25 because a study in Germany at the Max Planck Institute demonstrated that raw protein is absorbed twice as well.[1]

Then there's this from another study.

Cooking and other processing methods together can account for a 20–50 percent loss of many essential amino acids.[2]

To tell you the truth, I never bothered to count my protein grams. I just ate until satisfied, but since I was on a low-protein diet, it took a lot to satisfy me, which caused weight gain!

Though 25 grams seems ridiculously low, I realize now in retrospect that often it was all I got on my raw vegan diet. I am going to challenge the concept that 25 grams of usable protein is enough

for most people. My flabby thighs, thick and firm just a few years before, bore proof that this wasn't enough for me. Sure, it was enough that my nails grew. Sure, it was enough that I didn't have the signs and symptoms of protein deficiency that Dr. Vetrano warns about in my book *The Live Food Factor*. The enamel was not being dissolved off my teeth; I was not listless, with slow healing of wounds.

However, I was experiencing hair loss despite taking MSM supplements regularly, the vegan equivalent for gelatin. My hair length would not grow much until I later added a daily tablespoon of unflavored powdered gelatin to my diet. (This also did wonders for my knee cartilage.) But was my protein intake enough for peak insulin sensitivity? Was it enough to keep me from losing muscle mass? Apparently not.

Even the authors of *The CR Way*, who tout the benefits of a low-protein diet, claim you need 0.36 grams per pound of your ideal weight. Since my ideal weight is 120, I need 43 grams a day by that standard.

But that is only one way of calculating protein needs. Another way to calculate your protein needs is to get a certain percentage of your calories from protein, based on your metabolic type. Being a mixed type on some charts tells me I need 20 to 25 percent of my calories from protein.

Some diet books tell me I need to get as high as 100 to 120 grams of protein. Since I eat at least half my protein raw — even animal foods — let's say I can reduce this to 50 grams. This coincides with the amount that Nora Gedgaudas suggests, which is 45 to 55 grams per day for most adults.[3]

Bear in mind that 50 grams is conservative. On days that I am exercising to build muscle, which is several days of the week, I may need more, perhaps 60 grams or even more. In fact, if you go by the caloric ratios, 50 grams is a mere 12.5 percent protein for my diet of 1600 calories, my daily allotment for weight maintenance.

Protein has 4 calories per gram. Multiply 4 calories per gram by 50 grams to get 200 calories. Thus 200 calories is only 12.5 percent of 1600 calories. This may work if I am a carb type, but a mixed type needs about double that.[*] If I need 20 percent of my calories to be from protein, as many charts suggest, then I would need about 75 grams a day.

> *The big problem with most of the less-expensive seeds is that they are very high in omega-6 fatty acids.*

So 12.5 percent is a *bare minimum* of protein for most people. As you will see, it is difficult to get 12.5 percent on a vegan diet, especially a raw one that doesn't include legumes. If you need more, it can be nearly impossible to get 25 percent of your calories in protein on a healthful plant-only diet, as we shall see.

Now let's take a look at the pros and cons of some plant sources for protein. It is hard to get enough protein on a raw vegan diet without contributing substantially to the carb and caloric load, as well as creating imbalances in the omega-3 and omega-6 fatty acids. On a cooked vegan diet, soy is the usual staple, but as we will see in this chapter, it's toxic stuff. I even heard raw vegan David Wolfe say in a lecture that "you'd be better off eating a steak than soy."

With most plant food, you will also get antinutrients, poisons that evolved to keep predators away. Grains, nuts, legumes, and seeds all have them. In fact, one type of toxin is called a *protease inhibitor*, a substance that inhibits protein digestion by interfering with intestinal *proteases*, enzymes that break proteins down into their amino acid con-

stituents. Some of the foods with these toxins include soybeans, legumes, and millet.

Cyanogenic glycosides are produced by over 2,500 plant species, including common foods like cassava, bamboo shoots, flaxseeds, sweet potatoes, lima beans, and millet. These chemicals increase the need for iodine to such an extent that goiters may arise.[4] This can be prevented by adding some seaweed to the diet, kelp especially.

Even vegetables like turnips, cabbage, cauliflower, rapeseed (from which canola oil is made), onion, garlic, and mustard contain a variety of *goitrogens*, substances which increase the need for iodine and may cause enlargement of the thyroid gland despite adequate intake of iodine.[5]

Pyrrolizidine alkaloids, found in over 6,000 plant species, are thought to cause cirrhosis of the liver and liver cancer.[6]

Phytic acid and lectins, contained in grains, legumes, and other plant foods, bind minerals. Phytates contribute to osteoporosis by preventing absorption of minerals, such as calcium, iron, and zinc. *Even domestic, grain-fed pigs now get osteoporosis when breastfeeding.*[7] There is no evidence that humans, not even vegetarians, have adapted to phytates![8]

Furthermore, starch-based vegetarian diets promote the secretion of insulin. As mentioned previously in this book, a high serum insulin level is the number one indicator of accelerated aging.

Now let's take a closer look at plant sources of protein.

Nuts

To get 50 grams of protein from nuts, let's see how many nuts I would have to eat. Since nuts are commonly around 80 percent fat, that leaves very little actual protein in them. In all cases when I refer to nuts in this section, I mean unshelled.

Almonds are one of the higher-protein nuts, having about 6 grams per ounce. One ounce has 160 calories, including 14 grams of fat. So to get 48 of my 50 grams of protein, I would have to eat about 8 ounces by weight of almonds, making it 1,280 calories and 112 grams of fat.[9] To give you a visual picture, one cup has 822 calories but only 30 grams of protein.

---

[*]Wolcott and Fahey, *Metabolic Typing Diet*, say a protein-type individual needs about 40 percent of calories from protein. For mixed types, it is 30 percent; for carb types, it is 25 percent. These percentages seem high to me, and I believe they could be lowered on a raw food diet in which protein is better assimilated.

The above calories might not seem like a lot of calories for a teenage boy, but for a grown, middle-aged woman, that is two-thirds of my daily allotment of calories! And don't forget, the growing teen will need much more protein than my 50 grams a day. Another problem is that I may get bored eating only almonds.

> *It is hard to get enough protein on a raw vegan diet without contributing substantially to the carb and caloric load, as well as creating imbalances in the omega-3 and omega-6 fatty acids.*

My favorites, cashews, have only 5 grams of protein per ounce (160 calories). To get 50 grams, I would have to eat 1,550 calories of them, and that would be it for the day's food. I could add some greens, and that's all.

Brazil nuts, which I need for their selenium, come with 4 only grams of protein to 190 calories. I would have to eat two whole cups (240 grams) to get 40 grams of protein, giving me 1900 calories.[10] I would gain weight on that without even meeting my modest protein requirements!

Walnuts are about the same in protein content as Brazil nuts, only 4 grams per ounce (183 calories), so 2 cups give me 36 grams of protein and 1,530 calories. I have 70 calories left to get 14 more grams of protein, something I could barely do even with low-fat chicken!

Macadamia nuts have *only 2 grams* per 200 calories. Using them as a main source of protein, I would gain weight without even meeting *half* my protein needs!

Another issue with nuts: Unless you are eating walnuts or macadamia nuts, you are getting way too much omega-6 fats for the omega-3s present. Omega-6 fats compete with omega-3 fats for transport into cells and can crowd out the omega-3s. This keeps the body from being able to make use of the latter. This is why the ratio is critical, regardless of whether the diet is high or low in fat.

This imbalance has been implicated in weight gain and inflammation, leading to all sorts of diseases. The ratio is much, much worse with most seeds than with nuts. We need the right proportion of omega-3s to counteract the inflammatory properties of other fats.[11]

By the way, nuts and seeds should be soaked overnight and rinsed to get rid of their digestive enzyme inhibitors and phytates.* Amanda Rose, PhD, author of the e-book *Phytic Acid White Paper*, explains the intricacies involved.

> Reducing phytic acid in nuts and seeds is tricky. Soaking is recommended by such writers as Sally Fallon in *Nourishing Traditions*. The problem is that a nut like an almond has a small surface area. It would be better to grind the nut at least slightly before soaking it. I realize that you then have nut pieces which are not always nearly as interesting as the whole nut.[12]

A larger surface area allows more water to get into the nut and eliminate phytates.

Cooking the food reduces the phytic acid to some degree, but more effective methods are soaking in an acid medium, lactic acid fermentation, and sprouting.

Seeds

Now let's take a look at seeds, which tend to be cheaper than nuts and also lower in fat. To get 46 grams of protein from sunflower seeds, I would need to eat one and a half cups (about 192 grams, or 6.4 ounces), which would amount to 1,227 calories. This would cost about 25 percent as much as nuts, since they are cheaper, but that would consume two-thirds of my daily allotment of calories. That doesn't leave much for other meals.

I am also getting 108 grams of fat and 42 grams of carbohydrates. On a positive note, since seeds tend to be 30 percent protein, while nuts are only 10 to 20 percent protein, I am getting more protein for less money.

But this is the big problem with most of the less-expensive seeds: they are very high in omega-6

---

*See *The Live Food Factor*, page 320, for more information on deactivating enzyme inhibitors.

fatty acids. With that cup and a half of sunflower seeds, I get only 156 mg of omega-3 fatty acids but a whopping 49,402 mg of omega-6s! Yet, the ratio should be no more than 4 omega-6s to 1 omega-3. The ideal is 2:1 or even 1:1, which is what our paleo-ancestors ate.[13] The high use of safflower oil, sunflower oil, corn oil, and other vegetable oils instead of animal fat is largely at the root of our obesity and disease epidemics.

Flaxseeds may be a solution, as they have 9,931 mg of omega-6s to 38,325 mg of omega-3s per cup. The problem with flaxseeds is that they are toxic in more than very moderate doses. With all of the glamour attributed to flax, imagine my surprise when researching for this book to discover that flax can be toxic!

Flaxseeds can be toxic if more than a few tablespoons are eaten in one day.

Flax contains factors antagonistic to the vitamin B group. Several studies demonstrate that flax contains toxins that have caused medical doctors to advise against its consumption for pregnant and lactating women.[14] Human consumption of flax has even been *banned* in France and *limited* in Germany, Switzerland, and Belgium!

Major toxins in flax are *cyanogenic glycosides*, also found in lima beans, sweet potatoes, yams, and bamboo shoots. They metabolize into yet another substance called *thiocyanate* (SCN⁻), which over time can suppress the thyroid's ability to take up sufficient iodine. This means overconsumption of flax, in addition to being toxic, can actually indirectly cause us to gain weight by suppressing the thyroid, which regulates the metabolism.

I always wondered why I felt so tired after eating a bunch of flaxseed crackers. I used to think it was the excess fat, but this never happened with other seeds or nuts.

Nutrition expert Ann Louise Gittleman advises taking no more than three or four tablespoons of flax per day. She claims that baking or toasting the seeds deactivates the toxic cyanogenic glycosides but preserves the beneficial omega-3s when heated less than 300° F.[15] However, some researchers found that the free form of *secoisolariciresinol diglucoside*, one of its antioxidants, remained stable even in baked goods.[16]

Some of these toxins can be removed by soaking the flaxseeds overnight. However, flax tends to gel, making it very hard to rinse out the toxins. *The water you use to rinse the seeds just gets absorbed into the seeds.*

Gittleman points out that flaxseed *oil* is free of cyanogenic glycosides, but most flax oils are not raw, even when labeled *cold pressed*. They are usually heated at 160° F. And oil, being pure fat, is useless as a source of protein.

So now let's go to chia seeds. Americans need to create a demand for chia seeds. They were used in North America for thousands of years during the Aztec reign. The Aztecs even demanded that the nations they defeated pay them chia seeds as one of their tributes. Chia was one of the four main components of the Aztec diet, the other three being corn, beans, and amaranth.

I can get 40 grams of protein if I eat 8 ounces of chia seeds. The 8 ounces will cost me 1,096 calories and give me 96 grams of carbs and 72 grams of fat. The problem is, I have used up *two-thirds* of my daily caloric allotment! But compared to other seeds, I am getting more protein for fewer calories.

For each ounce of chia seeds, I am also getting 1,620 omega-6s, but a great amount of omega-3s: 4,915. The only problem is that these chia seeds cost about 6 *times* as much as the sunflower and flaxseeds. Nonetheless, if you are a vegan who can afford it, make chia seeds a primary source of protein in your diet.

Hemp has the best plant protein by far. With hemp seeds, chia seeds, and only moderate amounts of nuts and other seeds, we could feed the planet more efficiently.

Now let's look at the highly acclaimed hemp seed.[17] With half a cup, about 80 grams, I can get 44 grams of protein, which includes all eight essential amino acids. The best part: It is only 640 calories, which leaves me a bit more room for a more balanced diet — about 900 to 1000 calories. I am also getting 40 grams of fat and 18 grams of carbs. Hemp is the best plant protein by far. No wonder it is so popular in the raw vegan world. The ratio of omega-6s to omega-3s is also close to perfect, being about 2:1. This makes it an ideal source of protein for raw vegans.

With hemp seeds, chia seeds, and only moderate amounts of nuts and other seeds, we could feed the planet more efficiently. People would need only a small amount of meat to supplement for protein and nutrients not found in the plant kingdom.[*]

In the US, hemp seeds cost about as much as chia seeds, which is roughly five to six times that of the other common seeds (sunflower, pumpkin, flax, sesame). This is largely because it has to be imported. Unfortunately, politics and financial interests prohibit the growing of hemp seed in the US; otherwise, it would be much more affordable for Americans.[18]

With all the imbalances I had of omega-6 to omega-3 as a raw vegan, as well as all the calories, no wonder I was gaining weight. No wonder my memory deteriorated, since I had a hard time getting sufficient omega-3s (in relation to omega-6s) for making DHA for my brain. Nuts and seeds also contribute a bit to your glycemic load since they contain substantial carbs, especially my favorite nuts, cashews.

Do you see now why most nuts and seeds are best left as protein *supplements*? Unless you are eating walnuts, hemp seeds, or chia seeds, you can be skewing your balance of omega-3s to omega-6s. Flaxseeds can be toxic if more than a few tablespoons are eaten in one day. Nuts and seeds are also high in fat, which makes them very high in calories. To get enough protein from them, they would have to make up about half or two-thirds of your caloric intake.

Paleolithic man is thought not to have depended too much on seeds for food. Unless they are ground, many seeds are not digestible and pass right through the body.

Many seeds were tasty to attract animals to eat them. Then the animals would defecate at a different location. This was a method of seed dispersal for the plants. It wasn't until agriculture that much grinding, cooking, and food processing took place. Stone Age tools for grinding seeds have not been found.

Greens

Greens are often touted as a great source of protein, but to use them as a main protein source requires eating a lot, and I mean so much that it would cost a lot of money, and you would spend a large part of the day chewing them unless you blend or juice them, something our forebears didn't have available to them. Also prepare to be bloated if you eat too much of them (unless juiced so the fiber is removed). Our digestive tract is not like a gorilla's.

Let's look at spinach. It has one gram of protein to a cup (56 grams, or about 2 ounces). *One gram!* You would have to eat about 50 cups to get your daily allotment of protein. One cup also has only one gram of carbs. The calories are low, just 7 calories per cup, so they are not a great source of energy. You would obtain only 350 calories from those 50 cups! This would be the most expensive way to get protein for those of us on a budget. Organic, free-range meat would be a bargain by comparison.

A cup of kale (68 grams, or a little over 2 ounces) contains 2 grams of protein and 33 calories. It is higher in carbs than spinach at 7 grams. You would need to eat 25 cups to get enough protein. Again, this is cost prohibitive in terms of both time and money.

With mustard greens, you get 3 grams of protein per cup (56 grams, or about 2 ounces), with 3 grams of carbs and 21 calories. Again, you would be spending a lot of money and time to get your protein.

Are you starting to get the picture? While greens are a nutritious way to supplement your main protein source, they are not a good stand-alone source of protein. They are low in calories with little fat, but used as a main protein source, they would be inefficient in terms of both cost and

---

[*]See chapter 17.

time (chewing or juicing). You would also likely get bloated, if you are like me, from all that cellulose. We are not herbivores.

Soy: Hazardous to Your Health

Another vegan source of protein is soy. It's a bean that deserves discussion in a section of its own. Soy has been sold to the public as a health food to expand the soy market beyond its industrial and animal feed uses. Soy is about 23 percent fat by calories. Soy oil has been used for paint and glue. Chemical companies like DuPont that traditionally made paint, but now make soy food products also, wanted to find a way to use the rest of the soy, so they decided to market it as a health food product. Soy protein left over was soon added to many foods in the form of soy protein isolate.

A soy industry spokesperson said in 1975, "The quickest way to gain product acceptability in the less affluent society is to have the product consumed on its own merit in a more affluent society," and thus began the hype that led hippies and vegetarians down the soy trail.

Now you can find soy milk, soy burgers, soy ice cream, soy margarine, soy oil, soy flour, and tofu. It is almost impossible to eat any processed foods that don't contain soy oil or soy protein concentrates, texturized soy protein, or soy protein isolate, which is also used to extend meat in most processed foods and fast food joints.

Traditionally, Asians used cooking, long-term sprouting, and fermentation to eliminate the antinutrients in soy, and even then they ate miso, tempeh and tofu sparingly as condiments. Current American ways of making processed soy foods add numerous dangerous toxins without eliminating the antinutrients.

These soy foods are manufactured using chemical solvents, acids, alkalis, and aluminum-containing food additives. They are created in aluminum vats and stored in aluminum containers at the factory. Aluminum has been implicated in Alzheimer's disease.

An excellent book that thoroughly lists and documents the dangers of soy is *The Whole Soy Story: The Dark Side of America's Favorite Health Food* by Dr. Kaayla T. Daniel, PhD, CCN, in which *hundreds* of studies on soy are cited. Daniel gives us an in-depth look at the main antinutrients and toxins in soy, which I will briefly summarize here.

- Soy contains goitrogens that damage the thyroid.[*]

- Lectins in soy cause red blood cells to clump together and may damage immune system reactions.

- The sugars in soy, oligosaccharides, cause bloating and flatulence.

- Oxalates prevent proper absorption of calcium and may lead to kidney stones and *vulvodynia*, pain in the vagina.

- Phytates block absorption of minerals like zinc, iron, and calcium. Soy can thus contribute to osteoporosis. In one study, pigs fed soy protein developed reduced bone density and strongly elevated parathyroid hormone levels, another marker for bone loss.[19]

- Isoflavones (plant estrogens) in soy behave like hormones and affect the reproductive system, sometimes leading to cancer in that system.

- These isoflavones also wreak havoc on the brain and lead to Alzheimer's in some people.

- Protease inhibitors, such as trypsin inhibitors, interfere with digestive enzymes and lead to gastric distress, poor digestion, gas, bloating, diarrhea, and an overworked pancreas.

- Saponins bind with bile and may damage the intestinal lining.

- The heating of soy during processing creates *heterocyclic amines* (HCAs), toxic carcinogenic byproducts also found in cooked meat. These can lead to liver, lung, and stomach tumors, as well as lymphoma and leukemia.

- Soy reduces fertility in both men and women. It also reduces the libido in men.

---

[*]In *The Butcher and the Vegetarian*, the author tells of being raised vegetarian and developing thyroid problems without connecting them to soy. She became a part-time meat eater while still consuming tofu. Not until she gave up the tofu for a raw food diet did her energy return!

- The chemical process that breaks down the soybean's protein structure into free amino acids also releases the excitotoxins *glutamate* (MSG) and *aspartate*.

- Soy is one of the top eight food allergens. In some cases soy consumption even causes *death*.

Now, does that sound like "nature's perfect protein"? Pass the fish, please!

From 1991 to 1993, Dr. Lon White, a neuroepidemiologist with the Pacific Health Institute of Honolulu, completed diagnostic testing on 3,734 men using magnetic resonance imaging (MRI) on 574 and autopsies on 290. He and his team also analyzed 502 cognitive tests on women. They discovered that men and women who ate tofu at least *twice per week* experienced accelerated brain aging and diminished cognitive ability. They were *twice* as likely to be diagnosed with Alzheimer's disease.[20]

In one testimonial from *The Whole Soy Story*, a woman was found developing early Alzheimer's from eating just the minute amounts of soy present in everyday bread.[21]

One British study comparing the effects of vegan to omnivorous diets found low TSH levels and goitrogenic effects among the vegans. Vegans are especially vulnerable to thyroid damage if they are deficient in zinc and B_{12}, common conditions for vegans.[22]

Soy is touted for lowering cholesterol, which we have seen is often not a good thing. *Sterols* (waxy insoluble substances) in soy remove the cholesterol the body needs to synthesize hormones, such as estrogen and testosterone.

These sterols resemble natural hormones enough to clog receptor sites that genuine hormones need. The result can be devastating: birth defects, infertility, and higher risks of breast cancer, reproductive disorders, behavioral problems, and atherosclerotic lesions.[23]

I am reminded of a 2000 TV docudrama that I saw, *The Linda McCartney Story*. Linda and her Beatle husband Sir Paul McCartney were animal rights activists involved with People for the Ethical Treatment of Animals (PETA). Linda had it *all*: a very rich father, her own career as a photographer, a musical career with Paul, beautiful children, and wealth beyond belief. She declared she was experiencing "heaven on earth."

Then she was diagnosed with breast cancer. She expressed concern in the film that the public would no longer consider that her vegetarian diet was better for health than eating an omnivorous one. She died at the age of only 56. Could it have been all the soy she was eating? She even had her own company making frozen soy entrees. (Of course, eating lots of cheese, another contributor to breast cancer, didn't help.)

One of the most frightening things about soy is its impact on children. A pregnant woman eating soy jeopardizes the health of her child. *Hypospadias*, a disorder in which the opening of the urethra appears on the underside of the penis shaft and may require surgery, has been increasing in recent years and now occurs in one out of 125 males. Vegetarian mothers were found to be *five times* more likely to give birth to a boy with this defect.[24]

For female fetuses, the result of the mother's soy ingestion could be early puberty and even estrogen-dependent diseases, such as breast, ovarian, or uterine cancers.[25] Ieuan Hughes, MD, chairman of the British Committee on Toxicity of Chemicals in Food, Consumer Products and the Environment, said this.

> There is a clear association between child deformities and vegetarianism, and this is a cause for concern.[26]

Most tragic has been the great experiment of feeding babies soy formula. Its high levels of manganese create brain damage associated with learning disabilities, attention deficit, behavioral disorder, and violent tendencies. The high levels of plant estrogens put the infant's developing endocrine, nervous, and immune systems in danger. Feeding a baby soy formula gives him or her the hormonal equivalent of *three to five birth control pills* a day!

Soy formula's insufficient amount of the amino acid methionine doesn't enable babies to grow fast enough. It is so bad for babies that warnings are now placed on soy milk. At least cow and goat milks, though clearly inferior to human breast milk, contain the basic components of adequate amino acids, vitamins, and minerals to build the bone, muscle, and other tissues of a growing baby. In Asia, soy formula was never traditionally used. An animal's milk was used instead.

The government has a program that provides free infant formula to teenage and low income mothers. African Americans are often lactose intolerant and take advantage of this program. As a result, 48.3 percent of African American girls (as well as 14.7 percent of Caucasian girls) reach puberty by age eight![27]

Soy should be eaten only in its fermented state, such as in miso or tempeh, and only in moderation. In 1979, the average daily consumption of soy protein was a mere 150 mg (about ¼ tsp) per person, and an independent committee known as the Select Committee of GRAS Substances (SCOGS) reported to the FDA that they believed the nitrites found in soy protein were "generally recognized as safe." They did, however, recommend that studies be made to establish safe levels. Such studies were never done.

> *"Vegetarians and others who choose soy year after year as their principal source of protein are unwittingly volunteering themselves and their children to serve as guinea pigs in a truly long-term, unmonitored epidemiological study."*

Vegetarians today typically consume 100 times the former level of ¼ tsp, often with disastrous results, but even more often with slow accumulations of toxins that take years to show up. Many never make the connection to soy as the cause.

My editor met a woman expatriate living in Ecuador who suffered daily headaches. She was making the rounds of alternative healers looking for answers. She asked him what hygiene would say. He told her it was probably something she was doing or eating on a daily basis.

This woman was the town's supplier of tofu and tempeh for local restaurants and groceries. She cooked it up daily and ate plenty of it herself. She was unwilling to believe it could possibly be her favorite foods! She didn't make the connection even when it was pointed out.

Another time, my editor had a housemate whose quirky behavior proved him to be as crazy as a loon. He and his other tenants couldn't wait for the man to move out. That guy was a vegetarian who drank soy milk daily.

I had a friend who suffered from daily migraine headaches. He was eating soy ice cream every night. I suggested that he stop. When he did, the migraines ceased!

Listen to Kaayla Daniel.

Vegetarians and others who choose soy year after year as their principal source of protein are unwittingly volunteering themselves and their children to serve as guinea pigs in a truly long-term, unmonitored epidemiological study.[28] ...

The story of soy sheds light on the dirty little secrets of the modern food-processing industry, the power of public relations, the corruption of scientific inquiry, and the collusion of FDA and other government agencies that are mandated to protect us.[29]

Grains and Lentils

Let's now look at grains and lentils. Both contain substances called *lectins* (sugar-binding proteins, or glycoproteins), which the plants evolved to ward off insects and other animal predators. These lectins can bind with cell membranes from almost any tissue in our bodies and wreak havoc. The body can't digest and break them down, and they attach themselves to intestinal cells where nutrient absorption takes place.

Dr. Cordain explains what happens.

The lectins in wheat (WGA), kidney beans (PHA), soybeans (SBA), and peanuts (PNA) are known to increase intestinal permeability and allow partially digested food proteins and remnants of resident gut bacteria to spill into the bloodstream. (Alcohol and hot chili peppers also increase intestinal permeability.) Usually, special immune cells immediately gobble up these wayward bacteria and food proteins. But lectins are cellular Trojan horses. They make the intestines easier to penetrate, and they impair the immune system's ability to fight off food and bacterial fragments that leak into the bloodstream.[30]

Grains, wheat especially, also contain opioids, leading to brain fog in some cases so severe that it is diagnosed as schizophrenia. Wheat sensitivity sometimes leads to a form of dementia often misdiagnosed as Alzheimer's disease.[31]

Many people like seitan, a wheat gluten high in protein with the starch rinsed away, made into mock meat. In raw vegan circles, people usually think it is not so bad to cheat by eating something cooked if it is at least a vegan food. It is more important to be vegan than raw, they think.

So, in keeping with that spirit, I one day decided to try some of this stuff while dining at a vegan cafe. I must admit it tasted good, with a texture similar to meat, but my stomach soon bloated to the point where I looked four or five months pregnant. When I went to bed that night, I tossed and turned. I could not sleep due to a histamine reaction. Wheat is a common histamine-inducing allergen.

Wheat is not our natural food. It was introduced into the human digestive tract a mere 10,000 to 20,000 years ago. Nearly everyone has some degree of wheat intolerance. If you don't, count yourself lucky.

Brown rice contains phytates. You have to soak it overnight before cooking or sprouting it to get rid of most of the phytates. White rice has the phytates removed, but it loses 80 percent of its minerals as well when processors scrape off the bran.

Nutritional anthropologists have collected data from fossil records and other sources and discovered how much our health has changed since we began to cultivate grains. They found a 5 to 6 inch *decrease* in height, a shortened life span, and an increase in infant mortality, infectious diseases, dental disease, tooth decay, and bone diseases like arthritis and osteoporosis. This was true *even though* the grains were all organic and unrefined!

Today the situation is much, much worse, with genetically modified, sprayed, and refined grains. Refined grains stimulate insulin production even more. They lack nutrients found in whole grains.

Granivores, animals truly designed to eat grains, include birds, which have *crops*, or pouches, in their gullets where food is stored or digested. They swallow stones to mill the grain they swallow. Granivores have special digestive enzymes for grains and guts devoted to the digestion of starch. Their gut walls are full of micro-pits, and their pancreases have three ducts, one duct for each of the major enzyme groups. This complexity, which humans lack, allows for the proper digestion of grains.

Another problem with grains is that they are high glycemic when cooked, as they usually are, though not when sprouted and eaten raw. Richard Bernstein, MD, sounds the alarm.

> Corn and other grain products are transformed into glucose so rapidly that in terms of their effect on blood sugar and insulin requirements, they are just like table sugar.[32]

Grains, especially when refined but even when whole, contribute to deficiencies of zinc, selenium, carotenoids, folic acid, vitamin B_6, magnesium, potassium, biotin, vitamin D, and taurine. They also contribute to an imbalance of omega-6 fats to omega-3s.[33]

Nutritional anthropologist Geoff Bond cautions that grains also contain *alpha-amylase inhibitors*.

> [These] interrupt the activity of the starch digestion enzyme amylase and damage the pancreas. Worse, they are prominent allergens.

Then there are the *protease inhibitors*, which disrupt the digestive process and can lead to abnormal enlargement of the pancreas and cancer.[34]

Finally, grains have *alkyl resorcinols*.

> These disrupt a wide range of body functions, including disintegration of red blood cells, disruption to DNA maintenance, dramatic increase in blood-clotting, and the stunting of growth.

Bond notes that *no other primate* attempts to eat grains.[35]

Legumes, he warns, are not well digested. In extreme cases, some people get up to five gallons of flatulence per day, causing methane that contributes to global warming![36] Most legumes have a high percentage of indigestible oligosaccharides, notably *raffinose*.

Drs. Mary and Michael Eades point out that lectins from grains and beans cause leaky gut syndrome, which leads to a whole host of autoimmune disease conditions, including arthritis, multiple sclerosis, inflammatory bowel disease, systemic lupus, ankylosing spondylitis, ulcerative colitis, kidney inflammation, Crohn's, Type 2 diabetes, and more.[37]

One study found that lectins might even block leptin, the hormone that tells us to stop eating when we are full.[38]

Other phytochemicals from cereals, such as glycosylated* proteins, also were found to affect weight balance by affecting appetite and energy metabolism.[39]

If you look at many of the popular diets of recent years, you can see an underlying element they all have in common: eliminating or reducing grain consumption. The Maker's Diet, Dr. Mercola's No-Grain Diet, the Zone Diet, the Atkins Diet, the Paleo Diet, the Protein Power Diet, the various raw food diets, and many more diets will get results and make people feel better if for no other reason than they get people off these addictive, high-glycemic, fattening, and hard-to-digest grains!

Grains create opioids in the brain that are so addicting that there is even one theory that suggests that we settled down into agriculture just to nourish this addiction![40]

Wheat is no doubt the worst among the grains, since it has been crossbred so much for thousands of years that the body doesn't process it well and barely recognizes it as food. Wheat lectin has been shown in studies to increase the ability of foreign proteins to permeate the blood-brain barrier.[41] This pathologically increased permeability in the blood-brain barrier may trigger an autoimmune attack against the nervous system, resulting in multiple sclerosis.[42]

This property may explain why wheat has even been implicated in mental illness, such as schizophrenia. My husband's grandfather was in a mental institution for schizophrenia until he stopped eating wheat. Schizophrenia might not be an all-or-nothing disease: I recall getting a great deal of brain fog in my pasta-loving days that made it very hard to focus and interact with people. The wheat combined with all my mercury dental fillings made me so spacey that people often commented that I wasn't mentally present.

Wheat lectin also binds to the insulin receptor more intensely and longer than insulin does, causing insulin resistance.[43] Wheat lectin increases the breakdown of glucose and fat storage, but unlike insulin, the wheat lectin doesn't stimulate protein synthesis, so a person could end up losing muscle mass with a diet heavy in wheat.[44]

Many people eat concentrated protein powders, but this artificial practice is unnatural and thus less than ideal. One can end up getting excesses of some nutrients and not enough of others, resulting in nutritional imbalances. Take rice protein powder for example. Some people who eat it make too much histamine, which creates allergies. Histamine levels in some people can get so high that severe depression can develop.[45]

I was eating just a couple heaping tablespoons a day of raw rice protein powder and found that I became extremely depressed. I felt there was no point in living. Then I recalled what I had read about this several years earlier while researching for *The Live Food Factor*. When I stopped, I felt better within 24 hours.

A friend of mine had attempted suicide, so I told him it was due to eating excessive rice protein powder. Once he stopped the powder, he felt fine again. In *The Butcher and the Vegetarian*, Tara Weaver writes about also becoming depressed from eating rice protein powder.[46]

Dr. Price limited his studies only to peoples who exhibited superb health. Only a few of the cultures studied by Price ate grains. When they did, they were careful to prepare them traditionally. If you have to eat beans and grains, this is what chemistry professor Dr. Alsoph Corwin, PhD, advises.

> Sprout the beans. In this process, the germination produces an enzyme, phytase, which hydrolyzes the phytates and converts them into inositol. Phytates also occur in cereal grains and are converted into inositol by yeast in the leavening process. For those who can tolerate yeast, then, leavened bread is superior to unleavened bread.[47]

Spirulina

Spirulina is a single-celled oceanic blue-green alga. Like hemp, it contains all the essential amino acids. Since it is also very high in protein, a whopping 65 percent, and not overly expensive, it makes a great supplementary protein source. It is a great source of trace minerals and gamma-linolenic acid (GLA), an omega-6 fat that may reduce inflammation, unlike the other omega-6s that promote it.

---

*Glycosylation is the enzymatic process that attaches glycans (complex carbs) to proteins, lipids, or other organic molecules.

The taste is very bitter, however, and its B_{12} analogues (which come from processing it) increase the need for dietary B_{12}. It is also nearly impossible to find a raw version of it. Some people contend spirulina is neurotoxic.[48]

Fruits and Vegetables

Fruits and vegetables have very little protein and can only be considered supplementary protein sources. On the high end, relatively speaking, are asparagus, broccoli, cauliflower, and brussels sprouts, which all have 3 grams per 100 grams (about 3 ounces). If they are used as a major source of protein, you can count on loads of bloating and gas from the cellulose! Potatoes are also at the high end, with 3 grams of protein for the starchy part and 2 grams for the skin. But to get your 50 grams, you would be getting way too many carbs by eating 10 potatoes! Vegetables may thus only be considered supplementary protein sources.

It's Easy to Get Protein from Meat and Eggs

Meat is the superior choice for maximizing protein intake while minimizing calories. It is easier for most people to stay slim on chicken than on beans, grains, nuts, and seeds. Meat protein comes packed with fewer calories than found in the starchy beans and grains or in the mostly fatty nuts and seeds. You also don't get any carbs with meat.

With meat, it is super easy to get 50 grams of protein with a minimum of calories, especially if the meat is lean. For example, 100 grams of chicken, or a bit over 3 ounces, gives you 50 grams with only 340 calories. A steak filet of 100 grams gives you 56 grams of protein but only 380 calories! You have plenty of calories left for all sorts of other foods.

Eating eggs is one of the most economical ways to get protein, both financially and calorically. Two eggs have only 140 calories, but you get 14 grams of protein. A dozen eggs provides 72 grams of protein, about 6 grams per large egg.

Quality omega-3 eggs from organically fed chickens cost about $3.50 a dozen. So for about $10, 3 dozen eggs could give you get a total of 216

grams of protein. Each yolk also contains about 244 IU of vitamin A, 17 to 20 IU of vitamin D, and 0.6 mcg of B_{12}. You would have to consume too many eggs to get enough of those vitamins, however, which is why a diet that includes a bit of raw liver or cod liver oil is best.

What about the Fiber?

Attempting to convince the average dietitian that whole-grain cereal products are not a health-enhancing food is a task only slightly less difficult than trying to convert the Pope to atheism. Whole-grain cereals are repeatedly promoted as the holy grail of healthy eating, a concept completely unsupported by clinical evidence.
—Anthony Colpo[49]

When I embarked upon a very low-carb diet, I felt so satiated I rarely wanted to eat huge volumes of salads and vegetables, which I had eaten lots of on raw vegan diets, even though they are so low in calories that they do not contain large amounts of carbs. What I discovered, to my surprise, was that I now had the flattest stomach I'd ever had in my life. I was almost never bloated.

We have been conditioned to believe we need loads of insoluble fiber to have healthy colons. Insoluble fiber comes with carbs (especially grains and legumes), while meat, dairy, and eggs have no fiber at all.

Pharmacist and medical writer Konstantin Monastyrsky of Russia dispels this myth in his book *Fiber Menace*. He explains how fiber, especially the insoluble type in grains, interferes with stomach digestion and later clogs the intestines. Fiber can actually become addictive. The more you use, the more you need to get yourself unplugged. It becomes a vicious cycle.

Monastyrsky suffered for years with irritable bowel syndrome, constipation, hemorrhoidal disease, and anal fissures. Doctors ordered a high-fiber diet, and things only got worse. This prompted his research and shocking discoveries: that fiber (especially from processed, cooked grains) is actually the cause, not the cure, to these diseases and others, such as dysbacteriosis, diarrhea, appendicitis, bloating, gas, gastroesophageal reflux disease, dyspepsia, heartburn, gastritis, hiatal hernia, ulcerative colitis, Crohn's disease, colon cancer, and more.

As you increase the amount of animal products

in your diet, you will feel satiated more quickly and will naturally consume less fiber. Your stomach will shrink accordingly without such a high-bulk diet. Your stools will not be as large, but that is no problem. It is simply an indicator that you are eating more "zero-residue" food.

> Unlike indigestible fiber, protein- and fat-rich food — eggs, meats, fowl, game, seafood, and dairy — digest almost completely. Only minute traces of these foods reach the large intestine intact.[50]

Stools on a low-fiber diet are composed primarily of intestinal bacteria. They also contain water, mineral salts, coloring pigments, traces of fat, dead bacteria, and cellular debris shed by the body. If fiber were necessary, as Monastyrsky points out, why is there no fiber in mother's milk, yet babies have stools? How were the Eskimos so healthy on a diet nearly devoid of fiber? Also, people who fast or go on very low-carb diets may continue to produce stools without constipation despite no fiber intake, unless they had become very addicted to fiber, their colons having developed a dependency.

Dr. Ron Schmid has his patients eat a lot of fermented foods to restore healthful bacteria when they are transitioning to a diet higher in animal foods. Eating kefir, yogurt, and fermented vegetables increases beneficial bacteria that bulk up the stools, resulting in easy elimination even on diets with little fiber.[51]

The insoluble fiber hypothesis has been largely backed by the cereal industry. (As we have seen, those behind-the-scenes grain barons have power!) The scientific support for it, especially as regards grains, is weak except in certain epidemiological studies, as those with East African populations. Their fiber sources were vegetables, corn, and millet.[52]

Furthermore, six studies disprove the theory that fiber reduces the risk of colorectal cancer. Some studies even found that fiber actually *increased* the number of large *adenomas*, benign tumors that may progress to become malignant![53]

If we eat several servings a day of fresh fruits and vegetables, we get sufficient fiber, and evidence shows that their fiber is superior to the harsh insoluble fiber from grains, especially cooked grains.[54] The soluble fiber of fruits, vegetables, and nuts has been shown to improve blood lipids and glucose metabolism.[55]

Plant Protein Lacks Vitamins A and D for Protein Assimilation

Plant protein lacks what animal fat contains along with its protein: vitamins A and D. Fish, eggs, meat, and dairy contain these vitamins. (Cod liver oil is very rich in them.) These vitamins help with the assimilation of protein.[56] Dr. Price found that the diets of healthy, isolated people contained 10 times as much of these fat-soluble vitamins than the conventional diet of his day (the 1930s). And back then, people got a lot more vitamins A and D than we do now, since they ate more animal fats.

According to Dr. Price, without vitamin A from animal sources, neither protein nor minerals nor water-soluble vitamins can be utilized by the body. Vitamin A stimulates the gastric juices needed for protein digestion.[57]

GM Plant Diet: A Depopulation Trojan Horse?

It is fascinating that as we near 7 billion people, governments and food corporations around the world are endorsing soy and genetically modified organisms (GMOs). Corn is nearly all GM, soy is mostly GM, and GM wheat is now being introduced. To guarantee avoiding GMOs, you must purchase organic food.

The best book explaining the true agenda and politics behind GMOs is the highly researched *Seeds of Destruction* by historian F. William Engdahl. Of course, the most obvious agenda is to patent foods for profit. This way, a corporation like Monsanto can take monopolistic control over the food supply.

However, another side effect of many GMOs is infertility. Russian scientists have found, for example, that the fourth generation of hamsters fed genetically modified foods produce grandchildren unable to sire fourth generation offspring.[58]

Now, I am in favor of some world depopulation, mind you, but I think it should be done voluntarily, by educating people and lifting them to higher standards of living. The tendency is for more educated people to want and need fewer children. By restricting their family sizes, they feel they can afford to give their kids better food, higher education, and better chances at more opportunity in their lives. For most people in the world, children represent the only form of social security for the aged. In societies that provide for the elderly, families are smaller.

It turns out that there is a secret, sinister, dark side to this GMO research. Engdahl indentifies the culprits for you.

It was becoming clear why powerful elite circles of the United States, themselves enormously wealthy and largely untaxed thanks to Bush Administration tax cuts, backed the introduction of genetically modified seeds into the world food chain as a strategic priority. That elite included not only the Rockefeller and Ford foundations and most other foundations tied to the large private family fortunes of the wealthiest American families. It also included the US Department of Agriculture, as well as the leading policy circles of the International Monetary Fund, the World Bank, along with agencies of the United Nations including WHO [World Health Organization] and FAO [Food and Agriculture Organization].

The folks at the Rockefeller Foundation were deadly serious about wanting to solve the world hunger problem through the worldwide proliferation of GMO seeds and crops. Only their presumed method to do so aimed at a "supply side" solution rather than the "demand side." They were out to limit population by going after the human reproductive process itself.[59].

The author goes on to provide a documented case of deliberate depopulation via vaccinations: The World Health Organization oversaw a massive tetanus vaccination program in Third World countries. A Roman Catholic lay organization, Comité Pro Vida de Mexico, decided to test numerous vials when they became suspicious of the program's motives, since tetanus itself is so rare. The vaccinations were found to contain a totally irrelevant substance, *human chorionic gonadotrophin* (hCG). This is a natural hormone needed to maintain a pregnancy, but when combined with a tetanus toxoid carrier, it stimulates the formation of antibodies against hCG, thus inducing spontaneous abortion!

If this all sounds too incredible for you, read the highly documented book *Death in the Air* by Harvard-educated public health researcher Dr. Leonard Horowitz, which details several depopulation programs encompassing aerial sprayings and other vaccinations.

Another issue with Monsanto: Though it is pretty well established that one of their pesticides is destroying the bee population, this greedy company won't desist. Without bees, everyone will be living on a diet of mainly grains, one of the few plant types that don't rely on bees for pollination. We will all be constipated, diabetic, arthritic schizophrenics!

Is it any wonder that where I now live, in Ecuador, growing GMOs is unconstitutional? Now, if they will just do the same with pesticides.

Benefits of Plant Protein

By now you are probably thinking that I am not in favor of a diet rich in plant protein. Nothing could be further from the truth! The above discourse is just to show how hard it can be for many people to get adequate protein from plants *alone*. Including animal protein in your diet is also beneficial if you want to minimize the plant toxins we have discussed and also keep your omega-3:6 fat ratio in balance.

Plant protein should definitely be a staple in your diet. Eating it can be a slow but steady way to build muscles.[60] You also get a lot of free amino acids from plant protein, reducing the need to break foreign proteins down into small units before building them up into human proteins, as utilizing animal protein requires. A few steps are thus saved in the digestive process.

With plant protein, you are not in danger of overdosing on saturated fats like those found with most animal proteins. You also don't overdo methionine, an amino acid associated with atherosclerotic changes.[61]

Certain plants are important for their antioxidants. Leafy greens, especially spinach, help protect from Alzheimer's. So do cruciferous vegetables like broccoli, cabbage, and cauliflower.[62] A handful of almonds or walnuts a day can do the same.[63] Greens are very alkalizing. Nuts and seeds help increase our HDL and decrease our LDL cholesterol levels.

Again, variety and moderation are key.

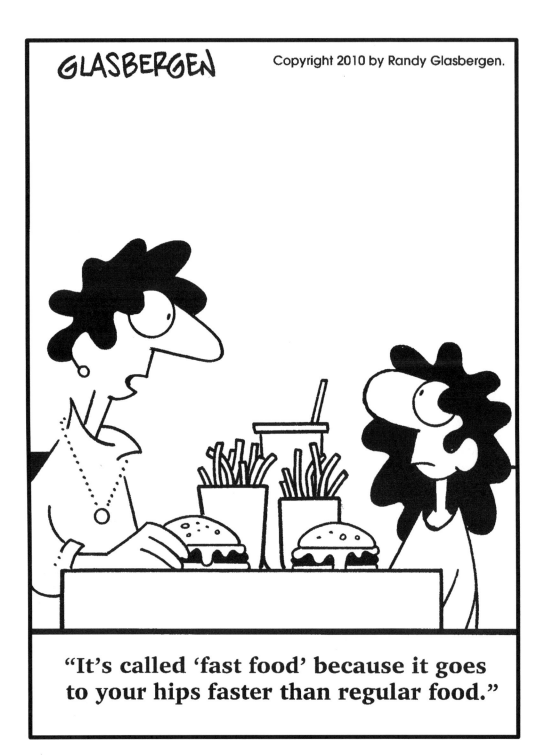

Chapter 16

Protein: Perils, Praise, and Myths

Extra protein, it turns out, sends "stop eating!" messages to the brain ... Protein's benefits go way beyond waistline trimming. The brain and its long spidery neurons are essentially made of fat, but they communicate with each other via proteins. ... Protein ... prompts the brain to manufacture norepinephrine and dopamine, chemical messengers that promote alertness and activity. —Carlin Flora, "The Protein-Hunger Connection," *Psychology Today*, January 23, 2006

Proteins have numerous functions. Some are commonly known, such as the formation of muscles, skin, and bones. Others are a bit more obscure, such as their use in performing enzyme-mediated biochemical processes, including cell signaling and hormone and antibody functioning.

Protein helps keep people satiated.[1] Protein causes the greatest release of a gut hormone (PYY) that reduces hunger.[2] Protein and fat are high in PYY, while carbs are low. This is why most people get hungry within a few hours of a high-carb breakfast, such as pancakes, muffins, or fruit.

Protein helps with losing weight and keeping the weight off. It can increase metabolism by 30 percent.[3] In one study, protein was the factor that made metabolism 100 percent higher even 2½ hours after eating.[4] It stabilizes blood sugar. It helps balance insulin release through the production of the hormone glucagon, which opposes insulin.[5] Protein has a preventive effect on atherosclerosis.[6]

According to Dr. Barry Sears, "Excess protein has the least efficient conversion into circulating fat because it requires about 25 percent of the dietary calories to convert it into circulating fat," whereas dietary fat requires only 3 percent, and carbs require 5 to 15 percent.[7]

Protein is needed for the brain to make endorphins and serotonin. Sugar will give you a rush of endorphins that lasts temporarily, resulting in cravings to replenish the supply by eating more, while protein consumption yields a steady flow of neurotransmitters.

Tryptophan is the amino acid precursor needed to make the neurotransmitter serotonin, an important factor in mood, sleep, appetite, memory, and learning. Most plant foods are low in it except for sesame, pumpkin, sunflower, and chia seeds, as well as lentils, beans, and potatoes. But eating a lot of seeds other than chia, hemp, or flax may skew your omega-6:3 ratio. Tryptophan is abundant in eggs, dairy, and meat.

Making endorphins requires 15 amino acids. With rare exceptions that include potatoes, only animal products have all 22 of the standard amino acids. Some people are not good at synthesizing the so-called "nonessential" amino acids and thus may need more than the essential ones. Nutritional psychologist Julia Ross, author of *The Mood Cure*, elaborates.

> Unless you are a very careful vegetarian, you can easily become deficient in the proteins you need to make your endorphins on typically low-protein vegetarian fare. ...

> Fats and oils also encourage endorphin release, making you satisfied with your meals. Fats are naturally combined with protein in most high-protein foods (like fish, eggs, and meats), so if you're on a low-fat diet, you may not be getting enough fat or protein to allow your brain to produce endorphins at optimal levels.

> For example, have you been throwing out the fat-rich egg yolks and eating only egg whites or removing the fatty skin from chicken? If so, you're reducing your endorphin levels too. Low-fat, low-calorie, and high-carb diets can definitely deplete your endorphin stores by reducing both protein and fat.[8]

Insufficient protein can cause B_{12} not to be absorbed. In order for the body to absorb B_{12} and bring it inside, it must combine with a digestive secretion called *intrinsic factor* (IF). IF is a protein. If your diet is too low in protein, your body stops making IF or makes very little. It's the same with other digestive juices (proteins), which can lead to other types of malnutrition.

Inadequate protein in the diet can also upset the proper acid-alkaline balance.[9] The pH at which IF combines with B_{12} must also be low. The stomach doesn't produce enough HCl to lower its pH enough when protein is lacking. So that's the second way B_{12} doesn't get absorbed when protein is too low.

Can a very low-protein diet (which by default is usually high carb) be conducive to health? Dr. Weston Price found some people on low-protein (10 percent or less), high-carb diets to be healthy. These were in the high Andes, Africa, and Switzerland. The thing these diets had in common was that the small amounts of animal proteins they consumed were of exceptionally high quality: insects, fresh and dried fish, shrimp, and eggs. Also, the carbs were usually fermented, making minerals more available and nutrients denser. Of course, those diets included no refined foods, as found in modern societies.[10]

Excessive protein intake is also not good. Find out what you need based on your metabolic type.[*] Whether plant or animal derived, protein metabolizes to produce the acidic waste product urea, which is harmful in excess, though this is less problematic when animal flesh is consumed raw, since the basic chemical ammonia present in raw flesh neutralizes the acidic urea. Nevertheless, Dr. Rosedale expresses a caveat.

> The more protein you eat, the more proficient you become at making glucose from the protein in your diet and from the protein in your muscle and bone.[11]

Protein poisoning results from overindulgence in very lean flesh. People in the arctic knew that if they didn't get enough fat along with their protein, they would suffer what is called *rabbit starvation*, so called because rabbits have such very lean meat. Those natives trying to subsist on rabbit meat would experience diarrhea, headache, fatigue, low blood pressure, low heart rate, and a vague discomfort and hunger that can only be satisfied by consumption of fat or carbohydrate.

Dr. Gabriel Cousens, MD, advocates going as easy as you can on protein for spiritual reasons.

> Excess protein, whether from animal or vegetable sources, slows the flow of the subtle energy in the system and decreases our capacity as superconductors.

It acts as a sludge to our body energy in general and specifically to the Kundalini energy.[12]

I ate too much protein one day and experienced the sluggishness from that sludge. I felt that heaviness and low energy.

Authors Fallon and Enig further explain the hazards.

> Protein requires vitamin A for its metabolism, and a diet too high in protein without adequate fat rapidly depletes vitamin A stores, leading to serious consequences — heart arrhythmias, kidney problems, autoimmune disease, and thyroid disorders. Diets too high in protein also cause a negative calcium balance, where more calcium is lost compared to the amount taken in, a condition that can lead to bone loss and nervous system disorders.[13]

It is not true that protein injures the kidneys unless excessive amounts are consumed or unless you already suffer from weak kidneys. The Nurses' Health Study concluded that "high protein intake was not associated with renal function decline in women with normal renal function."[14]

Another study compared renal function during weight loss induced by high- vs. low-protein, low-fat diets in overweight subjects. The conclusion was that moderate changes in dietary protein intake cause adaptive alterations in renal size and function without indications of adverse effects.[15]

It is also not true that low-carb diets, which tend to be higher in protein than high-carb, low-fat diets, cause mineral loss from the bones due to protein acidity. Some studies showed that high-protein diets cause urinary calcium excretion, but now some experts believe this occurs because calcium is so much better absorbed on diets rich in proteins (including animal proteins) that the body doesn't need it all and therefore excretes some of it.

The Framingham Osteoporosis Study investigated protein consumption in 615 elderly people over four years. They found that the people who consumed more protein had less bone loss, whereas those consuming less protein lost bone at the spine and femoral bones.[16] Another study demonstrated that protein intake for elderly women *above* current recommendations may be necessary to optimize bone mass.[17]

When you consider that protein is used in bone formation, doesn't this make sense? In fact, one

---

[*]Chapter 10

study showed that if protein intake wasn't adequate, taking extra calcium wouldn't help.[18]

Other studies have confirmed that protein doesn't cause osteoporosis, including one in which the short-term and long-term effects of a high-meat diet on calcium metabolism of four male adults were studied. The diet was found to significantly change neither calcium balance nor the intestinal absorption of calcium.[19]

In fact, studies have shown that a gradual increase in bone mass occurs with increasing protein intake, but there seems to be an *optimal window*, as protein that is over the basic requirements can contribute to bone loss. There are epidemiological studies that show eating *too much* protein is associated with osteoporosis. Some of these are cited in the book *Eat to Live* by Dr. Joel Fuhrman, MD. *Balance is key*.

Remember too that cooking meat makes it more acidic, thus causing the body to leach out important alkaline minerals like calcium and magnesium to neutralize the acid.

For most people, somewhere between 45 and 60 grams a day is enough protein.* Some experts consider over 100 grams of protein, typical in the American diet, to be toxic. One review suggests that if you don't make protein more than 25 percent of your caloric intake, you can avoid toxicity.[20]

Robb Wolf notes in *The Paleo Solution* that "as a stand-alone item, it is virtually impossible to overeat protein due to the potent satiety signal sent to the brain." He explains that this signal is because of a maximal ability of the liver to process protein when it is over 30 to 35 percent of the total caloric intake.[21]

Some people have speculated that plant food has a different effect on bones than meat, but this was not found to be the case. Vegetarians do not sport higher bone densities than meat eaters.[22]

Dr. Herta Spencer, MD, of the Veterans Administration Hospital in Hines, Illinois, noted that animal and human studies which correlated calcium loss with high-protein diet were using isolated, fractionated amino acids from milk or eggs.[23] When meat was instead used, no increase in calcium excretion or significant change in serum calcium was shown, even over a long period of time.[24]

Why the difference? Protein powders lack the fat-soluble vitamins D and A needed to assimilate calcium and protein.

It has been alleged that the Eskimos developed osteoporosis.[25] Actually, the study finding this was done in 1974 after the introduction of modern diets when the Eskimos began to drink imprudent amounts of alcohol. The fact is they did not acquire this disease condition until they began to consume modern diets that included alcohol.

Dr. Price visited the Eskimos before they left their traditional diets and observed this about them.

> In his primitive state, he has provided an example of physical excellence and dental perfection such as has seldom been excelled by any race in the past or present.[26]

One thing I noticed while scanning the studies on vegetarianism and osteoporosis is that vegetarians from sunny countries in Asia have no more osteoporosis than omnivores. Maybe it is because they get lots of vitamin D from the sun. I've been to Asia three times. You always see masses of people out on the streets. Some consume natto, the only known plant food with very significant amounts of vitamin K_2, needed for healthy bones. In Asia, many people are still eating traditional diets rich in nutrients.

Animal protein is also often blamed for ischemic heart disease, but a study on 80,082 women aged 34 to 59 at the onset of one study found otherwise.

> Our data do not support the hypothesis that a high protein intake increases the risk of ischemic heart disease. In contrast, our findings suggest that replacing carbohydrates with protein may be associated with a lower risk of ischemic heart disease.[27]

---

*These figures are taken from a protein chart at www.internet healthlibrary.com/DietandNutrition/Protein-tables_intake.htm, accessed 11-28-10. The chart is based not just on the RDA used in the US, but also on the Reference Nutrient Intake (RNI) used in the UK. The RNI is the amount of nutrient that is enough for at least 97 percent of the population. Research has shown that we do not need as much protein as previously thought.

Chapter 17

Meat: Correct Physiologically If Not Politically

Understand when you eat meat that something did die. You have an obligation to value it — not just the sirloin, but also all those wonderful tough little bits.
—Anthony Bourdain, American author, chef, and host of *Anthony Bourdain: No Reservations*

There is a hilarious scene from Woody Allen's 1973 movie *Sleeper* in which the owner of a health food store wakes up and finds himself in the future. Two doctors who revived him are discussing his case. The male doctor asks if the patient had requested anything special. The female doctor says he did in fact request odd items like wheat germ, organic honey, and "Tiger's Milk" (the original "energy bar").

The man laughs and says, "Oh yes, those were the charmed substances that some years ago were felt to contain life-preserving properties."

The female doctor, stunned, asks, "You mean there was no deep fat? No steak or cream pies or hot fudge?"

The male doctor replies, "Those were thought to be unhealthy, precisely the opposite of what we now know to be true."

Such irony is relevant to this book, at least for the steak and cream — certainly not for the sugar or deep fried fat!

Before I began to write this book, I spent months making recipes to jump-start my right brain and move through writer's block. I was inspired by the Meryl Streep movie *Julie & Julia*, in which the main character makes a different Julia Child recipe every day and blogs about it.

Then something funny happened. I ordered some wild meat off the internet. I started eating three ounces or so at breakfast. My obsession with food disappeared in just a day or two!

For nearly eight years, I had made intensely tasty, gourmet raw recipes. Now I had no desire for that. My cravings were suddenly gone, though I didn't know exactly what I had been craving. The protein and the nutrients in the meat stabilized my blood sugar so much that not only was I not hungry, but I had very little interest in food or in making tasty, spicy recipes. I had a lot more energy to put towards the more daunting task of writing this book.

Many people besides me have found nuts, seeds, and sprouted lentils very hard to digest, even when soaked and rinsed of phytates. I get fatigued when I eat more than a handful, but raw or lightly steamed meat goes through my system so gently that I barely notice it. It may take a bit *longer* to digest than plant protein, but it is so much *easier* to digest, because my ancestors evolved eating it as a staple in their diets.

In *The Live Food Factor*, I wrote about the time many years ago just after starting to go raw when I first experimented with raw meat for about a month.

I found that after eating raw meat, I maintained the light feeling that I had on a raw vegetarian diet. When I ate raw meat alone, it was actually easier for my body to digest than raw nuts, raw vegetables, raw sprouts, or raw seeds. I even slept better, with no disturbances, on the days that I had meat instead of the raw vegan food.[1]

As I stated earlier, it was my carb addiction as well as my philosophical desire to be in on the vegan movement that ended that experiment.

Even though wild or free-range organic meat is not cheap, I save money because I spend a bit less on food than before. I no longer need so many supplements, especially after adding cod liver oil to my regimen.

Again, when I eat nuts and seeds, I get fatigued and sluggish, even when they are sprouted; but when I eat raw meat, I feel light and energetic. It is so much easier for me to digest.

☞ If you have been eating a high-fruit diet, you may have temporarily lost some of your digestive ability because fruit is so easy and quick to digest. You may have to ease into eating animal products gradually.

If meat is so bad, why do I feel so much better when I eat it? Why do I sleep through the night every time I eat red meat, the "worst" *kind* of meat to eat?

I usually eat some free-range beef once a week or so. My moral programming says, "How can you eat a mammal?"

My spiritual programming haunts me: "Red meat will create the densest consciousness!"

My nutritional programming dictates, "Red meat gets stuck in your colon and causes cancer!" (Even though studies have shown this isn't true.)

My political programming screams, "Red meat causes water depletion and global warming!"

But my body's cells say, "This is great; it's what we wanted; it gives us carnitine, B_{12}, carnosine, and some other undiscovered ingredient(s) that makes me sleep more soundly than ever." The X factor might be tryptophan, but red meat often works better than tryptophan or 5-HTP supplements for inducing a sound sleep.

When I eat this at breakfast, I experience no hunger or cravings all day long. My blood sugar is stable. I have peak energy.

What Does Meat Have That Plants Lack?

Meat has been much maligned in recent decades while the myth of cholesterol and saturated fats was prevailing. There are also studies that "prove" that meat causes cancer. What do you expect when most of the studies used the meat of factory-farmed animals typically eaten in American diets? What do you expect when the meat is cooked at temperatures so high that toxic by-products are formed? What do you expect when it is heated in hydrogenated oils, man-made trans fats that our bodies cannot digest? What do you expect when meat is eaten in such high quantities as it has been in the West over the last century?

Over the past few decades, numerous studies purport to show the superiority of vegetarian diets, but usually the control group is eating the Standard American Diet (SAD)! That means they're eating cooked meat with all of its toxic by-products from animals that were factory farmed without exercise; improperly fed unnatural diets of grains too high in omega-6 fats, usually GMO grains full of pesticides; and injected with hormones, antibiotics, and vaccinations.

In processing after slaughter and butchering, meat is often infused with nitrates and other toxins for flavor or preservation, as with hot dogs and lunch meats. The newest destructive fad is to sterilize the meat by irradiation with radioactive nuclear waste materials. In addition, the consumer often eats twice as much meat as his body needs.

Um, hello? Just about *any* diet would be more healthful than *that*!

The China Study is often trotted out to make meat look inherently bad; however, the Chinese are known to deep fry much of their meat, making it full of trans fats. Furthermore, several of the conclusions drawn from the study are debatable, as will be discussed in chapter 19.

So where are the studies in which people ate the diets that we evolved on: meat from wild or at least free-running animals fed their natural, organic diets and not tortured with unnatural injections?

The largest experiment of humans eating meat lasted 2.6 million years. The meat was from wild animals, organically fed and free range. While some was cooked, *much* was eaten *raw*. While people often ate large quantities of meat after a kill, they also went days or even *weeks* with *no* meat, so meat was not overeaten as it is today by so many. The results? The skeletons of prehistoric man showed virtually no chronic disease, no osteoporosis, no arthritis, and no dental problems. Cancer, diabetes, heart disease, and all other chronic diseases became rampant mainly as a result of agriculture, not meat per se.

Factory farming of animals, the addition of nitrates to lunch meat, the feeding of grains to herbivorous animals in lieu of their natural foods, the barbequing and grilling of the meat — all of this made the meat toxic. In its natural form, meat is likely the highest quality super food on the planet, especially the meat of animals that have been wild or properly fed for at least three or four generations.[*]

Furthermore, Dr. Weston Price found that primitive peoples cherished meat and knew that it held

---

[*]*The Live Food Factor* describes instinctive nutrition more fully in pages 514–19.

powerful ingredients.

It is significant that I have as yet found no group that was building and maintaining good bodies exclusively on plant foods. A number of groups are endeavoring to do so with marked evidence of failure.[2]

The healthiest people he found didn't eat only the muscle meat. The organs were cherished above all. The entire animal would often be eaten: bones for soup, glands, and organs, all of which are very nutrient dense.

Skeletons of meat eaters were found to be much healthier than those of modern-day people: taller, stronger bones, no evidence of arthritis and osteoporosis. I doubt their health was perfect, and some probably suffered cancer because many of them cooked their meat in open flames. Plenty of studies have shown this creates carcinogenic by-products.[*] But the fact that they were nonetheless much freer of degenerative diseases than we are today reveals just how toxic grains and legumes can be as alternative sources of protein.

The American Dietetic Association believes a vegetarian diet is healthful when "appropriately planned."[3] But after researching for this book, I have come to the conclusion that even carb types, the only ones who thrive on vegetarian diets, would reach higher levels of health by becoming "flexitarians," vegetarians who occasionally eat meat.

From what I have seen, people who would rather die than eat animal products sometimes *do* — prematurely. Just as the toxic effects of cooked foods can take decades to show up, the correlation going unnoticed, so can nutritional deficiencies. The correlation likewise goes unnoticed because the effect is gradual. Rather than immediately killing people, these deficiencies shorten their life spans.

Now, let's take a look at what eating meat moderately can do for you. Dr. Stanley Bass told me that eating just 8 ounces a day (probably 6 for women) provides all the protein you need. Then you can eat plant food for the rest of the day's diet. If you eat the meat raw, as will be discussed in detail in chapter 24, even less is needed.

Vitamin A

True vitamin A is not found in plant food. Americans hold the common misconception that beta-carotene and vitamin A are the same, but they are not. Foods like carrots and pumpkins contain only the beta-carotene precursor to A, and it is hard for many people to make the necessary conversion. Children under five, diabetics, and those with thyroid or liver problems make the conversion very poorly, if at all.[4]

The conversion requires dietary fat, and the rate is often thought to be somewhere between 6 (World Health Organization) and 12 (US Institute of Medicine) International Units (IUs) of beta-carotene to make 1 IU of vitamin A. A review in the *Journal of Nutrition* reported studies which demonstrated that some people need *twenty-one* units of beta-carotene in foods to convert to *one* IU of true vitamin A![5]

The bioavailability of beta-carotene increases if a vegetable is cooked and if vegetables are eaten with fat, but blending or juicing are better ways to accomplish this. The problem with cooking is that you lose some of the nutrients, including the enzymes that help digest them. You also create some toxic by-products.[†] Lightly steaming is not as bad as grilling, as low heat is used, and the inside is still raw. If you are having trouble with all the cellulose in raw vegetables, lightly steam them and add butter or olive oil for increased absorption of beta-carotene. Better yet, eat some raw and some lightly steamed. Juicing is even better, but it is time consuming. Blending may also work for you.

Vitamin A is needed for eyesight and secretion of gastric juices for protein digestion, which assists with protein assimilation. It also plays a role in building strong bone, rich blood, and crucial *ribonucleic acid* (RNA) proteins. Vitamin A is needed to maintain normal skin.

Cod liver oil is a great source for this nutrient, as are other animal livers and liver extracts. Egg

---

[*]See chapter 9 and Appendix D of *The Live Food Factor* for proof that cooking creates toxins.

[†]See chapters 8 and 9 of *The Live Food Factor* for a full discussion of which nutrients are destroyed and which toxic by-products are created by heating food.

yolks also have some vitamin A. In traditional cultures, it was often known that blindness could be reversed by eating the eyes of fish, rich in vitamin A.

Excess vitamin A has been implicated in osteoporosis, but a closer look reveals that it may actually be a deficiency of vitamin D in relation to the A. Nutritionist Chris Masterjohn presents evidence that "high vitamin A intakes might be safe and beneficial when vitamin A is consumed in the proper ratio to vitamin D" and that a wide range of ratios between the two vitamins might be acceptable.[6] Sara Johansson of Uppsala, Sweden, also wrote her PhD thesis on this theory.[7]

Another reason to avoid supplements is that in natural foods, the nutrients come in the proper ratios in which we evolved eating them.

Dr. Weston Price observed that vitamin A from animal sources is needed for the body to utilize protein, minerals, and water-soluble vitamins. Vitamin A is needed to properly utilize iodine, which is essential for the thyroid. The robust people that he observed consumed about *ten times* the amount of vitamin A used in his era. Nowadays, with the use of vegetable oils and the drastic reduction of quality fats from grass-fed animals, we obtain far less vitamin A than in the 1930s and 1940s.

Chris Masterjohn points out the near-impossibility of attaining enough vitamin A from plant food.

> Eating liver once a week or taking a half teaspoon of high-vitamin cod liver oil per day provides the RDA of 3,000 IU.[*] To obtain the same amount with plant foods, one would have to consume two cups of carrots, one cup of sweet potatoes, or two cups of cooked kale every day. The presumed conversion rate, however, is just an average. ... People who convert carotenes poorly may suffer from vitamin A deficiency even if they eat large amounts of carotene-rich foods every day.[8]

The Weston Price Foundation recommends about 10,000 IU of vitamin A for an adult (about double the RDA) and 20,000 if pregnant or nursing.[9] This can be attained easily through cod liver oil supplementation. The foundation recommends supplementing with plant sources to get even more.

Let's revisit just how hard it is to get that amount from plant food alone. Assuming the person is a healthy adult (children and infants being poor at this particular conversion), then he would need 10 to 12 times that amount in beta-carotene according to the later research on conversion rates. For the sake of simplicity, let's go with ten. So you need 100,000 IU of beta-carotene to get 10,000 IU of vitamin A.

You would have to juice about 1 pound 10 ounces of carrots *every day* to get sufficient vitamin A, provided you could make the conversion. If your conversion rate is 20 instead of 10, as studies show that some people have, you would need over three pounds of carrots a day![†]

I believe this is the reason that vegetarians and vegans who juice are healthier than those who don't. Norman Walker, a mostly raw vegetarian, lived to 109. Few people would sit down and eat over two or three carrots a day, but juicing makes it possible to eat many more.

For those who are carb sensitive, however, ingesting that many carrots is not a good choice. At 21,383 IU per cup (nearly 4 ounces), carrots just happen to be the vegetable highest in beta-carotene. Spinach, for example, has only 2,464 IU per cup

---

[*]The standard adult US RDA is actually 5,000 IU. Perhaps Masterjohn was referring to the figure for children. Since the adult RDA is 5000 IU, his argument becomes even stronger, greatly increasing the amount of produce that we would need to consume in order to get the necessary precursors from a plant diet.

[†]"Yet in the 1990s, this view began to change. In 1994, Suharno and others observed that pregnant Indonesian women were consuming enough carotenes to yield three times the recommended amount of vitamin A based on the WHO's conversion factor, yet large numbers of them were suffering from marginal vitamin A deficiency. Subsequent intervention studies aimed at Indonesian school children and breastfeeding women in Vietnam found that the conversion factor for carotenes to vitamin A in vegetables was 26 and 28 respectively, and 12 when the carotenes were consumed in fruit. In 2002, the US Institute of Medicine (IOM) established a conversion factor of 12 for beta-carotene, 24 for other carotenoids with vitamin A activity, and 2 for beta-carotene dissolved in oil. West and others criticized the selective use of studies employed by the IOM and suggested that beta-carotene from fruits and vegetables in a mixed diet has a conversion factor closer to 21."[10]

(about 2 ounces), so to get 100,000 IU, you would have to eat 40 cups a day! One cup of pumpkin (about 4 ounces) might be a better choice at 12,231 IU. You would need "only" eight cups a day of pumpkin. Two cups of mangos would give you 12,850, along with a load of carbs.

So, it would be very unlikely for a vegan to get enough vitamin A without juicing and taking supplemental beta-carotene. But don't take a beta-carotene supplement: massive amounts of this supplement increase oxidative stress and stimulate the production of enzymes that degrade true vitamin A, which was shown to lead to cancerous changes in lung tissue even worse than those seen from cigarette smoking in one controversial study![11] Of course, whole-food supplements don't have this potential drawback.

Fallon and Enig have another excellent article about Vitamin A online, "Vitamin A Saga."[12]

B Vitamins

Meat is rich in folic acid, vitamin B_{12}, vitamin B_6, and choline. These nutrients lower serum homocysteine levels, which is considered desirable as already mentioned. Note that overeating meat will result in increased methionine levels, *raising* homocysteine levels, so *balance* is key. B vitamins are found mainly in beans and animal foods. Choline is highest in eggs, beef, organ meats, and fish. In one study, pregnant rats were given choline supplements and gave birth to babies that had superior brains with great memories their whole lives.[13]

B_{12} is found in nutritional yeast, but not naturally: the yeast is fortified with B_{12}. Nutritional yeast is not the best food if you are dealing with candida overgrowth. It also contains mycotoxins and is nearly impossible to find in an uncooked state.[14]

B_{12} is also made in the colon and therefore shows up in feces. According to raw vegan proponent Dr. Cousens, we cannot utilize the B_{12} made in the colon because it is absorbed only from the small intestine.[15] This explains why so many animals facing a deficiency condition sometimes instinctively eat their own feces.

☞ It may be that *some* people can access the B_{12} made in their digestive tracts, which could explain why some can remain vegan for decades without experiencing deficiency symptoms.

There is evidence that if we properly fertilized the soil with a proper balance of natural fertilizers, compost, and manures of diverse sources, that some B_{12} could be made available through plant food.[16] An Iranian vegan sect that fertilized their vegetables with human feces, and then did not wash the vegetables, managed to get enough B_{12}.[17] This concept would not work in developed countries, since sewage sludge contains so many toxic chemicals from sources other than human waste.

Natives of India who foraged for wild greens got sufficient B_{12}, but when they moved to England where they bought greens at the supermarket, they acquired deficiencies. They had previously been consuming insect eggs from unwashed greens.[18]

Currently, there is no plant source found in nature with reliably significant amounts of B_{12}. Raw sea vegetables may have some B_{12}, but not enough to raise the B_{12} levels in humans. Dried seaweeds often have B_{12} analogues that actually *increase* the need for B_{12}. Even those who eat cooked meat can develop B_{12} deficiencies, because B_{12} is heat sensitive.

> *Even those at the low end of "normal" for B_{12} experienced some of the worst diminution of their brain tissues.*

B_{12} deficiencies can be serious, possibly leading to irreversible damage to the nervous system, including blindness, dementia, and degeneration of the spinal cord.[19] Often people with dementia are found to have a B_{12} deficiency.[20]

British scientists at the University of Oxford found that brains low in B_{12} actually shrink! Over a five-year period, people with the lowest B_{12} levels had brain shrinkage *six times* more than those with the highest B_{12} levels. Shockingly, even those considered at the low end of "normal" experienced some of the *worst* diminution of their brain tissues.[21]

B_{12} deficiency can be hard to detect before irreversible damage is done, as test results can be fooled by high intake of folic acid. Eating high amounts of green leafy vegetables increases folic acid to the degree that blood assays of B_{12} may appear normal while deficiency may be progressing and damaging the neurological system. For this reason, some prefer the more definitive urine test.

In my case, I had a B_{12} deficiency with symptoms that wouldn't go away with injections, sublingual pills, and even eating two or three raw egg yolks a day. I finally ate meat three to five times a week, and the symptoms began to disappear. I was back to normal when I began eating a tablespoon of freeze-dried beef liver from Argentina every day.

After my recent move to Ecuador, where supplements are scarce, I now eat fresh raw liver, frozen for two weeks to kill parasites and then blended with orange juice to chug it down. Adding ginger reduces bitterness. Not the best food combining, but as the Mary Poppins song goes, "A spoonful of sugar helps the medicine go down." Since it is blended, I have no trouble digesting it even though fruit doesn't generally combine well with meat. Also, acid fruits have more capacity to combine with other foods as compared to nonacid fruits.

Vitamin C

Some organ meats have vitamin C provided they are eaten raw. This is why the traditional Eskimos were able to get sufficient vitamin C. Most modern people would rather just eat fruit.

Vitamin D

The RDA for vitamin D is only 400 IU per day. This is supposedly attained by being out in peak sunlight hours for 15 to 20 minutes with a fair amount of body exposure, more for those with dark skin, yet many experts conclude that this is not enough. Dr. Price noted that robust people attained ten times the amount eaten in the American diet of his day, which was considerably more than Americans obtain today. The Weston Price Foundation recommends getting vitamin D from cod liver oil in addition to plant sources and sunlight: 1,950 IU per day for adults and 3,900 IU if pregnant or nursing.[22] Dr. Mercola recommends 5,000 IU a day for adults.[23]

Cod liver oil varies in the amount of D, so you have to read the labels carefully. This is because some manufacturers are afraid people might overdose on D and A. It may be true for synthetic vitamins, which can be toxic in high doses and concentrated forms, but the natural forms found in cod liver oil are safe in moderate amounts. On the other hand, some people think it is best to take a cod liver oil that is not artificially concentrated in D, but has the same A:D ratio that is found in the cod.

To get this large amount of vitamin D otherwise, one may have to spend hours sunbathing at peak hours in a swim suit. For example, if getting 20 minutes of sun exposure gives you the minimum requirement, you might need 10 times that, or 200 minutes!

I lived in San Diego, often called "Sun Diego" for its 70° F temperatures and sunny skies year round, and I know of no one who has the luxury of time to do that, especially considering that you get more sun horizontally than vertically. Most people work during the day. When they go for afternoon walks, it is not in their swim suits; neither are they lying horizontally.

Foods rich in vitamin D include fish, especially fatty fish like salmon, mackerel, tuna, and sardines. Surprisingly, pork lard is also rich in vitamin D. Free-range pigs are out in the sun a lot. They don't have fur to block the sun's rays, and it's fat tissue that stores vitamin D. Tara Weaver writes about visiting the Prather Ranch, where the proprietors noticed that their customers would lose weight and gain a twinkle in their eyes through eating lard![24]

There is some evidence that UV-zapped mushrooms contain vitamin D_2, the precursor to D_3, but it is questionable as to whether dietary D_2 is very effectively utilized in humans.[25]

Dr. Sarfraz Zaidi, MD, cites studies in his book *Power of Vitamin D* in which D deficiencies were linked to cancer, heart disease, diabetes, high blood pressure, fibromyalgia, kidney disease, osteoporosis, asthma, depression, and much more. He believes we don't get enough from the sun and diet combined, so we should take supplements.

Vitamin K_2

Vitamin K occurs in two forms: K_1 and K_2. When animals ingest K_1 from green plants, they convert part of it into K_2. This ability to convert K_1 into K_2 varies widely among species and is known to be weak in humans. Humans cannot absorb the amount of K_1 needed to convert to adequate levels of K_2.* The maximal amount of K_1 absorbed is thought to be around 200 micrograms a day. However, large amounts of K_2 are readily absorbed. Evidence shows that to acquire peak health, humans need K_2 in the diet.

A great online article about this, written by nutritionist Chris Masterjohn, contains 81 footnotes with scientific studies to support the above information.[27]

Humans cannot absorb enough K_1 to convert to adequate levels of K_2.

Dr. Weston Price discovered evidence of a nutrient he called "activator X." The vitamin hadn't yet been discovered, but he observed its properties and knew it was in animal fats and organs alone, not in plant food. He observed that it was important for tooth health, growth/development, reproduction, protection against calcification of the arteries, and brain function. He knew that it worked synergistically with the other fat-soluble vitamins A and D.

We now know that this mysterious activator is vitamin K_2. Vitamins A and D tell the cells to produce certain proteins, but vitamin K_2 is needed to activate those proteins. Those proteins can only function after being activated by K_2. K_2 is preferentially used by tissue to place calcium where it belongs, in the bones and teeth, and to keep it out of where it doesn't belong, in the soft tissues.

Dr. Price knew this mysterious nutrient was present in butter, but butter varies widely in K_2 content, making it not an ideal source. So he combined cod liver oil with butter as his protocol for reversing dental caries. This not only stopped tooth decay, but caused the dentin to grow and remineralize, sealing the once-active cavities with a glassy finish. Nutrition advisor Aajonus Vonderplanitz writes about his experience with this in his book *We Want to Live*.

K_2 has also been used in the treatment of epileptic seizures and rickets. Vitamin K_2 also prevents fractures, including the dreaded broken hip common in old age.[28]

Vitamin K_2 is needed by the heart. A deficiency of K_2 causes calcification of the cardiovascular system, which nearly everyone has to some degree by age 65. K_2 protects against inflammation and the accumulation of lipids and white blood cells that are found in atherosclerosis.

Vitamin K_2 is needed by the heart and brain. Autopsies showed that K_2 made up 70 to 93 percent of the vitamin K found in the human brain, where it helps synthesize the myelin sheath of nerve cells, which contributes to learning ability. Children's learning capacity has been found to increase with the addition of K_2 to the diet.

Deficiencies of K_2 have resulted in fatigue, learning disabilities, and even epileptic seizures. K_2 supports the enzymes that produce sulfatides (lipids in the brain). Autopsies of brains in the early stages of Alzheimer's show up to 93 percent lower sulfatide levels than normal.

More and more roles of K_2 continue to be discovered. The highest concentrations of K_2 have been found in the salivary glands and pancreas, so no doubt this vitamin is critical for their functions. A deficiency of K_2 is also thought to be a factor in kidney stones. K_1 is preferred by the liver to activate clotting factors, but most tissues prefer to use K_2 to activate the other K-dependent proteins. For example, to maintain bone health, the human body prefers K_2 to K_1.

The only plant food known to contain significant amounts of K_2 is natto, an Asian soy dish with

---

* "Humans appear to have a finite ability to absorb vitamin K_1 from plant foods. In the United States, where the mean intake of vitamin K_1 is less than 150 micrograms per day, blood levels increase with increasing dietary intake until the latter reaches two hundred micrograms per day, after which they plateau. In the Netherlands, where the mean intake of vitamin K_1 is much higher (250 micrograms per day), plasma levels of vitamin K_1 have no relationship to dietary intake at all. These results suggest that humans do not possess the ability to absorb much more than 200 micrograms of vitamin K_1 per day from vegetables."[26]

a very strong odor. It is fermented for a long time to get rid of the antinutrients in the soy. Sauerkraut also has a little. Animal sources include goose liver paste, hard cheese, soft cheeses, egg yolks, butter, chicken liver, salami, chicken breast, chicken leg, ground beef (medium fat), bacon, and calf liver. Some is also produced by bacteria in the gut of healthy people,[29] but as stated earlier, humans have a hard time absorbing the amount of K_1 needed to convert to adequate levels of K_2.

Cobalt

A cobalt deficiency occurs most often in vegetarians. Cobalt is a molecule that resides in the center of the vitamin B_{12} molecule. This mineral works with copper to help assimilate iron.

Coenzyme Q₁₀

The chemical *ubiquinone*, also known as coenzyme Q_{10}, or CoQ_{10} for short, is an essential nutrient for the heart and for the production of energy by the body's mitochondria. It is produced in the body from precursors found in nuts and seeds. It is also found fully formed in meat, especially hearts and livers.

Vegans may not get sufficient amounts of dietary CoQ_{10} or its precursors, so this is a supplement they might consider taking. As people age, their bodies are less able to manufacture or assimilate it from foods, vegan and nonvegan alike.

It's a very expensive supplement, and unscrupulous suppliers dilute it, with the FDA looking the other way. Finding a reputable vendor is important if you wish to supplement.

Iodine

Vegetarians often become deficient in iodine, and so even do omnivores who are aware of the toxicity of table salt, which is supplemented with iodine. People who cut down on meat and eggs, moderate iodine sources, often become depleted if they don't eat enough seafood, plants grown in iodine-rich soils, or iodized salt. One can be vegetarian, even vegan, and get sufficient iodine by incorporating small amounts of sea vegetables, especially kelp and nori, into the diet.

Iron

Iron and zinc are often deficient on vegan diets.[30] Iron is found in meat, fish, liver, eggs, and to some extent in green, leafy vegetables, especially spinach.

☞ Some people say a myth was created that spinach is high in iron when actually someone put the decimal point in the wrong place![31] In some databases, it actually doesn't have appreciably more than other greens. One database shows one cup of spinach (56 grams, or about 2 ounces) containing 0.8 mg of iron, with chard at 0.6, mustard greens at 0.8, kale at 1.1, and lamb's-quarters at 1.3.[32]

On the other hand, the famous Firman Bear Report from Rutgers University in 1948 found that spinach and other vegetables varied enormously in their iron and other mineral contents, depending on the soils in which they were grown.[33] Our soils have only deteriorated since that study was published.

Iron from animal sources, called *heme* iron, is more readily absorbed by the body than the nonheme iron of plant sources. In addition, there is an as-yet-unidentified factor in meat that enhances its absorption.[34] While 10 to 30 percent of iron is absorbed from animal foods, only 2 to 10 percent is absorbed from plant foods.

One study showed that nonheme absorption for lacto-vegetarian women was 70 percent lower than for the nonvegetarians who ate beef.[35] Phytates and oxalates (prevalent in spinach and existing in various degrees in all vegetation) interfere with its absorption. Women during childbearing years may have problems getting adequate iron on vegetarian diets, while iron is common in animal foods, especially liver.

Note that iron deficiency can be masked by inflammation. Chronic inflammatory disorders like arthritis raise blood iron levels, indicating that there is no deficiency when there often is.[36]

Too much iron is thought to speed the aging process.[37] Excess iron buildup in the brain can lead to dementia.[38] Iron surplus is also implicated in heart disease. As with everything, balance is key.

Zinc

The ideal dietary ratio of the essential minerals zinc and copper is thought to be as high as 8:1 zinc to copper.[39] The best sources for zinc are eggs and land animals, especially those with red meat. Plant foods are rich in copper but poor in zinc, with the exceptions of wheat germ and pumpkin seeds, so vegetarians and especially vegans may develop a skewed ratio of copper to zinc. High levels of copper in relation to zinc cause chronic fatigue. Low levels of zinc can cause infertility in men by decreasing sperm counts. This is why oysters, very rich in zinc, are considered aphrodisiacs.

Nutritionist Ann Louise Gittleman saw so many people with chronic fatigue as a result of vegetarian and vegan diets that she wrote a book about it. She found that the high copper in relationship to zinc also made it increasingly difficult to digest animal protein.

Many people switch to a lighter diet because red meats and other types of animal protein feel "heavy" in their system[s]. Ironically, this feeling can develop from copper excess or zinc deficiency (or adrenal insufficiency...). Individuals with cooper-zinc imbalance have trouble digesting and absorbing fat and protein in particular, so they often opt for diets that avoid foods rich in these nutrients.

At first it might be only red meat that feels like a brick in their digestive tract[s], so they avoid it. Then, as their zinc deficiency or copper imbalance gradually worsens, they begin having trouble digesting other types of animal protein and usually eliminate them one by one – first poultry, then fish, then eggs and dairy products, on down the line. Yet the more an individual with copper imbalance eats a low-protein, high-carbohydrate diet, the more his or her metabolism will slow; then, as a consequence, the copper overload will worsen and digestion will further decline.[40]

Gittleman points out that the problem with vegetarian and vegan diets is that they often contain grains and soy that contain zinc-inhibiting phytic acid. She says that research has shown that high calcium intake along with high phytic acid synergistically decreases zinc absorption. So if a person combines dairy or sea vegetables (rich in calcium) along with soy, grains, bread, cereal, or pasta, they will increase the likelihood of zinc deficiency.[41]

Furthermore, plant proteins (soy, other beans, whole grains, nuts, and seeds) are rich in copper. You may need to eat lots of pumpkin seeds or wheat germ to get enough zinc to balance out the copper. But if you ate a lot of pumpkin seeds or wheat germ, you would get an excess of omega-6 fatty acids and skew your omega-6:3 ratio.

Phosphorus

Meat is the most concentrated source of phosphorus. Phosphorus intake is often insufficient in vegetarian diets, which is another reason besides high-carb intake and low K_2 consumption for vegetarians' more frequent dental and bone problems.

Complete Amino Acid Profile

Unlike plant foods, meat contains not only the 8 essential amino acids, but also all of the other 14 standard amino acids found in the human body. The 8 essential amino acids are phenylalanine, valine, threonine, tryptophan, isoleucine, methionine, leucine, and lysine.

Vegan diets are often low in the following amino acids: lysine, methionine, carnitine, taurine, and tryptophan.[42] Plant foods are also low in cystine and threonine.[43] Some people cannot manufacture the supposedly nonessential (meaning that they can be produced in the body from precursors) amino acids taurine and carnitine but must get them from meat in order to be healthy.[44]

In order to get the amount of methionine, a precursor to the major antioxidant glutathione, found in just 8 ounces of elk meat, you would have to eat 22 heads of lettuce, 127 bananas, 550 apples, or 46 slices of bread![45] But eating excessive amounts of methionine can shorten one's lifespan, so balance is key.

If you choose to eat legumes, you will have too little methionine, and if you choose to eat grains, you will have too little lysine. This is why every culture traditionally combines beans (lentils, soybeans, et al.) with grains (rice, corn, et al.). The grain/bean combo is difficult to digest because of all the phytates and lectins. They are not our natural foods and were only introduced to our diets after agriculture and cooking began. Eating large amounts of them will bind minerals and create bloating and uncomfortable amounts of gas. This can be reduced if they are soaked, rinsed, sprouted, and/or fermented.

Meat has a comprehensive amino acid profile. Although plant combinations of grains and legumes can bring you all the eight essential amino acids, the case has been made that another eight should also be classified as essential. These are glycine, proline, arginine, glutamine, tyrosine, serine, cysteine, and taurine.[46]

Furthermore, Lindeberg points out in his nutrition textbook an intermediate category besides essential and nonessential amino acids.

A third group [is] thought to be conditionally indispensable, i.e. they must be supplied under certain physiological or pathological conditions.[47]

Could You Use More Energy? Carnitine in Red Meat

Meat is the only appreciable source of L-carnitine. Red meat, especially mutton and lamb, is the richest of all. Chicken and turkey also have carnitine, but not as much as red meat. Tempeh, tomatoes, asparagus, eggs, orange juice, and avocados contain only small amounts of carnitine.[48]

The mitochondria are tiny powerhouses within all of our cells other than mature red blood cells. They are rodlike structures that handle much of the process of turning food into energy. They produce 90 percent of the energy used by our cells.

> *Mitochondria produce 90 percent of the energy used by our cells.*

When I think of mitochondria, I am reminded of the Gary Larson (Far Side) cartoon in which a medical student was put in a straightjacket and sent to a mental ward due to his frustrations in trying to memorize the complicated Krebs cycle, which explains how energy is formed by the mitochondria. I sympathize with the student in the cartoon, since I had to memorize the Krebs cycle in college.

Nearly all the energy you get comes from the mitochondria, so you will be tired if they don't get the ingredients to do their thing. If they are healthy,

you will be energetic. An active, energetic body has more mitochondria in its muscles, healthier mitochondria, less fatigued mitochondria.

Nutrition expert Robert Crayhon compares the mitochondria to "nonstop parties." As we age, we party less, and so do our mitochondria.

Liven up your mitochondria with the right nutrients, however, and you will slow the aging process. ... A fish rots from the head down. The cells of your body rot from the mitochondria out. You are only as young and energetic as your mitochondria.[49]

He compares the mitochondria to our hearts. Our hearts feed oxygen and food to our bodies and speed away waste products. Think of the mitochondria as the heart of each cell.

[Carnitine is] the most important nutrient for increasing mitochondrial energy and efficiency. Carnitine keeps energizing compounds coming into the mitochondrial party. It also acts like a bouncer and quickly gets rid of anything that could slow the party down.[50]

Carnitine is used by the mitochondria to clear their waste products to avoid free-radical damage as a toxic by-product of food oxidation. It helps the liver protect itself from toxins. The liver is the body's chief organ of detoxification.

Carnitine is critical for producing energy and having an active metabolism. Carnitine escorts fatty acids from the blood into the cell for them to be burned in the mitochondrial furnace. Weight-loss gurus Nicholas Perricone (*The Perricone Weight-Loss Diet*) and Ann Louise Gittleman (*The Fat Flush Plan*) recommend taking carnitine supplements even if you *do* eat red meat!

Carnitine helps prevent muscle loss during illness and aging, offers liver protection, and helps the immune system. But it doesn't work without adequate omega-3 fats, and it should not be taken at night, as it can cause insomnia. People who have a tendency toward mania or manic-depression should avoid taking carnitine supplements.

Gregory Westbrook and his family spent several years as raw vegans. When their health failed, they slowly added some animal foods to their diets. They finally ate red meat, which because it is from a mammal and because it has received so much bad press, always seems to be the last thing a vegetarian dares eat. All of them remarked at how much energy they suddenly had. It was likely the carnitine that made red meat give them such an energy boost.

Carnitine has helped stabilize my blood sugar. When I eat red meat, I go a long time without any hunger.

Carnosine for Antiaging

Meat is the only significant source of carnosine — especially chicken, pork, and red meat.[51] It is also in eggs, cheese, and milk to a lesser extent.

Carnosine has well documented antioxidant, antiglycating, aldehyde-scavenging, and toxic metal-ion chelating properties. It increases the synthesis of nitric oxide and decreases erroneous protein synthesis.[52] It also helps suppress Alzheimer's disease.[53] This nonplant-source nutrient is a powerful antiglycating agent, meaning that it slows down the formation of the advanced glycation end products (AGEs) that age a person.[54]

Carnosine is one of the most potent inhibitors of the accumulation of cholesterol in atherosclerotic plaque.[55]

Creatine

Meat and fish are the best sources of creatine, an amino acid used to form ATP, the fuel which powers our cells. Creatine helps bodybuilders and improves exercise tolerance in patients with congestive heart failure.[56]

Taurine

Terrestrial animals and certain seafoods are rich in taurine. Taurine is important for cardiac function, vision, the brain, overall nervous system, and bile acid conjugation. It is also a detoxifier.

Infants, unable to manufacture it, depend on milk to get it. Even some adults have trouble synthesizing it. It is rare in plant foods, though found in red algae in high concentrations.

The plasma taurine concentrations in the vegans were significantly reduced to 78 percent of control values. ... Although taurine is synthesized in humans, the current study suggests that the rate of synthesis is inadequate to maintain normal plasma taurine concentrations in the presence of chronically low taurine intakes. ... Long-term adherence to a strict vegetarian diet may lead to clinical manifestations of taurine deficiency.[57]

Studies have found that neonatal primates developed abnormal eye function after being fed a taurine-free diet.[58] Herbivores, unlike primates, have an ability *three times greater than humans* to synthesize taurine. The inefficient status of human taurine synthesis suggests a long dependence on dietary animal foods.

Taurine is also great in assisting in relaxation and sleep. I have talked to several former vegetarians who sleep better after going back to eating meat, and this may be one reason for that.

Fat Profile

Few realize this due to the anti-saturated-fat campaign, but the main fat in bacon and red meat is actually *monounsaturated*, the kind found in olive oil, nuts, and seeds that lowers your LDL cholesterol and raises your HDL cholesterol. If an animal is grass fed, its polyunsaturated fats will also be the good omega-3 fatty acids. Even the saturated fats, as we have seen, are critical for physical and mental health.

Don't worry about the fat in meat unless it comes from factory-farmed animals, in which case you *should* worry due to toxins and the omega-6 overload. Studies show that a high consumption of lean meat, including red meat, does not cause dyslipidemia, a disruption in the kinds or amounts of lipids in your bloodstream.[59]

Conjugated Linoleic Acids

Conjugated linoleic acids are available in the meat of ruminants: cows, buffalo, sheep, goats. These fats help with losing weight and keeping firm muscles, according to researchers at the University of Wisconsin School of Medicine. Grass-fed animals have three to five times as much CLA as grain-fed animals. CLAs have promising health benefits that range from favorable body composition to reducing the risk of cancer and diabetes and lowering blood lipids. Animal foods provide 97.6 percent of the total CLA consumed, with beef providing over one-third.[60]

One study in Finland showed that a diet composed of CLA-rich foods may protect against breast cancer in postmenopausal women.[61]

Brain Foods

Seafood contains a number of nutrients beneficial to the brain. Fish, sardines especially, are rich in DMAE, which helps with learning, attention, memory, and behavioral problems. DMAE reduces anxiety, stops mind racing, improves concentration, and promotes learning.[62] Fish and shellfish are rich in the five minerals needed for brain development and function: iodine, iron, selenium, copper, and zinc.[63] One study also found that while cooking other meats reduces their B_{12} content, the loss of B_{12} from cooked fish is not high.[64]

Organ meats and mackerel have an abundance of *phosphatidylserine* (PS), a phospholipid which helps with memory, learning, vocabulary skills, concentration, mood, alertness, and sociability.[65]

As discussed previously in this book, fish is high in DHA and EPA, needed for intelligence and mental well-being. We need 300 to 400 mg of both DHA and EPA a day for maintenance and double or triple that to correct a deficiency.[66]

Unlike Plant Food, Meat from Organic, Free-Range Animals Contains Few Antinutrients

A plant can't run away, bite you, or claw you, so it evolved the defense of poisoning you with antinutrients. But once you are able to catch the running or fighting animal, it won't poison you. The factory-farmed animal is the exception. Poisoned by greedy, ignorant humans, it gets its revenge by passing along these poisons to whoever eats it.

Eating meat allows people to grow taller because there are no phytates to bind minerals crucial for growth. I once had a boyfriend from Bangalore, India, who was 6'2" in height. This is very unusual for India, where the average male is 5'7". He attributed his daunting stature to having been raised on meat, since he was a Catholic.

When you add meat to a diet, it displaces some of the grain and legume combinations which would otherwise be used for protein. The phytates in those plant foods block mineral absorption. This is espe-

cially true in cultures that don't soak, sprout, and ferment these foods. Their people wind up being shorter.[67]

Phytates are a leading cause of poor growth, anemia, immune system incompetence, and other health woes in Third World countries where plant-based diets are the norm and mineral deficiencies common. ... Although it is widely assumed that these plant foods contain plenty of phosphorus for growth, anywhere from 50 to 75 percent is bound up in the phytates and not readily bioavailable.[68]

Unlike plants, meat does not feed candida, especially when raw or lightly cooked. This is why it is commonly used on anti-candida diets such as the Body Ecology Diet.

Meat Is Easier to Digest Than Most Plant Foods

One thing I noticed when I resumed eating meat is that I had no digestive problems. My bloating was gone. I no longer had to wear stretch jeans so that after I ate I could still button them at the waist. Give me more than just a cup of sprouts or broccoli, even steamed to break down the cellulose walls, and I will look pregnant for sure — for hours. I will also get uncomfortable levels of gas.

These are low-calorie foods. If you don't eat much, you certainly can't sustain yourself on them. So I would eat a lot of nuts and seeds, even though I could only eat them in small amounts, including when presoaked and rinsed, without experiencing bloating and fatigue in their digestion.

I have heard many others make the same comments about meat being easier to digest than many plant foods. But some people, after going without meat so long, might have to ease into eating meat more slowly. It could be hard to digest at first.

My stomach's hydrochloric acid returned quickly however. I am a blood type O, which is said to have more hydrochloric acid, so maybe there is something to that theory.

For people who have lost much of their hydrochloric acid production from vegetarian diets, or simply from aging, it helps to take a tablespoon or two of raw apple cider vinegar or lemon juice along with the meal. Digestive enzymes can also help.

I have a friend who was hooked on antacids.

When she turned 60, I gave her a card that said, "A child of the '60s turns 60. Want to drop some antacid?" When I turned her on to lemon juice, she was grateful to get off the toxic antacids. Antacids can even lead to kidney stones.

Meat Is Satisfying and Nonaddictive

Meat is filling and satisfying, keeping the blood sugar stable. Meat is "unbingeable." No one feels like eating meat past the point of feeling full unless it has monosodium glutamate (MSG), salt, or sugar in it. Carbs, especially refined ones, can easily pull one into an addictive nonstop eating frenzy. Unadulterated meat, no matter how good it tastes, does not override one's natural feeling of satiety.

Meat Needed to Slow Muscle Loss in the Elderly?

Loss of muscle mass in the later years is a significant problem. The elderly lose their independence with the progressive loss of strength. In a 12-week study of 19 men aged 51 to 69, it was found that the men eating meat experienced greater gains in skeletal muscle mass and fat-free mass during resistance training than the lacto-ovo-vegetarian group, those who ate dairy and eggs.[69] Other studies have confirmed this association.[70]

> A vegetarian diet is associated with a lower muscle mass index than is an omnivorous diet at the same protein intake. A good indicator of muscle mass index in women seems to be animal protein intake.[71]

Yet another study documented changes in skeletal muscles at the genetic level (DNA transcription) induced by short-term inadequate protein intakes, as low as 7 to 10 percent of calories, in older humans. The changes were the kind that might precede adverse metabolic, functional, and structural events, including muscle wasting.[72]

What about *E. Coli* and Mad Cow Disease?

Outbreaks of *Escherichia coli*, or *E. coli*, poisoning and mad cow disease represent further reasons to make sure your meat comes from a healthy source. *E. coli* is a normal constituent bacterium in feces. The variant known as H157:O7 is formed when cows are fed unnatural diets, such as grains. The pH in the stomachs of ruminants changes when they are fed grains instead of grass.

This results in a change of bacterial communities living in a symbiotic relationship with their hosts. Among the bacteria taking charge is variant *E. coli*, which can displace good strains, leading to the bad results we have seen reported in the news. The cows are then given antibiotics because their stomachs cannot properly handle grains.

Another factor in *E. coli* contamination is the extension of meat with genetically modified soy, as GM soy is thought to be even more dangerous than *E. coli* from the guts of commercially raised cattle.[73]

Bovine spongiform encephalitis (BSE), or mad cow disease, was thought to result from feeding cows dead animals, which is not one of their natural foods. However, Creutzfeldt-Jakob disease (CJD), which is the human disease from eating the beef of cows infected with BSE, never showed up in the Shetlands where feeding cows dead animals was a common practice.

There is much evidence that mad cow disease occurred as a result of farmers treating their cattle with organophosphate pesticides in a warble fly eradication program.[74] After all, wild vegetarian animals like deer and squirrels develop a similar brain wasting condition. They don't eat meat, but they are exposed to pesticides. In addition, a similar disease is found in animals and humans living in areas of volcanic soils, where diets are high in inorganic aluminum and manganese, known to be toxic to the nervous system.[75]

Some people like to play it safe and purchase beef from New Zealand, where no mad cow disease has ever been found. Sure, it has a high carbon footprint, but so does importing plant super foods from Asia or South America. *Sometimes our health is just worth it.*

Meat Cautions

Don't overdo red meat. Eating an excess of even *raw* red meat can give you too much iron, leading to oxidative damage.[76]

Don't overdo meat high in purines, such as

sweetbreads, anchovies, sardines, liver, beef kidneys, brains, meat extracts, herring, mackerel, scallops, and some game meats. Overeating these can result in gout, an inflammatory arthritis caused by caused by elevated levels of uric acid in the bloodstream.

Overeating meat is implicated in Alzheimer's.[77] This is because cooked meat creates toxic heterocyclic amines. Many cured meats also contain nitrosamines, also implicated in Alzheimer's.

This doesn't apply if the meat is fish or poultry. These meats can actually deter Alzheimer's.[78]

About three to four ounces of meat a day is sufficient for many people. For some, just a few times a week is enough. American diets average nine ounces a day, an overdose for most of us. The meat also consists mainly of toxic factory farmed meat cooked at dangerously high temperatures.

Chapter 18

Dairy and Eggs

Love and eggs are best when they are fresh. —Russian proverb

There are many people who can get by perfectly fine without meat if they eat adequate amounts of quality dairy and/or eggs.

Dairy Contains Unique Nutrients, but Use with Caution

Like all foods, dairy should be consumed raw so that valuable nutrients are not destroyed, such as enzymes and biophotons, and toxic by-products of cooking are not produced. Homogenization also creates toxicity. Raw dairy may be hard to obtain if you don't live in a raw dairy state like California, don't live in a state that allows owning cow shares, or don't know any Amish folk willing to sell you some of their unadulterated, raw dairy products.

The Good

Dairy contains CLA if sourced from grass-fed cows, but CLA is also available in the flesh of ruminants. These fats help with losing weight and keeping muscles firm. Vitamin B_{12} is also more bioavailable from dairy and fish than from terrestrial meats.[1]

The fermented milk product kefir contains vitamins B_1, B_6, B_{12}, and K_2, produced by fermentative bacteria. In Russia, kefir was once thought to be the fountain of youth. It also benefits the liver, kidneys, and nervous system.

Russian biologist Elie Metchnikoff won a Nobel Prize for discovering the immune benefits of lactic acid bacteria. He observed that people living in the Bulgarian mountains experienced great health as a result of drinking a fermented milk called *yahourth*, which slowed premature aging by neutralizing toxicity in the gut.

Butter from healthy, organic, grass-fed cows is also now known to be healthful. Talk about a turnaround! I recall my mother used to pour butter on the vegetables in the pre-margarine era. When I memorized the calorie book at age 15, I decided butter, at 100 calories per tablespoon, was a waste of calories. I never ate butter again, save with the occasional baked potato.

More recently, I've read that butter was prized by those traditional peoples observed by Dr. Weston Price, especially the rich yellow butter churned from milk produced during spring season. Butter and cream from grass-fed cows is rich in true vitamin A and vitamin D, though concentrations vary according to the mineral levels of the soil and the amount of sun the cows get. These vitamins help absorb the nutrients of the vegetables.

I now enjoy lightly steamed broccoli and cauliflower with raw butter on them.

The Bad

Despite the many benefits that can come from even raw, fermented dairy, it will for me at least always be that forbidden lover I was never permitted to marry. An occasional exciting flirtation or fling is all I am allowed; otherwise, I am visited with constipation and asthma. This doesn't apply to butter or cream, as they do not contain casein, its most aggravating dairy protein.

Dairy was not consumed in paleolithic times. It began to be widely consumed only within the past 10,000 to 20,000 years as man domesticated ruminants, such as cows and goats.

Most people cannot digest dairy well. This is because we gradually lose the ability to produce the lactase enzyme required to digest milk sugar after weaning. People of nonwhite races usually are the most lactose intolerant and get constipated from dairy consumption. Some people have acquired partial adaptation through a mutation that continues lactase production beyond infancy. These people seem to be able to handle dairy fairly well.

This is especially true for people of Northern European descent, since they have thousands of years of tradition in milking cows. This mutation occurred about 8,000 years ago and spread throughout Europe, reaching frequencies of over 95 percent in Denmark and Sweden. A similar mutation in 90 percent of the Tutsi, a cattle-raising tribe in East Africa, has also made them more lactose tolerant.[2] However, tolerance signifies only partial adaptation, since complete biochemical adaptation at the cellular level can take 40,000 years or more.

Lactose, or milk sugar, can pose other problems. In one study on baboons, lactose produced more pronounced atherosclerosis than fructose, sucrose, starch, or glucose.[3] This effect is thought to occur because the lactose breaks down into glucose and galactose (another sugar), and galactose has a great potential to bind to proteins.[4] This glycation happens during heating, one reason pasteurized dairy is so harmful. Galactose is also thought to be responsible for an increased risk of cataracts in milk-drinking populations.[5]

Casein, the predominant protein in dairy, can also create problems for many people. This nonfat portion of milk has been implicated in prostate cancer.[6] Casein may even contribute to fatty liver.[7] Casein has been known to cause more advanced atherosclerosis, insulin resistance, and lipotoxicity than other dietary proteins in animal research.[8] It can also be very constipating. Casein is used in making glue — that's how binding it is!

Because casein is so binding, I would relegate dairy protein to the "treat" category even if you are able to tolerate dairy to some degree. Casein is needed in cow's milk for calves to build hooves and horns. Calves get weaned after six months, so why do people still rely on cow's milk decades later?

The Masai, an African herding population that drinks raw milk mixed with animal blood as a staple beverage, were shown to have generalized coronary atherosclerosis (arterial streaking) but no plaque formation.[9] The study author attributed this to the amount of vigorous exercise they got, resulting in strong hearts and wide arteries. It may also partly have been because they fermented the milk, which reduced the lactose content. Their raw milk also has the benefit of being unhomogenized.

Dairy has been suspected of being a main causative factor in Type 1 and possibly Type 2 diabetes.[10] In one study, milk consumption was attributed to 94 percent of the international variation in Type 1 diabetes. Big milk drinking countries like Finland and Sweden were at the top of the list. Japan, where dairy wasn't used much until recently, was at the bottom.[11]

Dairy may also stimulate the release of excessive amounts of insulin.[12] Two components of milk have been demonstrated to contribute to insulin resistance in animals: lactose and casein.[13] Whey, another milk component, is also thought to increase serum insulin levels.[14] It is believed that the foreign proteins in cow's milk are confused with similar proteins in human pancreatic cells.[15]

The most notable human exception for drinking the milk of another species would be infants who can't be breastfed and thus need goat's milk.

The Toxic

Unfortunately, even dairy from good sources is tainted with dioxins. These carcinogens accumulate in the fat, yet the fat contains many of the nutrients. Dioxins, toxic carcinogens produced as industrial waste products, are found in the soil. This winds up in dairy fats. Dioxins have been implicated as immune disruptors, cancer causers, endocrine disruptors, and reproductive disruptors.

For this reason, some believe that animal fats cannot be eaten with impunity as they were in traditional diets. Dioxins are also found in meat fats, but if you eat low-fat meat such as turkey or from wild animals, the amount is not enough to worry about. Butter and cream, however, are *purely* fat and therefore contain enough dioxins to be a concern.

On the other hand, abundant ingestion of foods rich in vitamin A has been found to buffer the effects of dioxins. Nutritionist Chris Masterjohn tears asunder the vegan claim that we should avoid all animal foods due to dioxin contamination in an article citing numerous scientific studies.[16]

Masterjohn provides evidence that the premodern groups that Price studied — who thrived on animal products — likely consumed levels of dioxin rivaling our own, *because much of the dioxin contamination comes from nature itself.* Since our ancestors were very healthy and were subjected to dioxins, perhaps these are not as bad as we think, *at least if we consume ample vitamin A,* as explained previously.*

---

*Chapter 17

Also, studies show that phytochemicals found in produce impede the action of dioxins.

Masterjohn notes that many of the toxic effects of dioxin are similar to the symptoms of vitamin A deficiency.

It appears that the capacity of dioxins to produce both cancer and noncancer toxicity relates to their ability to deplete vitamin A reserves and oppose the actions of vitamin A in the body.

Masterjohn cites studies showing that many of the effects of dioxins can be reversed with vitamin A and also examines evidence that dioxin is not nearly as toxic as has been supposed.

In some cases, as in Greece, dioxins are found primarily in plant foods. Vegetarian diets do not offer sufficient true vitamin A for protection, providing only the precursor beta-carotene.

Pasteurization/Homogenization Hazards and Politics

Many of the problems people have in digesting dairy are due to pasteurization. This process destroys its food enzymes, inhibits the growth of symbiotic bacteria, and fosters the proliferation of harmful gut bacteria. A survey done by the Weston A. Price Foundation found that 82 percent of the people who could not tolerate *pasteurized* milk exhibited no signs of lactose intolerance with *raw* milk.[17] Since most people stop making the lactase enzyme, they need to have it in the milk.

Pasteurization destroys the milk's own lactase enzyme content, which supplements whatever our bodies might also produce for digesting lactose. It also destroys the enzyme *phosphatase* that allows the body to absorb the calcium from the milk; the beneficial *lactobacillus* bacteria that produce B-complex vitamins; the "Wulzen factor," a cortisone-like chemical that prevents stiffness in the joints; the colloidal minerals; and enzymes needed for the absorption and utilization of the sugars, fats, and minerals in the milk.[18]

David Gumpert, author of *The Raw Milk Revolution*, notes the following.

More health and medical authorities are questioning whether the ever-widening use of sanitation techniques, including pasteurization, irradiation, the overuse of antibiotics, and even including sanitizing soaps and wipes, could be eliminating beneficial bacteria that not only keep pathogens at bay, but also boost the nutritional value of foods.[19]

Perhaps even more frightening than pasteurization is homogenization. This process breaks dairy fat into tiny droplets that are so small that they can actually get absorbed by the villi lining our small intestines. They make their way from there into our arteries, leading to all sorts of cardiovascular difficulties. Companies do this only because customers don't like to see the cream float to the top!

A book published in 1905 by Dr. Charles Porter, MD, *Milk Diet as a Remedy for Chronic Disease*, recommended raw milk as a cure for everything from asthma to rheumatism and high blood pressure. Milk "fasts," diets consisting only of raw milk for a period of time, often brought amazing results. This is thought to be due to the immune-boosting power of the amino acid *glutathione*, rich in raw milk and raw egg whites, which is destroyed by heat.[20]

A forerunner of the Mayo Clinic also praised the use of milk as an antidote to many illnesses. Much of the research demonstrating the health benefits of raw milk never made it into databases like PubMed because those studies were done before the 1960s, as far back as the databases reach.

Raw dairy's beneficial bacteria enhance the immune system and protect against allergies. Naturopath Ron Schmid explains in *The Untold Story of Milk* that the friendly bacteria in raw milk displace the potentially "bad" ones like salmonella and mutant *E. coli*.* He points out that raw milk from cows, goats, sheep, and camels was consumed for centuries without problems.

The Organic Pastures Dairy Co. has a relevant statement on its website.

It has been estimated that about 70 percent of the strength of a healthy immune system is made up of the diversity of living bacteria found in the intestines. Raw milk provides a perfect source for the 'seeding and feeding' of these diverse populations of living

---

*See chapter 5 of *The Live Food Factor* for a detailed explanation that it is really the biological terrain, or inner environment, that determines one's level of health. Bacteria are truly not to blame. In a suitably alkaline terrain, pathological bacteria do not proliferate.

bacteria. The average American diet is practically devoid of living bacteria. ... Our immune systems have suffered as a direct result. Consuming raw milk and dairy products is an important step towards regaining immune strength and overall health.[21]

Milk began to be pasteurized because factory farming and unsanitary conditions around the milk after it left the cow gave rise to the spread of tuberculosis, typhoid fever, and diphtheria via milk.

Now, however, conditions are more sanitary. In fact, you have *ten times* the chance of getting sick from *lunch meat* than from raw milk![22] Even pasteurized milk sometimes carries infection. Salmonella outbreaks can come from pasteurized milk, for example.[23] Yet state governments insist on pasteurization except for the states of California, Pennsylvania, Connecticut, Maine, Washington, New Mexico, Arizona, and Utah.

Why is this? Pasteurization persists due to dairy processor lobbying. For the shelf life of milk to be long, the bacteria — even the good ones! — have to go. But once that bottle is opened, pasteurized milk begins to decay and putrefy rapidly, whereas raw milk will remain good for a couple of weeks.

Since the small farmer cannot afford costly pasteurization equipment, the large dairy processors enjoy monopolistic influence over farm prices, profits, and politics. If the food production industry told us the truth, that pasteurization and irradiation is for *their* benefit though it compromises *our* health, we would not be happy campers. It is more convenient for them to lead us to believe that such practices are for *our* health rather than for *corporate* well-being.

Eggs: Surprising Super Foods

No animal dies when you eat an egg, unless it has been fertilized. Eating a fertile egg is tantamount to "chicken abortion" according to some. Most fertile eggs are so labeled. You will likely see a dot of blood in the yolk as the embryo forms.

If you are concerned about the conditions the chickens are subjected to, visit the source where you get your eggs. If you live in the country, raising your own chickens would be the ideal way to obtain eggs that you know come from organic, free-range cruelty-free chickens fed a diet rich in omega-3

foods.

A four-year experiment on mice was performed by Dr. Stanley Bass in which he subjected them to various versions of vegetarian diets. He found that raw diets were best, but not vegan ones, which turned them into cannibals, eating their babies![24] The ones fed raw egg yolks fared best. This report is available at his website, www.drbass.com.

Eggs are a super food. Dr. Eric Berg, DC, calls them "nearly the perfect food for health and weight loss." Eggs have a very high protein-efficiency ratio (PER). PER is based on the weight gain of a test subject divided by his or her intake of a particular food protein during the test period. In other words, eggs convert efficiently into muscle mass.

Chicken eggs have protein in almost exactly the proportions humans require. Dr. Richard Wrangham of Harvard University stresses the importance of that fact.

The match gives eggs a higher biological value – a measure of the rate at which the protein in food supports growth – than the protein of any other known food, even milk, meat, or soybeans.[25]

He cites a study done in Belgium in which cooking eggs increased the protein absorption by 40 percent, since raw egg white, which contains nearly half the protein, is poorly utilized. But since the yolks lose many of their valuable nutrients when heated, I advise cooking only the whites, which are unappetizing when raw and also contain the antinutrient protein *avidin*, which is neutralized by heat.

Avidin can neutralize the body's reserves of biotin, one of the B vitamins. Furthermore, lightly cooked egg white proteins do not get as badly coagulated as the proteins in cooked meat do.[26]

In recent years, the saturated fatty acid content of eggs, especially the palmitic and linoleic acid content, has decreased, while the omega-3 content has increased. Clinical studies show that the consumption of such omega-3 rich eggs has decreased the risk of cardiovascular heart disease.[27] Eggs that are from free-range chickens fed chia, hemp seed, flaxseed, or fish are best. The eggs should display "Omega-3" or "DHA" on the carton.

Eggs have numerous health benefits:

- The white contains 55 percent of the egg's protein, but most of the micronutrients are in the yolk.

- Egg yolk is a great source of lecithin, a fat emulsifier. Lecithin is the chemical phosphatidylcholine, which prevents the oxidation of cholesterol, protecting both the liver and arteries.

- Egg yolk is rich in vitamin B_{12}, selenium, and DHA (if the chicken was fed a diet rich in omega-3s).

- Egg yolk contains some vitamin A, vitamin D, vitamin B_2, niacin, folic acid, and choline, important for the nervous system and memory.

- Egg yolk also has the carotenoids *lutein* and *zeaxanthin*, which reduce the risk of cataracts and age-related macular degeneration. In one study, older subjects with low macular pigment ate four eggs a day for five weeks. Their macular pigment concentration went up, along with their HDL levels![28]

Eggs have been given a bad reputation for decades due to their cholesterol content, but Dr. Mark Hyman says this is not a problem.

Eating cholesterol does not raise your cholesterol. Nearly all the cholesterol in your blood is manufactured from saturated fats and sugars or refined carbohydrates.[29]

One man ate 25 eggs a day for 15 years and was found to have normal cholesterol levels![30]

Eggs themselves are not high in saturated fats, containing only two grams (the omega-3 eggs even less). Our bodies need the "good" cholesterol (known as HDL). Our livers make about 75 percent of the cholesterol we have in our bloodstreams, and they need lecithin to do it. Eggs are high in lecithin.

In fact, a study published in the *Journal of Nutrition* showed that including eggs in a calorie-restricted diet actually raised the serum HDL. The men in the study were eating three eggs a day.[31]

Like any other food you put into your body, eggs should be eaten raw or rare for optimal nutrition. For those of you who are old enough to remember, you used to be able to eat nearly all eggs raw before all the horrible factory farming came about. Back then most chickens were healthy!

In the movie *Rocky*, the boxer even chugs a bunch of raw eggs down. I recall in the late '70s when the restaurant chain Orange Julius came out,

making the smoothie a popular drink. They would add a raw egg to a smoothie of orange juice, bananas, and a little honey.

Nowadays you have to watch out for salmonella poisoning. You have to get raw eggs from a reputable source, and they should be labeled that they are from "organically raised free-range chickens." Often they will boast how much DHA each egg contains. These are top-dollar eggs, but they should be if you are going to eat them raw. The yolk should be bright orange, not a pale yellow commonly found in the factory-farm eggs.

Dr. Ben Kim recommends four measures to spot an egg healthy enough to eat raw: an intact shell, no bad odor, a white that is gel-like and not watery, and a yolk that is round and firm. The darker the yellow or orange color, the better. He warns not to overdo eggs, as one can develop an allergy to them by doing so. He says to eat three to five servings a week. Note that most people consider two eggs to be one serving.

I recommend not eating raw eggs until you know your immune system is in good shape. Keep some strong probiotics (beneficial bacteria) on hand, as well as charcoal, just in case you do get too much of the wrong kind of salmonella, resulting in digestive upset symptoms, such as cramping, vomiting, or diarrhea.

All the hype about the dangers of bacteria is often used as an excuse to pasteurize and irradiate everything. With a strong immune system, I would much rather take my chances on some *E. coli* or salmonella than on man-made chemicals, irradiation, pasteurization, or GMOs. Humans have lived with bacteria, viruses, parasites, fungi, and yeast throughout our existence. Man-made contamination has mushroomed only within the last century.

I have eaten *thousands* of raw egg yolks over the years. I got a touch of salmonella poisoning only *once*. I had bought the eggs from a new source at a farmers' market. I woke up in the early morning with painful abdominal bloating, which went away fairly quickly after taking some charcoal tablets. On a raw diet, we are filled with "good" bacteria that crowd out the "bad" bacteria. If you get a touch of "bad" bacteria, no big deal; just consume some probiotics.

People are amazed when I tell them I eat raw

egg yolks. Most find the idea *revolting* and scrunch up their foreheads in disgust. I tell them they could put the yolks in their smoothies, and they taste remarkable. For me, a yolk by itself is actually one of the most delicious foods I have ever eaten. Think of a soft-boiled egg; then multiply by many times the creamy texture and rich taste.

Certain people may have difficulty at first, such as the sick, the elderly, or those new to raw food diets. Also, if you suffer from high blood pressure, significant fluid retention, or inflammatory conditions like arthritis, bursitis, asthma, allergies, or skin rashes, Drs. Michael and Mary Eades advise limiting yourself to about six eggs a week. This is not because of the cholesterol issue, but because egg yolks are rich in arachidonic acid, one of the fatty acids that lead to the production of the "bad" eicosanoids that can worsen these conditions.[32]

Chapter 19

The Vegetarian "Conspiracy" and the China Study

Cooking meat can also cause many problems, and I believe it is in large part responsible for many of the valid findings Dr. Campbell observed. Unfortunately, it is also quite clear Dr. Campbell failed to appreciate the major dangers of meat and milk are related to cooking them. He makes the invalid assumption that raw and cooked (pasteurized) milk and meat are equally harmful. This is simply untrue and not at all addressed in his study or book.

—Dr. Joseph Mercola, MD

If you have read everything so far, you may have these questions: How did the idea that vegetarianism is more healthful become ingrained in our minds? And what about the China Study?

Is there a Vegetarian Conspiracy?

We know that the meat industry has been guilty of its share of hype and propaganda, but few people realize that the profit margin is so low that even factory-farm meat producers do not have the money to play with that the grain merchants do. Grains can be stored cheaply and are not as expensive to maintain as animals, so they create larger profits.[*]

By now you've seen how we were lied to about meat, saturated fats, and eggs — told that they were the culprits behind heart disease and obesity, when carbs and omega-6 fats from vegetable oils played a huge part.[†]

We were lied to about soy — told that it was the "health secret of the Asians" — when in fact Asians eat soy only fermented and only as a condiment. Eating soy the American way leads to cancer of the reproductive organs, thyroid problems, and Alzheimer's.

We were lied to about margarine — told that it was more healthful than butter when really it was a deadly trans fat.

We were lied to about grains, told that we needed 6 to 11 servings a day and that we needed the fiber from grains. Grains were even put at the base of the food pyramid, but now we know they are the base of many of the diseases of civilization, not to mention shrunken and arthritic skeletons.

Do people *really* take that government food pyramid seriously and eat 6 to 11 portions a day of grains? Or perhaps they do, which is why we have an epidemic of obesity and diabetes.

For me, it was the last straw when we were lied to about agave. I was so convinced that this was a health food that I ate it daily and even recommended it to others in my weight-loss e-book! But it turned out to be a more expensive form of high-fructose corn syrup. Use it in moderation in a raw dessert, if at all.

> *Grains are responsible for many of the diseases of civilization, not to mention shrunken and arthritic skeletons.*

How long is it going to take before we realize that we cannot trust any nutritional advice that comes from the corporate-controlled media? I finally decided to look to man's dietary history to find some answers, as detailed earlier in chapter 6. When I did, I was *shocked*. Have we been lied to about the nutritional "benefits" of a vegetarian diet?

History reveals itself in the bones, teeth, fossilized fecal matter, and tools, as well as in the spear dents in an animal's bones, indicating that man has been eating meat as long as he has been human, and his predecessors for 2.6 million years. That is

---

[*]See chapter 11.

[†]See chapter 12.

100,000 generations. If meat were so deadly and so unnatural for our digestive tracts, wouldn't we have figured out by now that it is inherently bad? Wouldn't we have become extinct by now?

But no, it is the rise of agriculture that appears to have brought on the shrinking of our brains, the rise of chronic diseases, and the extinction of many species. (If GMOs continue, this may include man.)

This brings us to the question, why did people ever think vegetarianism was superior? In reality, I doubt there was some conspiracy per se to make the masses strict vegetarians, but rather a series of misconceptions, lies, and philosophies that led to this idea.

The biggest misconception is that meat causes cancer. As we saw in chapter 6, it is not the meat *itself* that causes cancer. We have eaten it for 2.6 million years, plenty of time not only to adapt, but even to gain a *dependency* upon it.

Instead, three things happened with meat in the last century: *cooking temperatures* increased, *quality* deteriorated, and *consumption* increased to unhealthful levels in developed countries.

Meat that is heated will have cancer-producing chemical by-products called heterocyclic amines. The longer and higher the temperature at which it is heated, the worse it becomes.[1]

In the 1930s and 1940s, people started using more cooking gadgets. This may be in part because women joined the work force while men were fighting World War II. Cooking at high temperatures grew ever more popular with gadgets like barbeque grills, microwaves, pressure cookers, and even turkey fryers to deep fry your turkey!

It was around this time too that factory farming was in its rudimentary beginnings. Everything was becoming industrialized, mechanized. Food was becoming more processed, fractionated, and chemically adulterated.

Our way of eating meat has become toxic through factory farming: feeding animals unnatural diets, injecting them with chemicals, and preventing them from exercising. No wonder meat was thought to be toxic: meat in certain forms certainly *is* deadly!

The vast majority of modern meat is rich in omega-6 fatty acids instead of the omega-3s found in healthy, properly fed, wild animals. These omega-6s are at the root of many modern-day diseases, such as heart disease, insulin resistance, cancer, diabetes, and obesity.[2]

While some saturated dietary fat, as we have seen, is healthful, excess is known to be dangerous. Modern meat is full of saturated fat because the animals do not get proper exercise. Wild meat is extremely low in fat, and the unsaturated fat it does contain is mostly the omega-3s that our bodies and brains so desperately need to keep healthy.

> *If meat were so deadly and so unnatural for our digestive tracts, wouldn't we have figured out by now that it is inherently bad? Wouldn't we have become extinct by now?*

Even pigs that are allowed to roam in forests are found to have only 2 percent body fat, with a ratio of polyunsaturated fats to saturated fats of 2 to 1. A modern pig is about 40 to 80 percent fat with a ratio of polyunsaturated fats to saturated of 1 to 5.

Lunch meats and hot dogs are filled with cancer-causing nitrates and nitrites that have been proven to be ten times likely to induce bacterial illness than unpasteurized dairy. They also often contain soy-based meat extenders.

Also, as meat became cheaper with the factory farming, people started overdosing on it. The fast food industry created nations with some people thinking nothing of eating a couple pounds of meat daily!

Most of the experiments that "proved" meat causes cancer simply proved that factory-farmed, omega-6, fatty meat cooked in trans fats (typical at restaurants) caused cancer. I know of no experiment showing that cancer comes from eating moderate amounts of raw or lightly steamed wild meat or from consuming the flesh of 100 percent free-range animals pastured on organic feeds of their natural biological adaptations.

I have heard so many people, including several raw diet leaders, claim that meat in itself causes cancer. Yet the Eskimos had nearly no cases of cancer before they started cooking and eating Western diets that included grains and starches. People often associate meat especially with colon cancer, yet no one has been able to document one case of colon cancer among the traditional Eskimos.[3]

In an article written in 1952, three physicians from Queen's University in Ontario wrote this.

> It is commonly stated that cancer does not occur in the Eskimos, and to our knowledge, no case has so far been reported.

Yet their diet was nearly 100 percent meat much of the year. On the other hand, cancer has often been found in vegetarian populations like India.[4]

If meat were so toxic, why is it that people have been healed of diseases by diets high in meat and low in carbs? This is accomplished routinely by Drs. Stanley Bass and Ron Rosedale. I personally know a woman who was healed from advanced cancer using a raw organic meat diet. It should nevertheless be noted that appropriate raw vegan diets can also reverse cancer.*

☞ Just remember the 3 Q's: (good) *quality*, (low) *quantity*, and *quitting* (cooking) — or heating only at low temperatures.

· On the other hand, some people believe there *is* a sort of political conspiracy to restrain the intensely passionate activism of fervent young rebels via veganism. Former vegan Megan Mackin explains.

> It begins, eventually, to look like a very effective way to co-opt a movement: take the most passionate activist-minded, girls especially, and get their focus on a way of living that drains energies and enforces conformity in others. The Big

"It begins, eventually, to look like a very effective way to co-opt a movement: take the most passionate activist-minded, girls especially, and get their focus on a way of living that drains energies and enforces conformity in others. The Big Boys still run things, but now even more freely – without much interference."

Boys still run things, but now even more freely — without much interference.[5]

The blogger Natasha claims this is what happened to her. After years on a vegan diet, she recaps the results.

> I began to lose the will and the energy to do the vital work I had so loved. I no longer had the mental clarity to write my famous scathing exposés, or the physical energy to teach, organize, and build solidarity. I was sputtering out, grinding to a screeching halt. I realized that veganism, my choice to buy "cruelty-free" foods, was quickly becoming my only avenue for activism. It was the only thing I really had energy for anymore.[6]

The China Study

I quoted excerpts from Dr. T. Colin Campbell's book *The China Study* in *The Live food Factor*. For example, Dr. Campbell reached this emphatic conclusion.

> Nutrition [is] far more important in controlling cancer promotion than the dose of the initiating carcinogen.

When asked if he could make specific dietary recommendations for specific disease conditions, Campbell replied that he had come to see two truths from his decades of research. First, diseases all have "impressive commonalities." Second, the same good nutrition benefiting the body in disease prevention can also nourish a sick body back to health. In addition, *The China Study* implicates dairy in Type 1 diabetes, MS, osteoporosis, prostate cancer, breast cancer, and other diseases.

These are valuable observations consistent with hygienic principles of health.[†]

---

*See pages 55, 213, and 218 of *The Live Food Factor* for testimonials from people who partially or completely reversed cancerous tumors.

[†]The physiological Laws of Life that pertain to all life forms
(continued in the next column)

I also agree with him that overeating dairy casein is a factor in many of these cancers and with his conclusion that a plant-based diet is best for many people. However, when it comes to his idea that everyone can benefit from a strictly vegan diet, I have to part ways with Dr. Campbell.

Dr. Campbell's book is often used by vegans to prove the superiority of their diets, since lower rates of cancer and heart disease were found in those Chinese populations eating plant-based diets. But close examination of the actual China Study research data on which Dr. Campbell based his vegan conclusions paints a rather different picture, as we shall see.

Participants likely consumed cooked animal protein and pesticides abundantly

A main issue with the China Study is that the Chinese, like Americans, eat nearly all of their meat cooked. Colin Campbell admitted in an e-mail to my editor that his interviewers made no attempt to find out how much, if any, of their meat consumption was raw. He assumed it would have been a rare practice and so didn't think it was an important question to ask.

I learned while in acupuncture college that the Chinese are not even close to being raw fooders. They believe in a mostly cooked diet. We already know that the cooking of meat is a significant cause of disease.

The other problem with meat, both cooked *and* raw, is that the higher up on the food chain you eat, the higher the concentration of pesticides, heavy metals, and other industrial contaminants you are eating and accumulating in your own fat tissues. Some pesticides actually become "activated" — more carcinogenic — by heat, and most meat is eaten cooked.

Folks didn't have to worry about this in paleo days, so they could get away with more meat in their diets. We *do* have to worry today, even with naturally raised animals. You can't control the air pollution, water pollution, and often low-quality feed. Today's environment is so much more polluted that the lower you can healthfully go on the

food chain, the better your chances of avoiding degenerative disease conditions.

Another concern with conclusions drawn from China Study data is that China does not have the constraints that we have here regarding the use of extremely toxic pesticides like DDT. When I was a practicing acupuncturist, I always obtained my Chinese herbs from US sources for this reason. Since pesticide toxins collect in animal fats, my hypothesis for why the study showed cancer increasing as cholesterol consumption increased is that it involved the consumption of such tainted animal fats.

It is true that in the first part of the study, many of the farmers likely did not use pesticides, but as China opened up to trade in the '70s and grew more prosperous thereafter, pesticide use expanded to levels unseen in most countries.

How healthy were those eating extremely low-animal-protein diets?

Dr. Campbell says that there is a "myth" in the US that health problems can arise if cholesterol levels get below 150 mg/dL.[7] He says that 85 percent of rural Chinese have such low cholesterol. But the study apparently did not test for *psychological* health, which is affected by low cholesterol, as we saw earlier in chapter 11. Studies link extremely low serum cholesterol levels to depression, irritability, and even violence and suicide.

In a country like China, where there is strong social cohesion and peer pressure, we may not expect to see much violence, because a person knows he could be executed for it. However, it would have been interesting to test the people in the experiment for depression and irritability. What was their happiness quotient on a scale of 1 to 10?

I also wonder if they compared the intelligence of those with low quantities of animal products to those with higher intakes, since our brains evolved on animal foods like eggs and fish. A person can be free of cancer and heart disease, but it is hard to have healthy intelligence and emotions without brain food.

Yet Dr. Campbell insists that "eating foods that contain any cholesterol above 0 mg is unhealthy." That would exclude nearly *all* of the most potent brain foods! What good is cardio health if you lose your intelligence and happiness?

---

are explained in Appendix F of *The Live Food Factor*.

Furthermore, a lack of observable disease does not imply health. Dr. Price reported that he could not find a vegetarian population with superb health. Did the "healthy" China Study subjects demonstrate the robust levels of health Dr. Weston Price found in traditional omnivores?

In fact, they did *not*. Campbell points out that the rural Chinese may not have had cancer, the "disease of affluence," but they often had pneumonia, tuberculosis, intestinal obstruction, rheumatic heart disease, and many other "diseases of poverty" caused by "nutritional inadequacy and poor sanitation."[8]

Studies show that one's immune system can be lowered by consuming insufficient quantities of *methionine*, an amino acid that has been found to play an important role in immune function. It occurs abundantly in flesh, as well as in nuts and seeds.[9] For example, G. Martin got infections easily when he was vegan.[*] Other nutrients are difficult for some people to get on a plant-only diet.[†] Many other nutritional deficiencies can be avoided in some people, but only if the "veg" diet is carefully planned.[‡]

So take your pick:

- diseases of poverty/*deficiency*: very low animal protein diet,

- diseases of affluence/*excess*: high animal protein diet, *excess*), or

- peak health/*balance* — moderate but adequate animal protein diet.

I know what my choice is.

Is there an Asian advantage favoring agricultural adaptation?

The China Study subjects were of similar genetic stock. For example, we know that most Japanese do well on high-plant diets combined with fish. They are mostly of blood type A. When people used to ask me what I thought of the blood type diet, I would dismiss it with the comment that there weren't enough studies.

Then I read the book *The Answer Is in Your Bloodtype* by Dr. Steven Weissberg, MD, and Joseph Christiano, APPT. This study involved 5,000 people, which is enough to give some credence to a theory. Interestingly, 36 percent of the group of 5,000 proved to be of blood type A. This coincides nearly with the 25 to 33 percent that are estimated to do well on a high-carb diet — those who do not easily get resistant to insulin.

If the blood type theory has validity, it appears that I do need some animal protein, since I have the most prevalent blood type, type O. Dr. Mercola has blood type A and fared poorly on vegetarian diets, so not *every* individual will fit the blood type profile. This theory could just reflect a tendency if it's valid at all. I do know three leaders in the raw food movement who are a type O and do well without animal products, though they take a lot of dietary supplements.

For some reason, it does appear that Asians do better on vegetarian or at least high-carb diets than most people. The Hunzas, known for their superb health, were from India and ate nearly vegetarian diets, eating meat only once every two weeks or so, though they did consume dairy regularly.[10] When I looked at studies on vegetarianism and osteoporosis, the studies I encountered in which people's bone densities fared best on meatless diets were in Asia.

My theory is that Asia, the cradle of civilization, has long been overpopulated. They have had less room to raise animals as a result. Eating less meat for thousands of years has given them more time to adapt. Agriculture in China is thought to have begun as early as 15,000 years ago. This clearly gives many Asians a slight evolutionary edge over other ethnicities when it comes to adjusting to carbs and grains. Anthropologist Geoff Bond claims that agriculture didn't catch on in the British Isles until as recently as 2,000 years ago.

Another factor is that rice makes up a large component of the Asians' carbohydrate allotment. Cooked whole rice is moderate on the glycemic index, much better than all the high-fructose corn syrup, sugar, and refined wheat eaten by Americans and Asians who dine at American restaurants. Several experts on various metabolic types indicate that Asians are in a category of their own by doing well

---

[*]Chapter 5.

[†]See chapter 17.

[‡]See chapter 26.

on low-fat diets.[11]

Where are the Chinese vegans?

Campbell makes the point that a diet low in animal products can be healthful. He includes an eating chart in his book which merely suggests minimizing animal products because he realizes most people won't become strict vegans out of habit. But in his commentary on the previous page, he reaches this conclusion.

> So it's not unreasonable to assume that the optimum percentage of animal-based products is zero. ... My advice is to try to eliminate all animal-based products from your diet.[12]

I'm all for plant-based diets, but it is folly to say that *zero* animal products — or the less, the better — is even *more* healthful. Such logic would require one to think that since *excess* oxygen is toxic, we should strive to live with *zero* oxygen.

The fact is, *none* of the people in the study group were *100 percent* vegan! They simply ate diets very high in plant food and low in animal products. I cannot argue with that, but to take it to the extreme of eating *no* animal foods is just as radical as eating no *plant* foods — perhaps even more radical. At least we do know of a race that survived and thrived on very little vegetation: the Eskimos.

Campbell has a chart that demonstrates that Americans typically get 10 to 11 percent of their calories from animal protein, while the Chinese typically get only 0.8 percent of their calories from animal protein.[13] Yet you will see upon closer examination an asterisk by the 0.8 percent, indicating that this is the *nonfish* animal protein. They could be eating a great deal of fish, definitely an animal food as well as a brain food, and yet we wouldn't know it from this chart! Yet he urges people to go vegan, which means not even

eating fish.

It's ironic that a study done in China is supposed to prove that vegan diets are superior. Having a master's degree in Chinese medicine, I am well aware that animal products are considered super foods in Chinese medicine. Among the hundreds of medicinal potions, it's the animal products that are cherished the most. Used are such ingredients as silkworm, antelope horn, male seal genitalia, geckos, clamshells, seahorses, pipefish, and tiger bones among their healing pharmacopeia.

Most Chinese cannot afford to eat animal foods freely because of overpopulation, but were someone set on becoming vegan, his doctor would sternly warn that he has enough *jing* (vital essence) stored up to last only a few years. The Chinese did not know about vitamins thousands of years ago. No one did. But they and most of the traditional peoples Dr. Price observed were correct in the observation that the human body can store the various nutrients found only or primarily in animal products for about two to ten years. After that, the person may develop deficiencies.

Campbell claims, "There are virtually no nutrients in animal-based foods that are not better provided by plants."[14] But as we have seen, many people are not efficient at converting plant-based precursors into those end products found only in animal foods: vitamins A and K_2, DHA, EPA, et al.

Interestingly, another study done in China seems to prove the opposite of Campbell's claim. An extensive study found that in a region in which large amounts of whole milk was consumed, half the rate of heart disease was found compared to the rate in an area in which only small amounts of animal products were ingested.[15]

> *I'm all for plant-based diets, but it is folly to say that zero animal products – or the less, the better – is even more healthful. Such logic would require one to think that since excess oxygen is toxic, we should strive to live with zero oxygen.*

> *Animal products are considered super foods in Chinese medicine.*

What other critics have to say

One of the criticisms about the China Study is that it was only epidemiological, noting correlations without corresponding verification tests. Correlation does not prove causation. Dr. Michael Eades explains that observational studies only provide data on which people can form hypotheses, which later need to be proven in rigidly controlled studies.[16]

An example of "correlation never proves causation" would be the following: Suppose a study shows that in a certain population, eating mustard correlates with constipation and brain fog. People conclude they need to stop eating mustard. In reality, it may be the wheat in their sandwiches causing those health issues because everyone in the population is putting mustard on bread.

Probably the biggest criticism of the study is that Dr. Campbell cherry-picked his correlations and was caught by Chris Masterjohn and Anthony Colpo.[17] Both point out that Campbell cites a study by Dr. Lester Morrison as proving that a low-protein diet helped reduce heart disease. Yet the study in fact had the patients eating several ounces of meat a day — low by American standards, but nowhere close to vegan!

There is even more. Campbell apparently ignored information from data that disproved his case, data from both the study on Chinese people as well as from his rat studies.

Masterjohn cites another indication of Campbell's having selected only the evidence favoring veganism in two tables.[18]

In the first table, variables are correlated with cancer *occurrence* in Chinese households. It shows highly significant correlations between *total* protein consumption and cancer incidence (+44%) and also between *animal* protein consumption and cancer incidence (+42%). In this table, fish consumption is *negatively* correlated with cancer incidence (-15%), yet Campbell apparently ignores this when he says we should minimize animal protein in our diets and strive for veganism.

The second table shows the exact same variables correlated with overall cancer *mortality* in China, but it shows different numbers. This table shows an *insignificant* correlation between total protein consumption and cancer (+12%) and an even *less* significant one between animal protein and cancer (+3%).

In the second table, ingestion of carbs is more significantly related to cancer (+23%) than total protein (+12%), animal protein (+3%), fish (+7%), and other meat (-20%) — all put together!

What both tables also agree upon is that cancer correlations were -36 percent (Table 2) to -42 percent (Table 1) in hot climates. No doubt it was the vitamin D from soaking up sunshine.

Masterjohn even went to the source data that Campbell used for the conclusions in his book. He found that many animal foods were not even covered by the survey! These included organ meats, insects, bone, and bone marrow, all of which the Chinese eat.

Additionally, the autumn dietary survey did not take into account foods that were not in season at the time. So the people could have been eating several animal products that were not listed on the survey. This means they may have been getting significantly more animal foods than were reported.

The Chinese could have been eating several animal products that were not listed on the survey. This means they may have been getting significantly more animal foods than were reported.

The questionnaire also did not distinguish between fish and shellfish despite their very different nutrient profiles. It didn't cover nutrient differences among foods grown in different soils.

I would add that the survey also left out those super foods used in traditional Chinese medicine, which include obscure but highly nutritious items like silkworm, antelope horn, male seal genitalia, geckos, clamshells, seahorses, pipefish, and tiger bones.

Dr. Price found that those on low-protein diets could do well only when the animal protein consumed was of very high quality.

After studying Campbell's raw data, Masterjohn drew this conclusion.

It is interesting to see ... the general picture that emerges. Sugar, soluble carbohydrates, and fiber all have correlations with cancer mortality about seven times the magnitude of that with animal protein, and total fat and fat as a percentage of calories were both negatively correlated with cancer mortality.

In other words, carbs correlated with cancer seven times more than animal proteins did, and low-fat diets correlated positively with cancer!

In other words, carbs correlated with cancer seven times more than animal proteins did, and low-fat diets correlated positively with cancer!

Supporters of the China Study will often cite studies by Drs. John McDougall and Caldwell Esselstyn that allegedly confirm its results.[19] Masterjohn examined those studies. Neither had control groups. McDougall's patients were on low-calorie diets and lost an average of seven pounds. This, and not the low animal protein, could have been what helped their arthritis.

In Dr. Esselstyns's case, half of the patients (11 of 22) dropped out during the ten-year study. Since there was no control group, did the high drop-out rate come from patients that felt their low-fat vegetarian diets made them feel less healthy? We don't know. Furthermore, the results were successful — decreased blood vessel occlusion — only in 5 of the 11 patients who remained in the study.

Masterjohn points out other flaws in *The China Study* book, including the following: In the rat studies, Campbell lumps milk protein casein in with other animal products as "nutrients from animal-based foods." The oft-quoted conclusion that we should eat no more than 5 percent of our calories in animal foods was "proved" by a rat study in which the protein used was isolated casein. In other words, a *dairy* product not even whole, but *fractionalized,* and no doubt *heated* in its processing is *generalized* to include *all* animal proteins!

On top of that, casein is known to be implicated in cancer from various other studies.[*] If whole eggs, chicken, or fish had been used raw, there would very likely have been much different results.

Dr. Campbell makes this farfetched generalization.

The finding: casein, *and very likely all animal products* [my emphasis], may be the most relevant cancer-causing substances that we consume.[20]

This is a huge flaw since many, including myself, who can digest *meat* well, will have problems with *dairy*.

As Masterjohn points out, the casein used in the cited experiment was extracted from whey, which is known to have some protective effects against cancer. Furthermore, he adds that the true vitamin A found naturally in whole animal foods is known to have many protective effects against cancer.

Dr. Campbell stresses in his book that the rat study "proves" that animal (actually fractionalized dairy) protein leads to cancer, while plant protein (wheat) does not. But blogger Denise Minger dug up one of these studies. She found that when the amino acid lysine was added, the plant food lost any advantage.

This is important because no one eats just wheat or other grains low in lysine. To make complete proteins, all vegetarians and vegans instinctively seek out complementary proteins that contain lysine, such as beans. In other words, Campbell's argument only applies to *incomplete* proteins, which doesn't happen in human diets.

The rat study that Denise found added lysine to the wheat.[21] When lysine was added to the wheat protein, it had the same detrimental effect as casein! The study implies that the only reason wheat protein didn't promote cancer was that it was *not a complete protein*. This seriously jeopardizes Campbell's claim that animal protein correlates with cancer while plant protein seems protective of cancer.

Things get even more bizarre. Masterjohn analyzed several of the rat studies performed by Campbell et al. that were never cited in the book because

---

[*]See chapter 18.

they did not prove his point.

In one of them, the 20 percent casein diet got spiked with double the amount of the toxic aflatoxin that the 5 percent casein group got (5 ppm as opposed to 2.5 ppm) because "5 ppm was found to be lethal for this dietary group."[22] *What?* Wasn't the low-protein diet supposed to protect them from cancer? Apparently not in this case. It made the carcinogen more deadly!

Masterjohn notes the results of one study.

Twenty percent casein diets promoted the growth of precancerous lesions when they were fed to rats already dosed with aflatoxin, but protected against the formation of precancerous lesions when they were fed to rats before, during, and soon after the dosing period.[23]

In other words, this dairy protein can actually be *protective* against cancer, unless eaten after precancerous lesions have already formed!

Dr. Mercola points out that Dr. Campbell never had a practice and *never saw real-life patients*. Mercola, on the other hand, has had 25,000 patients and witnessed many of them grow unhealthy on the type of diet proposed by Campbell and regain their health on diets that included some meat.

In many cases, the data (presented in arduous detail in the book *Diet, Life-Style, and Mortality in China*) do not show statistically significant correlations between animal protein consumption and disease such as cancer at all. On the contrary, it would seem that sugar and carbohydrates are correlated with cancer — not animal protein. In addition, the data indicate that fat is negatively correlated with cancer mortality, which again contradicts the claim that meat is harmful.[24]

In that same article, Mercola explains that he himself went on a raw vegan diet loaded with fruits and vegetables and saw his fasting triglycerides shoot up from 100 to nearly 3,000!

Another critic of the China Study is Professor Cordain. He wrote a paper found online that refutes the low-protein theory. He cites studies showing that animal protein is needed and nontoxic in amounts above what Campbell recommends. Cordain's conclusion:

Accordingly, the fundamental logic underlying Colin's hypothesis that low-protein diets improve human health is untenable and inconsistent with the evolution of our own species.[25]

The subtitle of *The China Study* boasts *The Most Comprehensive Study of Nutrition Ever Conducted*. Yet Dr. Weston Price's epidemiological study lasting many years covered several continents displaying a myriad of genetic variations. I would argue that his book *Nutrition and Physical Degeneration* deserves that subtitle. He found no evidence of a vegan or vegetarian people with robust health in any of the populations he examined.

Major Flaws in the China Study: A Summary

- The China Study was observational in nature (correlation doesn't prove causation).

- The idea that animal protein causes cancer dismisses the evolutionary science of anthropological nutrition. It fails to take into account all the evidence that man has eaten meat for 2.6 million years and that our brains depend on seafood nutrition, proven in countless studies. These were carefully controlled studies.

- The China Study was interpreted by someone with no actual clinical experience in dealing with the unique nutritional needs of individual patients.

- It was done in China where strictly vegan diets are neither practiced nor encouraged, making it highly unlikely that anyone was close to being vegan — though Campbell concludes that veganism is superior, based on data from this study.

- The food eaten was largely cooked, and we know that cooked meat is toxic.

- A corroborating rat study used isolated casein, which lacked protective factors in whey and the vitamin A contained in whole dairy foods.

- The survey questionnaire ignored several animal foods customarily eaten by the Chinese, including medicinal super foods used in traditional Chinese medicine. This makes it likely their animal protein consumption was significantly higher than estimated.

- People were not tested for mental health and intelligence, in which cholesterol plays a role. Lack of cancer does not indicate robust health.

- Rat studies that did not support Campbell's thesis were omitted.

- Those on very low animal protein diets often died of diseases related to immune deficiency, possibly due to insufficient methionine. But they likely suffered other deficiencies as well (chapter 17).

Part 4

Morality, Spirituality, and Sustainability of Eating Meat

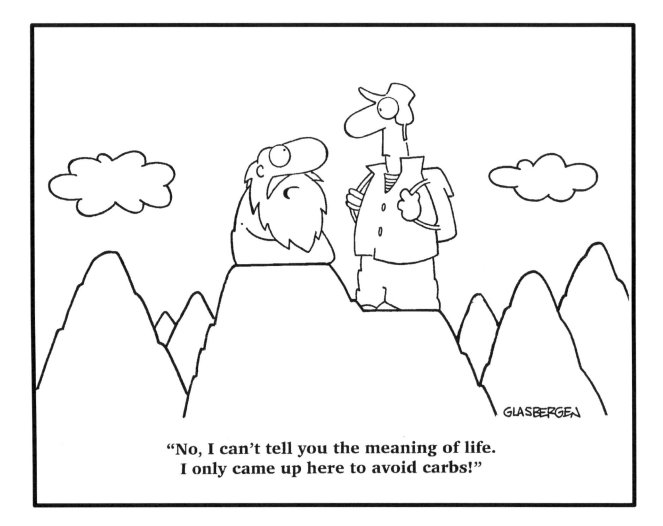

"No, I can't tell you the meaning of life.
I only came up here to avoid carbs!"

Chapter 20

The Morality of Eating Meat

No matter how cute Wilbur the pig may be, if it comes to me or him, he's going down.
—Tara Weaver, *The Butcher and the Vegetarian*

Throughout human history, people have eaten animals. It is the way of the earth. Animals eat other animals. Only herbivores are nearly vegans, and some of them even have several stomach sections to digest the cellulose. They also inadvertently consume insects.

Philosopher Frederick Ferre notes this.

Except for the green plants ... all life on earth feeds on other life for its very existence. From the broadest biotic perspective, life is cannibalistic upon itself. An ecological ethic must begin with the affirmation of this nutrient cycle.[1]

Dr. Bass told me that often he gets vegan patients who won't eat eggs even when their health depends on it, insisting it would be immoral. Dr. Bass will ask them, "If it is immoral, then why would God or the Universe set things up so that most of the living creatures on this planet depend on eating other creatures for their existence?"

"In the strict scientific sense we all feed on death – even vegetarians."
—Mr. Spock, "Wolf in the Fold"
Star Trek episode

We cannot deny that on this planet, at this time, it's a creature-eat-creature world. Benjamin Franklin was vegetarian at age 16. It didn't last long. He went on a fishing voyage and smelled the fish frying. He debated about whether he should eat any. Then he noticed that when the fishes' stomachs were opened, there were tiny fishes inside them. He then reasoned that if these fish eat *one another*, there was no reason he shouldn't be eating *them*!

Compassionate carnivore and sustainable farmer Catherine Friend makes a further point.

Acknowledging that livestock animals have personalities and emotions doesn't mean, for most of us, that we can't eat them. Instead it means we must work harder to ensure that their lives are better than they are now. Better lives mean happier animals.[2]

I have heard many say, "I would rather die than eat an animal!" Examine that thought. It is truly a noble thing to sacrifice your health or your life for a worthy cause, but is this cause truly worthy? Are you really willing to sacrifice your health and your vitality for your philosophy, beautiful and idealistic though it may be, in order to avoid eating animals, or even eggs or dairy? What about the animal that is nearest and dearest to you, *your own body*?

People tell me, "I'm a vegetarian because I love animals." Sometimes it's said with an insulting implication that I *don't* love animals because I eat meat. In fact, I adore animals. But my favorite pet happens to be my own body, which functions better with meat.

If a vegan or vegetarian diet is ruining your health, consider that it might also ruin the health of others. What if everyone on the planet became vegan or vegetarian and half were healthy, but the other half grew emaciated (often happens to men), overweight (sometimes happens to women), or nutrient deficient? Is that such a great cause, for people to have poor health in order that some animals live a bit longer?

Vegetarians think that we, unlike other animals, are capable of moral decisions and thus should not eat animals, since we have other food options. I argue that most of us would reach mediocre levels of health at best without a bit of flesh. I was a raw vegan for about six years. For about a year after that, I secretly ate raw eggs and some raw dairy (kefir and goat cheese) before I came out of the nonvegan closet.

This was because the nutritional deficiencies of vegan diets often take years to show up. When I began to eat a little raw meat, just three to six ounces a day, I felt better than ever. My blood sugar stabilized, and I never had food cravings. I was no longer bloated, often a sign of high blood insulin levels or gut fermentation. I slept better than ever, often not waking up once throughout the night.

Yet I knew I could not tell anyone but my husband and my omnivorous friends. Within the social circles I frequented, this would have been likened to a steadfast Christian announcing to her pastor and churchmen that she had decided to "switch teams" by becoming a Satan worshiper. The shock effect would be no less. "Meat is murder" goes the slogan.

Animal activist Peter Singer argues that we must choose between "a lifetime of suffering for a nonhuman animal and the gastronomic preferences of a human being."[3] I would argue that it is not a matter of satisfying the taste buds. Indeed, for most of us, it is *carbs* that are much more tantalizing! Rather it's that most humans really do need at least some meat for optimal health. Furthermore, it is now possible to purchase meat from free-range facilities where animal suffering is minimized.

If you think no one died for your vegetarian meal, you are mistaken. Think of all the animals that are now extinct — entire species gone forever — due to clearing land for farming.[*] Sally Fallon elaborates.

> Not a single bite of food reaches our mouths that has not involved the killing of animals. By some estimates, at least 300 animals per acre — including mice, rats, moles, groundhogs, and birds — are killed for the production of vegetable and grain foods, often in gruesome ways. Only one animal per acre is killed for the production of grass-fed beef, and no animal is killed for the production of grass-fed milk until the end of the [useful] life of the dairy cow.[†]

> And what about the human beings, especially growing human beings, who are suffering from nutrient deficiencies and their concomitant health problems as a consequence of a vegetarian diet? Or does only animal suffering count?

---

[*]Fruitarians argue that orchards do not cause any animal death, and in fact may add new animals. But as shown elsewhere in this book, very few can live long-term on a fruitarian diet. Nonetheless, increasing fruit and decreasing grains would be an improvement over most diets.

[†]This is true unless new land is being cleared for raising cattle, as unfortunately happens in Amazon rain forest clearings.

Of course, we should all work for the elimination of confinement animal facilities, which do cause a great deal of suffering in our animals, not to mention desecration of the environment. This will be more readily accomplished by the millions of meat eaters opting for grass-fed animal foods than by the smaller number of vegetarians boycotting meat.[4]

Journalist Michael Pollan reminds us that many mice, woodchucks, and other animals die in the tractor, and songbirds are killed from pesticides.

If our goal is to kill as few animals as possible, people should probably try to eat the largest possible animal that can live on the least cultivated land: grass-finished steaks for everyone.[5]

There Is No Death

In my worldview, shaped by an insatiable appetite for uncovering what happens after death, *there is no death*. There is also no birth. There is only a switching of dimensions. This view is now backed by a new scientific theory called *biocentrism*.[6]

The absence of death, in the sense of extinction of consciousness, applies to all life forms, not just humans. This view is well known to be held by Hindus, but it is not limited to Hindus alone. The Inuit believe that when they kill an animal, the soul departs into the universal spirit to be reborn in a new body. Many other aborigines hold the same belief.[7] Plenty of books have been published with accounts of people seeing the ghosts or spirits of their deceased pets.[8] Do we really think we are so superior to other species that the afterlife would be limited to humans? We are, after all, animals biologically. Simply having bigger brains doesn't mean we get to live on, and other animals don't.

Would a loving God, Nature, or Universe be guilty of the same speciesism that vegans abhor, the same speciesism condemned by animal rightists?

All is consciousness, patterns of energy. Energy is neither created nor destroyed but simply changes form. So if you devour an insect, that insect's body is converted into energy for you. But the insect's consciousness simply goes into a parallel universe. Perhaps it will choose to be born here again, or not.

For at least some people, the reincarnation of humans is a proven fact. Just read *Old Souls* by

Tom Shroder if you want the scientific evidence. Shroder documented the work of Dr. Ian Stevenson, MD, who spent 40 years examining reincarnation by applying scientific methods to the study of children who vividly recalled past lives. He took children to the cities where they remembered living in past lives and systematically verified the details that the kids had previously remembered. The children remembered names of people, locations of items, and secrets that only their former incarnations could have known. Upon meeting her husband from her past life, one little girl even became angry at him for remarrying, citing his promise never to do so!

The *Journal of the American Medical Association* wrote of his thousands of case studies that he "had collected cases in which the evidence is difficult to explain on any other grounds [besides reincarnation]."[9]

The real issue behind the "meat is murder" argument is fear or denial of death, which is so rampant in our culture. Death is supposed to be bad, when actually many believe it is the *greatest liberation*.

> *The real issue behind the "meat is murder" argument is fear or denial of death, which is so rampant in our culture. Death is supposed to be bad, when actually many believe it is the greatest liberation.*

About half of people's medical expenses occur in the last six months of their lives as they are hooked up to machines or getting toxic drug treatments such as chemo-"therapy." Why are they spending their last months in such horrid pain? Why are they squandering their children's inheritances for a few months of wretched existence that can only loosely be considered life? It's because they are afraid of death and in denial of its inevitability.

If material life were all that existed, and this life were just some fluke of accidental chemicals coming together for a blip in eternity, then death would be the ultimate calamity. I can assure you that this is not the case. Don't trust me, though. *Do the research for yourself.* There are currently numerous books proving the afterlife using standard scientific methods, just as much as science can "prove" anything.[10]

Rules of the Game

I compare death to getting knocked out in the game of dodgeball, the childhood game in which anyone who is in the circle and gets hit with the ball is out. Try to remember this game: You get knocked out and then have to sit on the sidelines. You are really pissed off at first, but then you surrender to it and socialize with the others who are out. You also root for the ones still in the game. Then you reincarnate into a whole new game and get another chance. Of course, we think of death as much more serious than this, but a second grader takes getting knocked out of the game very seriously, no matter how much you plead with him or her that it is *only a game*, and it really *doesn't matter* in the grand scheme of things.

If I am hiking in California and a hungry mountain lion eats me, is he being unethical? Of course not! Being a carnivore, he needs meat to live.

Will I die? My body will die, but I am not my body. My awareness, my being-ness, will simply flip to a different dimension. Now, I might be annoyed that I did not get to finish certain goals, say goodbye to certain people, but I am sure I would get over it. And I would sigh with wonder and awe, "*Le saqué el jugo!*" — a Spanish expression which means, "I got the most out of it!" (literally, "I squeezed out the juice!").

By the way, that lion would get a very healthy profile of omega-3 fats from me! And I would be happy to be recycled, even if I didn't get to die surrounded by loved ones.

If I eat that lion instead, he will die, but he is not his body either. We are just here visiting this dimension temporarily. While here, we have to eat to feed our "spacesuits." Sometimes we even have to eat the "spacesuits" of other species! These are the rules of the game. At some point they may change with evolution.*

Most philosophers would say that if the lion were capable of moral decisions and were our evolutionary equivalent, it would be morally wrong to eat him. So cannibalism is a taboo unless there is a starvation issue and one eats someone already dead for survival purposes. This was the case with the survivors of an airplane crash in the Andes mountains in 1972. The survivors managed to stay alive until their rescue by eating those who had died in the plane crash.

This reasoning may also be why so many people boycotted tuna when dolphins were caught in tuna-fishing nets. Dolphins have been found to be as moral and intelligent as humans, even to the extent of saving people's lives. Some believe them to be our evolutionary equivalent, exploring oceans instead of land.

Some vegetarians say it is wrong to eat anything with a face, assuming that only beings with faces have similar consciousnesses. But when you look at the studies done on plants and their sentience and consciousness, you could just as well say that "no face, no crying-voice discrimination" is on a par with sexism, racism, or homophobia. True, their consciousnesses are different from ours, but does that make them any less valid or inferior to ours?

Plants have been found to feel loneliness, love of music, and prefer certain kinds of music.[11] Plants have been hooked up to galvanometers to measure

If your child's health depended on eating meat to get better, I am sure you would come up with a way to justify it.

their minute movements and chemical reactions. They have been found to feel "horror" if a nearby plant is being burned. They have even been able to read people's minds.[12]

Some vegans think it is OK to eat insects — but not poultry, fish, or mammals — because we cannot hear them cry. If we were to peer deeply into the psyches of insects, I am sure we would find a vast intelligence unlike what we could imagine.

We live in a creature-eat-creature-for-energy world. Unless we can come up with alternate forms of energy, we are fighting against nature itself. If we deny what our bodies have genetically evolved to depend upon because of our philosophies, we are sacrificing optimal health for the sake of a lower species. Noble as it may be, it defies the order of nature. It is a creature versus creature world. Don't blame me. I did not make the rules. I didn't invent this game. Whoever did was very creative, you have to admit. It sure makes for interesting conflicts.

Another point for all who shun meat for moral reasons: If your child's health depended upon eating meat to get better, I am *sure* you would come up with a way to justify it. So why not justify it for your *own* health, your own 30 to 70 trillion "children," the very cells that make up your body?

With this book I am outing myself. It is quite reminiscent of the 1970s when I was attending some fundamentalist, rather dogmatic churches. I woke up to love and forgiveness. I realized that God would have infinitely more love than I do and that this love and compassion would extend beyond the grave. I realized that the concept of a vindictive, judgmental, jealous God was a projection of our own human traits.

I finally got the courage to tell my friends that I believed it was a misconception that people would spend eternity in hell just for not believing in the "correct" religion. They immediately expressed concern for my soul. In their minds, I was no longer part of the group. Nor did I feel comfortable in the company of dogma. The whole ordeal was painful, but I realized that being true to myself was what mattered. New, like-minded friends eventually

---

*In my opinion, based on research as well as information from people I have met, there may be other possible means of deriving energy: from prana, or even from sunlight. I have met quite a few people who profess to do so. Yes, most of them do eat a bit of food here and there for pleasure but not enough to sustain them: maybe 200 to 400 calories a day. So there may be an alternative to eating plants and animals. A good book on this, by a scientist who became a breatharian and allowed experiments on his body, is Michael Werner's book *Life from Light*. Be that as it may, it is nevertheless hard to write about what one is not experiencing, and I haven't gotten there yet.

came into my life to replace the old ones.

Just as people once asked me, "How can you forsake the 'one true' religion?" people now consider me a dietary heretic. People think I have fallen, lost my way, and will surely die of cancer or heart disease! I will also not enter the higher spiritual dimensions where only vegans can go.

I have to admit, there are times I wish the rules of the game were different. I was feeding a pair of wild ducks at a parking lot one day. My husband told me later that a couple grabbed the ducks to take them home and eat them just as we left. I was thinking *how horrible*! Why can't they just buy their meat at the store like most people do? These were tame ducks — *how terrible to break their trust*! Then it dawned on me that in traditional farming, the animals are also tame and trusting. That's just the way life is. Why struggle against nature? After all, we are in an economic depression. Was it really so awful that the couple snatched the ducks instead of buying them at the grocery store?

The Covenant among All Life Forms

There is really a covenant among life forms, an agreement to eat and be eaten, if not by animals, then by worms, bacteria, and plants that feed off the soils enriched by our remains. The Mayans call this *Kas-limaal*, which author and musician Martin Prechtel translates roughly as "mutual indebtedness, mutual insparkedness."[13]

One of the Mayan elders explains it to Prechtel.

> Everything comes into this Earth hungry and interdependent on all other things, animals, and people, so they can eat, be warmed, not be lonely, and survive. ... The knowledge that every animal, plant, person, wind, and season is indebted to the fruit of everything else is an adult knowledge. To get out of debt means you don't want to be part of life, and you don't want to grow into an adult.[14]

The Native Americans knew the value of nature and keeping things in balance. A Native American named Elk of the Black Moon, a revered Sioux medicine man, appeared to Aajonus Vonderplanitz in a vision. Aajonus was deteriorating after being a raw vegan for 11 years. He felt so bad that he decided to just starve himself to death. Elk told him raw meat would heal him, but Aajonus objected to

eating animals. Elk's reply:

> When someone only kills to eat, it is according to the goodness of Nature. It is an agreement among all species. Death is quick in the hunt. Suffering is a lifetime in disease. You choose.[15]

Later, when a pack of coyotes killed a rabbit for Aajonus to eat, he could *see the rabbit's spirit leaving its body* just before they killed it.[*]

The history of domestication indicates that it was a two-way street between man and animals. Animals benefit from their relationship with man, receiving shelter from the cold, food, and protection from predators. If you let a dog go, do you think he is going to suddenly "enjoy" his freedom? No, he will likely come back quite willingly. Mice have come to depend on people, living in garbage cans or house walls. If you catch a mouse and put it in a forest, it will find another house, be eaten by a predator, freeze in winter, or starve to death in the woods.[16]

There are symbiotic relationships found throughout nature that were not invented by man. Anemones on the back of a crab protect it while also feeding from the bits of food that float by as the crab tears apart some meat. A hippopotamus allows a bird to enter its mouth to eat parasites.

Vegetarians sometimes claim it is okay to eat an animal that died naturally, but it is wrong to kill it in midlife. They liken it to when a human dies as a child or in the prime of life. (If someone dies after 50, most people don't think it is quite as bad as dying younger.) The fact is that most animals have little concept of future outside of instinctive events such as mating, migrating, and feeding. They lack the advanced frontal lobes in the brain that enable elaborate planning and goal setting. They don't feel the pain of unaccomplished dreams or never living to see their grandchildren.

Michael Pollan offers this argument.

> Predation is not a matter of morality or of politics; it too is a matter of symbiosis. Brutal as the wolf may be to the individual deer, the herd depends on him for its well-being. Without predators to cull the herd, deer overrun their habitat and starve — all suffer, and

---

[*]See chapter 2 for the rest of the story.

not only the deer, but the plants they browse and every other species that depends on those plants.[17]

Pollan wonders if the quarrel that animal rightists have isn't really with nature itself. He argues that their concern with the individual animal comes from a culture of liberal individualism, but how much sense does this make in nature? A vegan utopia can only thrive in a world "where people have lost contact with the natural world."[18]

Our domestication of animals could also be interpreted as their adaptation to us. In fact, Stephen Budiansky, former US editor of *Nature*, argues that they may have chosen domestication as much as we did.[19]

Why were sheep and cows domesticated, while gazelles and antelopes were not? There seem to have been certain characteristics of the animals that allowed us to domesticate them, because other animals have not submitted to domestication. If you have a pet wolf or chimp, for example, they go wild during adolescence and are not safe to have around.

> If we come to see the domestication of animals not as a crime against nature, but as a product of nature, we will in the process confront something much more fundamental about man's part in nature. ... If life with man was a better evolutionary bargain for domesticated animals than was life in the wild, then it makes no sense to say that nature (really just another word for evolution) ends where man's presence begins.[20]

As far as evolution goes, domesticated animals have benefited from their partnership with us. There are 100 million dogs in the US, while wolves are nearly extinct. There are over a billion sheep and cattle, while their wild counterparts teeter on the brink of extinction.[*]

Domesticated animals raised on traditional farms also lose much of the fear that is common in

wild animals.[21] Life without fear is certainly a more pleasant existence.

Hunters, according to Budiansky, know that animals are neither *things* (the Descartes view) nor *people* (the Animal Liberation Front view). They know "the contract that was sealed when man and domesticated animals cast their lot together ten thousand years ago."[22]

> *When farm animals agreed to domestication, one can be fairly certain that factory farming was not what they bargained for.*

Yet hunters have often been forced to give up their rights due to the animal rights movement and wildlife management. When we remove man from the animal food chain, it doesn't always work out for the animals either. Many deer have starved to death, slowly and painfully, because of overpopulation when man is prohibited from hunting them.

In Kenya, elephant populations dwindled down to 19,000 in 1989. However, when controlled hunting was introduced, native farmers and villagers were motivated to set aside land for the elephants and thus increased their population to 30,000 because foreign hunters paid $30,000 for the privilege of hunting one elephant. Villagers made 15 million dollars a year from sales of the ivory. When the animal welfare groups put a trade ban on ivory, the natives had no incentive to protect the elephants from poachers or to set aside farm land for them.

Philosophy professor Tom Regan has written several books arguing that animals have rights, but other philosophers, such as Carl Cohen, argue that they have no rights, not being capable of moral decisions themselves. On the other hand, an infant or retarded person incapable of moral decisions has rights by virtue of being the same species that we are. It is part of nature for members of a species to give priority to their own.

Though we certainly have ethical obligations to treat animals without cruelty, we don't have to give them the right not to be eaten. Cohen gives us

---

[*]Of course, it can be argued that man messed everything up by overpopulating and clearing out lands that wolves and other wild animals once inhabited. These animals would not be on the brink of extinction if not for man. But remember that man, an animal, is also part of nature. That doesn't justify everything humans do, but it puts it in the context of nature. At any rate, the point is not diminished that animals domesticated by man have an advantage over wild animals in terms of avoiding extinction.

this example: If you see a lion attacking a baby zebra, you would not interfere, but if you saw a lion attacking a human baby, you would probably shoot the lion because the human baby has the right not to be eaten.[23]

The Real Morality Issue: Factory Farms and Slaughterhouses

If farm animals indeed agreed to be domesticated, one can be fairly certain that factory farming was not what they signed up for. The desire of corporations to satisfy stockholders and consumer demand for cheap meat no doubt overpowered the traditional small farm model, with its longstanding humane treatment of farm animals. Photos of animals cramped into tiny stalls in which they can't even turn around will often get the greatest meat enthusiast to "go veg." Animals are not allowed to express their animal nature, run, be social, and enjoy the sun when raised in such conditions. Usually, they are not even allowed to nurse or care for their young.

British chef, farmer, author, and food activist Hugh Fearnley-Whittingstall notes that the time-honored tradition of animal husbandry has been violated by the industrial system that neglects animal welfare for high yield and cheap prices.

> This isn't husbandry; it's persecution. We have completely failed to uphold our end of the contract.[24]

He is among many who feel we should pay twice as much money for half as much meat if that is what it takes to get better treatment of animals and higher quality food.

The unspeakable cruelty of slaughterhouses is no doubt responsible for converting many people to vegetarianism. At www.youtube.com, you can watch slaughterhouse scenes set up by hidden cameras. Even kosher and halal slaughters, which in theory are designed to minimize suffering, are often horrific for the animals involved. The karmic "revenge" of the farm animals translates into poor health to all who consume their desecrated meat.

Tara Weaver visited a farm on which friends had a factory-farmed cow and asked the organic farmers to slaughter it. Their custom was to compost the blood and entrails to enrich their soil, but the remains of the factory-farmed cow *did not break*

down. Three months later it looked the same. Even the microbes refused to eat it, yet humans are eating this kind of meat all the time!

Animal rights people accuse slaughterhouses of skinning and cutting animals alive because they still move after being hit by the stun gun. A person who runs such a slaughterhouse assured author Michael Pollan that this movement is just reflex kicking and that most of the animals are already dead or at least unconscious. If the head is not flopping, they stun the animal again, realizing it is still conscious.[25]

Nonetheless, the high quotas for animals killed per hour often mean that the unskilled, underpaid and stressed-out workers resort to violent measures to keep the line moving. Sometimes this means dismembering or skinning animals that are still struggling and kicking.[26] The meat is also ruined because adrenaline and lactic acid are released, and the muscles get tense, making the meat tough with an off flavor.[27]

While animals in slaughterhouses may not die surrounded by loved ones, their attack in the wild is supposedly much scarier and more painful than being killed by humans. At least there is not the long, drawn-out chase in most cases.

This is especially true in about half the slaughterhouses in the US, which use a method created by an autistic woman named Temple Grandin. She could sense the fear of cattle about to be slaughtered and empathized with it. This led her to designing a narrow tunnel that the cattle could walk through single file. Once a cow exits, it is immediately stunned in the head. The cattle following behind have little idea what is going on, minimizing their fear. The movie *Temple Grandin* is all about this remarkable woman and her work in animal husbandry.

We should raise animals on farms in natural sunlight, letting them express their animal beingness. It is said, "Let them have only one bad day in their lives," the day in which they die. This day is unavoidable, domesticated or wild. Such animals on a traditional farm will live longer than they do in the wild and suffer less torturous deaths.

British philosopher Roger Scruton explains how animals should be killed.

There is a distinction between sudden death and death preceded by terror, and to the conscientious farmer, who has looked after animals from day to day ... this terror is not merely unwelcome, but a betrayal of trust. ... Livestock farmers therefore prefer to see their animals dispatched suddenly and humanely in the place where they have lived, by skilled slaughterers.[28]

He explains that health and safety regulations are destroying these humane practices, and this is what should be protested.

Professor Frederick Ferre explains that if people cared enough, we could demand slaughter under total anesthesia. (Of course, residues of those chemicals would remain in the meat we eat, but at least we wouldn't get the animal's adrenaline.) If we get rid of animal cruelty, he points out, it may mean the end of the cheap hamburger.[29]

I would argue that those who eat the omega-6, factory-farmed, charcoaled burger cut with soy would be healthier to be vegetarians anyway. Or they could at least switch to free-range poultry.

It is said among vegetarians that they should not eat meat unless they can look the animal in the eye and kill it themselves. Many traditional people did this, and they did it very consciously and prayerfully, speaking to the spirit of the animal and thanking it.

I had a roommate who was very spiritual, yet any time an insect invaded our home, she thought nothing of smashing it. She would pray, "Into the light!" while killing the creature, as she was sure that the astral realms of the afterlife are not limited to those with the human form.

Most people would kill an animal if their families needed the food, but I don't think most people could keep the animal locked up for life on a factory farm. I could never do that, and I do not think it is wise to support this cruel industry that keeps animals trapped in small pens where they can get no exercise or social life and are separated from their offspring. Quite often they can't even turn around or lie down!

Tara Weaver explored alternative options in her book *The Butcher and the Vegetarian*. She found that it is possible to own a share of a cow and have some say in how it is raised. It is then legal to have it killed outside the slaughterhouse. She was

warned that this privilege might be lost soon.[30] She also interviewed a woman who simply raises her own meat in her backyard and kills the animals herself: goats, rabbits, chickens, and turkeys.

The answer to this moral dilemma is to spend money only on free-range, organically fed animals free of steroids, hormones, antibiotics, and (if possible) vaccinations.

Best is wild game that got to live free lives and were quickly shot by hunters. Such wild game has the best ratio of omega-3 fatty acids to omega-6s. It costs the most, but just eat less of it. Of course, if you can hunt, all the better in terms of saving money.

If you cannot afford this, buy free-range poultry that was organically fed and kosher if possible.

Philosophy professor R.G. Frey argued in his book *Rights, Killing, and Suffering: Moral Vegetarianism and Applied Ethics* that people switching to vegetarian diets would not stop the factory farming. Twenty years later he revisited the issue and found he was right. The millions who "go veg" barely put a dent in the industry and don't even make up for the increasing demand for meat by others. He estimates the number of factory-farmed animals to be as high as 25 billion annually.[31]

Since most people crave meat — biologically, not just to appease their palates! — the solution is to increase awareness of factory farming ills and for everyone to find compassionate farmers to patronize, preferably local in order to support those in your area and leave less of a carbon footprint.

Tom Frantzen is an example of a farmer who switched to a free-range hog farm after visiting one in Sweden. He found that in some ways it was actually *more* cost efficient. Once he created a "hoop house" for them, he set them free to run.

> They ran all day long, and they must have run around all night long too, because when I went out to the building the next morning, I will never forget what I found. ... I peeked into the hoop house to see 180 pigs in one massive straw nest — snoring. I laughed until I cried. Their stress was gone, and so was mine. I know I'll never go back to confinement. Once you cross that road, there is no way you can go back.[32]

Small farmers who raise animals with compassion usually don't sell to stores. They have to be sought out by the consumer. They do not receive government subsidies like the big factory farms. They need our support. The tide will turn as more of us switch.

A great book to read on this topic is Catherine Friend's *The Compassionate Carnivore*. Catherine is a farmer who raises sheep compassionately.

I don't need my meat to come from animals that lived an entire life without pain or fear, since I now know that's almost impossible to deliver. What's more important to me is that domestic livestock be raised as living, breathing creatures with emotions and needs, not as inputs in a widget factory.[33]

Chapter 21

The Spirituality of Eating Meat

I cannot see a vegetarian who gorges him/herself on huge plates of pasta marinara having a stronger sense of spirituality than one who consumes modest amounts of meat with humble gratitude of the prey's sacrifice.

—Gene, blogger

The main quandary I had at first about my return to eating modest amounts of meat revolved around its spiritual suitability. There is a concept in various spiritual communities that by not eating meat your consciousness becomes "lighter" and your body "purer." However, I can assure you that simply abstaining from eating meat or animal products is no guarantee of higher spiritual evolution, though for some people it may facilitate meditation. I have come to realize that eating animal products is not incompatible with spirituality. Many highly spiritual people throughout history have eaten meat or other animal products.

Nonetheless, this proved to be the biggest challenge for me in adding "dense" foods to my diet, which had been nearly 100 percent plant. Here is an e-mail a friend sent me after learning that I was straying from the party line. She got this from a site in which a woman claims to channel her dead son.

Now, then, animals becoming vegetarians will be a process of their choosing that kind of diet because it is more appealing, just as it will be for Earth's human residents. As the light intensifies in all bodies at cellular level, humans and animals alike naturally will choose foods that have light properties, and *severed animal flesh does not* [emphasis added]. Without the current food chain, animals will not overcrowd the planet; instead, they instinctively will reproduce more slowly or not at all.

So, according to various New Age paradigms, I will not express my full "light potential" if I eat any animal foods. At least the channeler in the e-

"He who gives up meat-eating but does not alter his nature and thoughts, thinking to gain in spirituality, may flatter himself and perhaps make a fetish of his denial, but will certainly thereby make no spiritual progress."
—William Q. Judge, 19th century theosophical author

mail says I won't go to hell.

There absolutely is no "condemnation by God" for eating meat and seafood, but expressing gratitude for the animals that provide these foods is most appropriate.

For the record, I am not saying that this can't happen in the future, but I am living in the present where such evolution has not occurred in my body.

By far the most influential spiritual teacher in my life was Robert Adams, a fully realized sage whose talks have been transcribed in the book *Silence of the Heart*. He gave *satsang* (sitting in silence and then talking about the highest truths) in Los Angeles in the 1990s. He said, "No one ever got enlightened by eating meat." And he never ate meat.

My husband Allen and I took him out to eat a few times, and he always ordered a vegetarian salad. Yet, he died while only in his 60s after a long battle with Parkinson's disease. Parkinson's disease is now known often to be caused by a deficiency of vitamin B_{12}, which is reliably found only in animal products.

Dr. Gabriel Cousens also became a raw vegan for spiritual reasons. He felt it helped him maintain his high level of spiritual consciousness. On the other hand, Dr. Stanley Bass has been practicing meditation for over 40 years and has found no difference in his results after going back to meat eating.

My husband is also very sensitive and claims if he eats meat, he can feel the suffering that the animal he is eating went through in its slaughter. Sometimes, for health reasons, he will eat some smoked or raw wild salmon. He just doesn't pay attention to the suffering vibration. On the rare occasion that he eats wild meat, he doesn't even feel the suffering, however. The animal has usually been killed quickly.

I once asked another person in the raw food movement who had been vegan for several decades if he thought being vegan was really necessary to ascend to the greater spiritual heights he had been saying we were evolving toward. He said absolutely, only vegans would inherit this consciousness. *Yet he was losing his eyesight!*

My husband and I noticed he had to be led around, apparently not able to see clearly. He also would look only in your direction, not right at you, when addressing your question.

DHA, found prominently in animal products, is necessary for the retina. Also, true vitamin A is found only in animal products and not manufactured in our bodies efficiently. Without enough vitamin A, we become blind. It takes an immense amount of the plant precursor beta-carotene to convert to vitamin A, and it happens only in very healthy bodies, not at all in infants or young children. Or was it vitamin B_{12} that was missing? A deficiency of B_{12} can also cause the optic nerve to degenerate.[*]

Was this raw food adherent, as well as my spiritual teacher Robert Adams, trading health for spiritual advancement? If so, it might be a good trade because the spirit is the only part that lasts. But is it really necessary? Would I be "cursed to stay in the lower dimensions," equivalent to the Christian idea of "going to hell," unless I were to eat a vegan or vegetarian diet?

Ask yourself this: In a benign universe, would it really be necessary to trade optimal health for spiritual progress? Do you really think that God, Nature, or the Universe intended for us to sacrifice health for divinity?

On the contrary, I find that for me at least, healthier physical states facilitate higher spiritual awareness.

No doubt it is nice for us to be considerate of animals, but our physiology evolved with animal food dependencies. Our bodies need about 40,000 years to make significant genetic changes, and only if there is *selective pressure*, some particular biological advantage that results in those having favorable genetic adaptations that result in breeding more viable offspring than the rest of the herd.

For most of us, our consciousnesses are evolving faster than our bodies. We should listen to our bodies, in my opinion, and not eat beyond our physical evolution.

I asked Aajonus Vonderplanitz, a raw meat eater, what he thought about the spiritual question of eating meat. I knew from reading his autobiography that he had a strong and deep spiritual background, and I wanted to know how he reconciled his controversial diet with his philosophy. He told me he is calmer and less emotional than when he was a raw vegan for 11 years.

Aajonus told me that one time a bunch of vegetarians were yelling at him and telling him how bad he was to eat animal food. He patiently listened, then held up a mirror and said, "Look at who is being verbally violent. Look at who is acting mean and crazy. Whose diet produces calm and tranquility?"

A few of them got it. Vegan and sometimes even vegetarian diets lack sufficient amounts of good saturated fats, as well as DHA, EPA, B_{12}, and tryptophan, which are crucial for the brain and emotional well-being. Also, unless you are a carb type, eating a high-carb diet rich in fruits can cause blood sugar swings.

Vegetarian researcher Tom Billings writes on his and Ward Nicholson's website www.beyondveg.com that he has been a vegetarian for 40 years and has experimented with every sort of vegetarian diet, including raw vegan and *fruitarian*, which he defines as getting at least 75 percent of calories from fruit.

When I experienced the "light" mental feeling one gets on a fruit diet, I thought it was pretty neat, and an indicator of spiritual progress. Since then, I have had the opportunity to do real spiritual work (yoga) on a different raw vegan diet, and I can vouch that, from direct firsthand experience, the "light" mental

---

[*]See chapter 17.

feeling one gets on a fruit diet is not a real spiritual feeling. The light feeling of a fruit diet is ungrounded, airy, a feeling of apathy and not being connected. (Such "light" mental feelings may actually be a symptom of a zinc deficiency. Further, in Ayurvedic terms, it may indicate a *vata* imbalance in the nervous system.) A spiritual feeling is warm, grounded, secure, loving, and one retains interest in things around them. It is not "spacey" like the light mental feeling of fruit; instead it is blissful.[1]

Interestingly, this is confirmed by Dr. Carl Curt Pfeiffer, PhD, MD.

> The light-headed feeling of detachment that enshrouds some vegetarians can be caused by hidden zinc hunger, rather than by some mystical quality of the brown rice or other food consumed.[2]

From my own personal experience, I do not believe that the only spiritual benefit to a raw vegan diet is a zinc deficiency. Eating any kind of diet *raw* — even omnivorous — will decrease the need for your digestive system to work as hard as it used to. This extra energy goes up to the higher chakras (energy centers) and increases the amount of energy available for mental and spiritual pursuits.

I see raw diet author Natalia Rose advising people to eat meat in order to get rid of their candida, but she herself wrote a book about how she is practically in another dimension because the only animal food she eats is goat cheese.

> Rose writes that when you reach a certain spiritual phase, the body's real fuel is electromagnetism. Anything that stands in the way of this is detrimental to the body. She goes on to list vitamin pills, whole grains, animal products, soy products, and packaged foods as detriments.

She concedes that some are worse than others.

> Raw goat cheese is an animal product, but it is not going to infringe on your electromagnetism as much as a sloppy joe or deli meats.[3] ...
> If you eat flesh, try to limit your flesh to no more than once a day (preferably at dinner) and stick with low-density fleshes like seafood.[4]

In my case, eating animal protein in the morning works best. The lack of carb overload and the high protein keep my blood sugar steady, keep hunger at bay, and keep me mentally clear all day.

In conclusion, the spiritual argument may have some validity for being vegetarian for some people.

Even then, being vegan is definitely not necessary, as the most spiritual people I have met or known personally were not vegans, though often vegetarians.

> *"What you think matters more than what you eat. We line up our vibrations through our thoughts, not through food."*
>
> *–Graham Cook, blogger*

I conversed with my husband, who has devoted more of his energy to spiritual practice than anyone I know. Bear in mind, as he defends the vegetarian view, that even he eats raw dairy, raw eggs, and occasionally raw or smoked wild fish and land animals.

Susan: I am learning that we are designed to eat meat. This is my next book.

Allen: Are you sure you want to write a book telling people to eat meat? Your readers don't want to hear that. Vegetarians think meat is murder. They don't want to eat animals, especially mammals!

Susan: But we evolved eating meat! We have been eating it for 2½-3 million years, or 100,000 to 150,000 generations!

Allen: Well, maybe we're evolving out of it.

Susan: But agriculture, which gave protein sources to vegetarians, is only about 10,000 to 20,000 years old, or 500 generations. It takes 2,000 generations, about 40,000 years, for even minimal changes to evolve.

Allen: Well, maybe we are evolving at an accelerated pace these days.[*]

---

[*]Some anthropologists, such as the authors of *10,000 Year Explosion*, do believe evolution is happening at an accelerated pace. Some scientists even believe we are actually on the brink of a quantum evolutionary leap, like David Wilcock, a professional lecturer, filmmaker, and researcher of ancient civilizations, consciousness science, and new paradigms of matter and energy.

Susan: Do you think eating meat can interfere with one's spiritual progress?

Allen: Being a vegetarian may be a phase in which people learn compassion, but once they get it, they can go back to eating meat because *nothing really matters*. There is no birth, and there is no death. So once you get compassion, you can go back to eating meat if you need to for health issues, as long as you eat it with awareness and sensitivity.

Susan: So why do you think Robert Adams didn't eat meat?

Allen: He wanted to be an example for us.

☞ My husband has found that whenever he does eat flesh, it helps ground him and make him less susceptible to "picking up other people's negative energy" — something he has been complaining about for years. But he nonetheless eats little of it at a time and just a few times a week.

Now, I am all in favor of any alleged evolutionary leap that could make us successful vegans or even potentially minimal eaters getting by on extremely low-calorie diets. I personally believe it is possible. But to switch your body to this alternative fuel takes a great deal of mental focus and spiritual discipline. It doesn't just happen because you decide to transition by eating a vegan diet, to be followed by a diet of fruit only. It hasn't happened in my body yet. You might want to keep close track of your own body, since deficiencies can take years, even a decade, to show up.

Paul Nison: A Biblical Perspective

Many vegans use Genesis 1:29 as a reason to shun meat.

And God said, Behold, I have given you every herb bearing seed, which is upon the face of all the earth, and every tree, in which is the fruit of a tree yielding seed; to you it shall be for meat.

But there is more to the scriptures than that. Raw food advocate and author Paul Nison is no longer vegan. Here is his story in his own words.

For fifteen years, I ate a strictly raw, vegan diet. After being diagnosed with a deadly affliction (inflammatory bowel disease), I began to research natural healing methods, and I was convinced a raw, vegan

diet was the way to go. Because I was in this position, I understand the raw-vegan mentality, and I'm not saying that way of eating does not work for a certain time. I felt great and think the vegan diet is a wonderful cleansing and healing diet.

However, the issue is that it is highly unlikely that raw vegans are receiving all of the nutrients their bodies need. The soil our food is grown in today lacks vital nutrients because of years of depletion and damage. Raw vegans can take supplements to obtain the missing nutrients that they are not getting from their food, but many vegans often shun even doing that.

After years of research and experience, I have decided that there is nothing wrong with including some nonvegan products in the diet to help obtain these vital nutrients in an easily absorbable and economic way. Let me tell you my story.

After being on a 100% raw, vegan diet and knowing that one of the most toxic foods for man is pasteurized cow's milk from the supermarket, I was convinced vegan was the way to go. In fact, I healed from inflammatory bowel disease (IBD) by avoiding processed dairy, so eliminating all animal products from my diet was easy, and I felt great.

After about 10 years on my raw-vegan journey, I began to question whether this diet was sustainable long-term. I had written five books on this topic and interviewed numerous people living this way. I was also the chef of the world's biggest raw food restaurant in NYC. I soon began reading the Bible and became a believer in the message of the Scriptures. The reason I first picked up a Bible was because someone told me it contained information about health.

After studying the Scriptures, I was confused because I always thought the diet of the Bible was a vegetarian diet, but after actually reading it and not listening to what others had to say about it, I saw that God allowed man to consume animals with certain restrictions. Also, after reading that God was going to bring the children of Israel to the land of "milk and honey," I thought to myself, "Why would God give them something so unhealthy and toxic as milk?" And why would God refer to the Promised Land as "milk and honey" if it was not desired and healthy?

This piqued my interest enough to do more research, and I found that although store-bought milk that is pasteurized and loaded with chemicals is not healthy; raw, fresh milk from a goat or sheep is delicious and full of absorbable nutrients. It's not the milk that is bad, but what man does to it.

During this process of discovery, my wife had our first baby, and she began breastfeeding. I found out breast milk is the best food for a newborn because you simply can't get everything from vegetation. Now I love green vegetable juices, but no baby is going to be healthy on green juices alone; they need milk.

Finally, I had to try for myself to see if milk was going to cause an issue. This was very scary to me because my condition from IBD could have come back, but I had to try it and see. So I tried some raw goat milk fresh from a local farm and felt just fine. I didn't feel amazing, but I was told if I ever went back to eating animal products, then I'd get sick. Well, I didn't get sick. This led me to try raw goat cheese, and again I felt okay. I still was a raw foodist, but no longer "vegan" and had no issue about it.

Over the years, I've done blood testing to monitor my health and have seen improved results since adding animal products. But more important to me, God said it was okay, and if it's okay for Him, it should be okay for me.

It had been more than 15 years since I had eaten any meat, but when Passover came that year, I decided to eat some grass-fed organic lamb to see how I would feel. I ate it cooked, the first cooked food I had eaten in about 15 years. I only had a very small amount and didn't get sick. This opened my eyes to a whole new way of thinking. I've even met people who eat raw meat. I haven't done that yet, but I can say I do have a more open mind now than I ever did, so let's see what the future holds.

As of now, I still consume mostly raw vegan foods, occasionally raw eggs, goat milk, and on a very rare occasion, some meat. I've been adding some fish to my diet as well. I feel fine on a lacto-vegetarian diet, but after doing research, I am convinced a complete vegan diet is not ideal or practical for most people. Some people have said they have an ethical issue with eating meat, and I say that's their issue and their decision. I also see ethical issues with how animals are treated on certain farms, but as long as the products I consume are not from a factory farm and kosher, I don't see any ethical problems. My advice is this: If people are not ready to consider consuming animal products, consider getting your blood checked and taking supplements to fill in any nutritional gaps. To everyone, I say, have an open mind, and trust that God is smarter than we are.[5]

An Indian Swami Speaks about Vegetarianism and Spirituality

Swami Narayanananda, author of a multitude of spiritual books, has some interesting comments on diet in his book *The Secrets of Mind-Control.*

In India, some narrow-minded and bigoted people have much hatred for nonvegetarian diet. The very idea of meat eating is galling to them and puts them off their moorings. They can never tolerate meat eating.

He goes on to explain that in some parts of India, there are people who are forced to eat meat because plant food is scarce and expensive, yet the vegetarian bigots nonetheless consider them heretics.

Take the case of the great spiritual and moral giants, the great law-givers and the founders of great religions of the world. ... All these great Prophets sprang from the nonvegetarian class. Manu, Rama, Krishna, Buddha, Mahavira, ... Moses, Jesus, Mohammed, Nanak, Lao-Tze, Sinto, and Ramakrishna were all nonvegetarians. If religion forbids fish and meat eating as sin and limits its followers to vegetables alone, were these great men nonreligious? ... Can anyone dare deny the highest spiritual attainments of these great men?[6]

Is eating meat equivalent to the sin of murder? The swami addresses this.

Killing is a sin without doubt. Even to injure another in thought and word is also a sin. Not a single recognized religion asks its followers to kill mercilessly or to be unkind to any living being. In its code of moral conduct, every religion lays much stress on love and compassion for all living things.

But then in this world, one life subsists at the cost of other lives. The lower life serves as food to higher life. In water, air, etc., there are innumerable living things which are invisible to the naked eye. In mere breathing, walking, talking, drinking, and eating vegetables, grains, and fruits, one kills millions and millions of microscopic organisms.

Taking all this into consideration, it would be clear that one can observe perfect Ahimsa [the Hindu practice of harming no living creature] only in Nirvikalpa Samadhi, in which state the body becomes almost a corpse devoid of breathing, moving, and thinking. Apart from this state, life can continue only at the cost of other lives.[7]

Eating Meat Can Be a Very Spiritual Experience

Raw diet author Zephyr (Ano Tarletz) writes in his book *Instinctive Eating* that he once found his body craving something he hadn't been giving it. An inner voice told him to eat raw meat, and this turned out to be the missing link that liberated him from backsliding into cooked foods. He claims that certain states of consciousness are activated and nourished by eating and even killing animals.

Zephyr talks about the spiritual experience he had in killing a chicken. At first it seems rather appalling that the little creature trusted him, yet he slit the bird's throat. But as he goes on to experience this primal, very natural event, the very foundation of life eating life, it becomes a spiritual experience. He describes it as a power surge, and a feeling that he was "tasting God."

Our animal essence has no charge about the idea or morality of eating raw meat. It can only have a here/now experience. Humans tend to have overreactive intellectual and moralistic charges about killing. The other animals lack this charge. The origin of the charge comes from being broken from the natural instinct of killing *only* for food and protection of young. Most of us do not commune with, and are unable to identify, our own killer instinct.[8]

Zephyr claims that eating raw meat brought a feeling of peace to his body, ended food cravings, and filled him with a sense of power. He felt "strong, passionate, primal, and driven."[9]

Though I have never killed an animal, I came close to the spiritual euphoria Zephyr describes the first time I tasted wild buffalo meat. I had dehydrated it overnight at 105° F, so it was raw but dry and rare in the middle — like a jerky but with more moisture. It had very little fat, and there was a sense that this creature got to live life in nature and was killed quickly and relatively painlessly.

I gave thanks, and my spirit felt awe and euphoria as I felt the essence of this magnificent creature merging with my consciousness. I thanked the being for nourishing not only my body, but also my brain with omega-3 fatty acids. I had never in my omnivorous or vegan life tasted anything so great, so *primal*.

I connected with all Native Americans, realizing that they probably never took this animal for granted, relishing the treat of their meat while also fully respecting the buffalo spirit. The rest of my day was spent with stable blood sugar, a focused mind, mental clarity, and a high energy level.

I dance with delight whenever I have the chance to eat raw, wild buffalo meat. I am so thankful we didn't let this creature get extinct, which almost happened when I was a child. I don't experience the same ecstasy and intense flavor when I eat raw buffalo meat that is free range but not wild. Only the wild buffalo makes me feel this way.

I refuse to let my body's dependence on small amounts of animal food limit my spiritual life. Surprisingly, I would say it has greatly *enhanced* it! I am no longer a "foodie," obsessed with what I will eat for the day. I spend very little time even thinking about food — apart from researching and writing for this book. I don't crave any complicated recipes.

I realize now that it was difficult to satisfy my instincts with dishes lacking animal foods. I got very creative within the limitations of fruits, vegetables, nuts, and seeds. There are so many delicious combinations with just those four items, but I stay so satisfied now that I no longer need to make recipes. I mostly eat just whole foods. My cravings and voracious appetite, very typical on vegan diets, are gone — especially when I have a high-protein animal food at breakfast, usually eggs.

It is said that the path to breatharianism (living on prana instead of food) is a vegan diet followed by a fruitarian diet, followed by a liquidarian diet. Ironically, the opposite seems to be true with me. By eating meat, I feel less attached to food than ever and find it easier than ever to stay close to 100 percent raw. I actually feel emotionally closer to letting go of food altogether — if such a thing is possible.

Chapter 22

The Sustainability of Eating Meat

If the world were merely seductive, that would be easy. If it were merely challenging, that would be no problem. But I arise in the morning torn between a desire to improve (or save) the world and a desire to enjoy (or savor) the world. This makes it hard to plan the day.

—Elwyn B. White

I used to belong to a club that was all about "eco-eating," "saving the planet," "being kind to animals." I've now switched teams in the minds of many; but honestly, what good would I do for the planet were I unhealthy?

Man as a species has sacrificed wild animals to make space for agriculture and thus no longer has enough wild animals to feed the population our original diet. But we *as individuals* can choose not to suffer for what our ancestors did and can resume a healthful diet. We can even do it without adding to planetary destruction.

Environmental Issues

A sustainability issue that frequently arises involves the environmental impact of increased global warming from raising animals. Remember, however, that a larger number of bigger mammals once roamed the earth before humans hunted them into extinction. These creatures also emitted methane, urine, and manure, but they were not factory farmed and locked up in tiny jails. They were also free to eat their natural diets.

When animals are free, fed properly, and not injected with toxic hormones, antibiotics, and vaccinations, their excrement is a benefit. Their waste products nourish the soil, making it fertile and mineral rich for crops. Don't blame the animals when it is the factory farm that causes environmental destruction.

Here is what a *Time* article had to say.

Of all the animals that humans eat, none are held more responsible for climate change than cows. Cows not only consume more energy-intensive feed than other livestock, they also produce more methane, a powerful greenhouse gas.

But grass-fed cows may have the opposite effect.

Grass is a perennial. If cattle and other ruminants are rotated across pastures full of it, the animals' graz-ing will cut the blades, spurring new growth, while their trampling helps work manure and other decaying organic matter into the soil, turning it into rich humus. And healthy soil keeps carbon dioxide underground and out of the atmosphere.[1]

Eliot Coleman, author of *The New Organic Grower*, claims in an article that if he butchers a steer for his food and that steer has been raised on grass on his farm, he is not responsible for any increased CO_2.

A vegetarian eating tofu made in a factory from soybeans grown in Brazil is responsible for a lot more CO_2 than I am.[2]

According to one report, raising cattle on well-managed pastures has the following advantages: decreased soil erosion and increased soil fertility, improved water quality due to decreased pollution, improved human health due to reduced antibiotic use and more omega-3 fats, improved farmer and farm worker health, improved animal health and welfare, and more profit per animal for producers.[3]

Furthermore, the issue of global warming is not without controversy. Sure the earth has been warming, but so have the other planets. They do not contain humans that drive cars or raise cattle![4] The entire solar system has been heating up due to the sun's solar flare activity. Why isn't this in mainstream news? Certain political figures would love to use global warming as an excuse for a "carbon tax."

Then there is also the issue of spending our scarce fresh water on animals. OK, so it's bad to eat them, but not cruel to deprive them of water? Sally Fallon, bestselling author and founder of the Weston A. Price Foundation makes this point.

If a sheep drinks one gallon of water per day — which is a lot — the animal would only need about 600 gallons of water to yield almost eighty pounds of meat. That's less than eight gallons of water per pound, much less than the water required to produce a pound of wheat.[5]

Nonetheless, vegetarians do have a point when it comes to sustainability. What about all the water required to irrigate the grain or grass the sheep eats before slaughter? If it takes 200 days to raise the sheep, and it eats 4 pounds of feed per day, you are feeding it 10 pounds of feed to produce that 1 pound of meat. At 8 gallons of water per pound according to that quote, that's 80 gallons per pound to raise the feed plus the 7.5 gallons the animal drinks. The meat has about 3 times more calories than sprouted wheat, so on a calorie basis, the 87.5:8 ratio reduces to about 30:8 in favor of the grain using less water if people ate that feed instead of sheep.[6]

But does this analysis even matter? All the water on the planet is constantly recycling anyway!

Former vegan activist Natasha's perspective has changed.

I now realize that the statistics I used to quote about environmental devastation, grain and water consumption, pollution, and ill health, were all based on numbers from factory farms, not from the realities of traditional land-base-specific farming, which is the only kind of farming that can heal our planet and us.[7]

Feeding the Planet

A chief reason used by vegans to stop raising farm animals is that the animals can then be free. OK, so we set those animals free. Where will they go? They will soon become extinct, just like the tens of thousands of species that have already become extinct as man clears out more and more land for agriculture and cities. I really don't see a lot of people being able to afford pet cows, pigs, goats, and chickens.

The other reason, of course, is to use the land to raise crops for people to eat, as it is more efficient to feed people the food that would be fed to animals. The problem with this, as Lierre Keith discovered, is that raising these crops depends on our limited supplies of fossil fuels. We need that for fertilizer and for running farm machinery.

Lierre was determined to grow her own food. She learned that plants eat animals — they need the nitrogen from dead bones, manure, or fossil fuel (which experts claim is dead prehistoric animals). Where was she going to get this manure? It would have to come from oppressed farm animals.

"As I learned while sitting at the metaphorical feet of the world's leading revolutionary ecologists and food rights advocates, the only way for humanity to survive in any meaningfully sustainable way is for us to live entirely within our local food systems, eating the plants and animals that naturally live on our immediate land base."
—former vegan activist Natasha

That agriculture is ultimately unsustainable is argued in depth by many authors, including Lierre Keith and Thom Hartmann, author of *The Last Hours of Ancient Sunlight*. We have created an artificially large population by using fossil fuel for fertilization and for running farm machinery. We have grown surplus crops, but to grow these crops, we have destroyed topsoil, taken away the habitats of wild animals, and even sold these crops to Third World countries so cheaply that the local farmers have been forced out of work, leaving them no option but to live in squalor in large cities.

Vegetarians often don't realize that we need animals to graze on rotated land in order for the soil to be fed with the animals' excrements. This is in harmony with nature. The alternative is to use toxic synthetic fertilizers which require a lot of energy use and leave toxic pollutants like fluoride as byproducts.

We could use *human* manure, but that presents its own set of problems and controversies. For one thing, we would have to be sure the humans donating to the fertilizer were not taking drugs, prescription or recreational. Their sewage would also have to be separated from toxic chemical wastes that also end up in the sewers presently. Even if we could recycle our human wastes successfully, widespread adoption of this practice to move us to vegetarian diets would result in the near extinction of farm animals and lead to human dietary deficiencies, as previously explained in chapter 17.

The late Mark Purdey of Somerset, UK, was an organic farmer who wrote about sustainability. He resisted the order to spray his cattle with organophosphates for warble fly and went to court over it. No cows born in his herd developed mad cow disease, thought by many to be a result of those toxic sprays.

In his article "The (Vegan Ecological) Wasteland," he argued that the biggest threat to sustainable mixed farming is the fanaticism of various vegetarian pressure groups that don't really understand the ecology of mixed farming. If they had their way, he said, soil erosion, cash cropping, prairiescapes, and ill health would escalate. He argues that we need the livestock for fertilizer. Without them, we will have to use chemical and biotech agriculture.[8]

Mark explained how going back to traditional farming is much more efficient energy-wise than feeding everyone a vegetarian diet.

One of the most nutty, stereotype fallacies emanating from the vegetarians is their claim that crop husbandry is less energy and chemically intensive than livestock farming. Whilst this is true in consideration of the intensive, grain-fed livestock units, the traditional mixed farming unit raises livestock for meat and milk off extensively managed, low-input grassland systems; and each acre of well-managed grassland can produce four harvests a season of high-protein forage utilizing its all-inclusive clover plants as a green manure for fixing free atmospheric nitrogen into the soil. Whereas, an arable cropping system will only yield one or two crops per season and will largely remain reliant on the inputs of artificial fertilizer for its nitrogen source, one ton of which requires ten tons of crude oil in the manufacturing process.[9]

He claimed that vegetarians simply lack an understanding of the relationship between soil fertility and the ecosystems on earth. They would prefer to use up our limited fossil fuel for agriculture than to use manure from livestock!

Furthermore, the argument goes, we could be feeding people 20 pounds of grain instead of feeding that to the cattle from whom we get only one pound of meat. But what informed health seeker in his right mind would want to eat those grains? Or would want to eat cattle fed those grains? *In nature, cattle and humans do not compete for food.*

What if everyone in the world were to join hands and make a solemn vow to never again eat animal products and to divide all food equally so we could all be fed? Well, first of all, there would be many people, probably a majority, who would have shortened life spans and compromised health. If everyone were eating grains and beans, it would be equal diabetes and arthritis for all!

Even if we sprouted the grains and beans, this restricted diet would make some of us so bloated that we couldn't eat enough to get sufficient calories with it. Cooking makes it easier to eat more; plus it increases caloric absorption. A diet consisting of only sprouted beans and grains without some animal foods is unlikely to create health in most people. They make good *supplements* but not the *base* of one's diet.

While it may be noble of us to sacrifice health for animals, is it really in our best interest to have an overpopulated world of undernourished, sick people? I say that because I really believe very few of us can be sustained on strictly vegan diets.

> *I question whether sustainability can be had simply by feeding everyone a diet that is not sustaining health.*

I am sure governments all around the world would dance with delight. Finally they have what they want — tax paying laborers who die at midlife and never need to collect retirement or social security benefits, people who never live to the age when most people catch on to how corrupt the government really is and how much their hard-earned savings have depreciated. And since these people would be deficient in DHA, they would be less intelligent and easier to control. Talk about efficiency and maximum profit!

I admit the vegetarians have a point that we would get more calories to feed the world if we used the land for produce to feed us instead of for cattle. Yet I question whether sustainability can be had simply by feeding everyone a diet that is not sustaining health. Most of the crops grown are things that people have no business eating if they want to be healthy. Grains — and that includes hybrid corn — are at the root of the chronic diseases of civilization.

Grains are high in phytates, which prevent our bodies from absorbing minerals. When refined and cooked, they wreak havoc on the blood sugar, spiking serum insulin levels — high insulin levels being at the root of most disease.[10] They increase the body's ratio of omega-6 to omega-3 fatty acids, leading to obesity, cancer, and depression. So why are we growing these crops? Because they can be stored a long time and are therefore very profitable to the food companies. Because food companies and grain merchants lobby the government for farm subsidies.

For true overall sustainability, you need to have sustainability in the microcosm, with each individual being healthy. What works for the macrocosm has to work for the microcosm. If a dietary plan is not sustainable for each individual, it is not sustainable for the planet. If we feed the people grains, soy, and corn, we will have an arthritic, diabetic, cancer-ridden population with chubby or obese bodies and dull minds.

I have been to India three times; I know what a diet of beans and rice does. I have seen the extreme thinness of the majority of the population, which is barely getting enough calories from these high-carb foods, even though they are high in calories per pound. The middle classes, who can afford more food, tend to be somewhat overweight after the age of 40 when insulin resistance is greater. This is also true in South America, where much of the population is economically forced to be mainly vegetarian, living on beans and rice.

What about creating a raw vegan agriculture?

Granted, if we were to grow fruit and nut trees everywhere and make everyone eat a grain-free, high-carb raw diet that included plenty of greens, nuts, and seeds (with some seaweed for trace minerals), this would be a *tremendous* improvement. But for many, many people, including myself, this would nonetheless not result in peak health. Some of us just don't attain peak health on vegan or even vegetarian fare. *Raw*, yes. *Vegan*, no!

For the individual to have perfect health, we need to go back to a high-raw hunter-gatherer diet. For most people, even only three ounces of meat a day would be enough to get the nutrients that are hard or impossible to get from plants. But where are we going to find the wild game to hunt? Where are we going to find wild fruit that has not been hybridized and improperly grown such that it contains too much sugar relative to the minerals needed for the body to properly metabolize it? There might be a bit here and there, but definitely not enough to feed 7 billion. Good luck trying to reproduce the wilderness that we spent 10,000 years destroying!

The average hunter-gatherer needed five square miles to feed himself.[11] With that ratio, the US would support only about 600,000 hunter-gatherers! Our current population exceeds 300 million.

We could certainly improve the plant part of our diets by using heirloom seeds and permaculture and by increasing the mineral content of our soil. But wild animals still need room to roam.

So, as we gather and hunt at the grocery store, we simply have to do the best we can. We shun factory-farmed meat. We seek out meat from wild or compassionately raised animals, even if we have to order online. Or we get clean meat from animals that are free range and fed organically their natural foods right up to slaughter, with no steroids, antibiotics, and preferably no vaccinations.

We buy poultry, which is more eco-friendly than mammals, using less space and resources per pound of meat. We reserve beef or lamb for once every week or two. Even then, the price is high, so we don't eat a lot of it, just enough to get the nutrients we need.

We also try to find animal products with the labels *kosher* or *halal*, even if we are not Jewish or Muslim, because these animals have supposedly been more compassionately slaughtered in such as way that they didn't even realize they were going to be killed.

Now I am sure some of you are going to ask, "But is it economically feasible for everyone on the planet to eat enough meat?" I would argue that with planning, this can be done. Most people in a modified paleo diet don't need meat every single day and can use eggs as their main animal protein.

Professor Loren Cordain argues that we need

to eat about half our diets in meat.

When accompanied by sufficient amounts of alkaline fruit and vegetables, high-protein diets do not promote osteoporosis. Instead, they protect you from it.[12]

To that I would say: *No way!* Fruit nowadays is picked before it is ripened (at least in the US). It is therefore not as alkaline as it should be. If you eat a diet which is half meat, not only will it be very expensive if you get the high-quality, clean meat, but it will be very acidic to eat so much protein (if cooked). Very few people need that much protein. There may be some who need this much *temporarily* — while they are trying to get their insulin sensitivity back and restore depleted nutrient reserves.

A normal diet in which 10 to 30 percent of the calories are protein is adequate for nearly everyone. It is not necessary to eat that much meat, since we can get much of our protein from plant foods (especially greens, hemp seeds, and nuts, with the occasional tempeh). For many people, eating three to six ounces of meat or fish once a day is sufficient; for some, two to five times a week would be enough. Some carb types might need it once or twice a month, as the Hunzas. This is especially true if the meat is raw or rare, as the nutrients and protein are better absorbed. And you might need even less if you eat a considerable amount of organ meats, which are much more nutrient-dense.

At the root of all sustainability issues is population. I once saw a headline saying, "India is requesting that Americans stop eating meat, as it is destroying the environment." I couldn't help but think (at the risk of offending my Indian friends, ex-husband, and former boyfriend!) that we should tell *them* to stop increasing *their* population! Wouldn't it be much more effective if we all joined hands and promised not to have more than one child each rather than pledge never to eat any meat?

As our population grows, competition for high-quality meat or even quality produce will grow fierce, driving prices up even more. You think I don't care about sustainability because I eat animal products? At least I never had any children. If you care about the planet, not having children is one of the best things you could possibly do. Or just have one, and give him or her the best education, the most love, and the most healthful diet possible.

Nonetheless, the Indians were correct to say that we eat too much meat in the US. According to an article in the *New York Times*, we eat about eight ounces a day, which is twice the world average.[13] Factory farming has made meat cheaper than ever in the US. By 2005, our consumption was 200 pounds a year per person, which is about *nine* ounces a day.[14] Yet the USDA recommends only four ounces per day.[15]

Another sustainability consideration is the *locavore* consideration of eating locally grown food to minimize the use of fossil fuel ("carbon footprint"). Unless you are living in a warm climate, it is *nearly impossible* to be a very healthy vegan without a large carbon footprint. Fruits, vegetables, nuts, seeds, and especially super foods, are usually imported from all over the world. It is usually not possible to eat seasonally on such a restricted diet either, unless you dehydrate or can food thoroughly.

Reporter Steven Shapin addresses the sustainability issue in a *New Yorker* article.

A recent report by the U.N.'s Food and Agriculture Organization reckons that at least eighteen percent of the global-warming effect comes from livestock, more than is caused by all the world's transportation system. It has been estimated that forty per cent of global grain output is used to feed animals rather than people, and that half of this grain would be sufficient to eliminate world hunger if — and it's not a small if — the political will could be found to insure equitable distribution.

Yet the energy-cost argument is formidably complicated and cannot by itself support refusing all forms of meat in favor of all forms of plant matter: shooting and eating the deer chewing up the tulips in your garden may turn out to be more environmentally virtuous than dining on tofu manufactured from Chinese soybeans, and walking to the local supermarket for a nice hanger steak cut from a grass-fed New Zealand steer may be kinder to the planet than getting into your Toyota Prius to drive five miles for some organic Zambian green beans.[16]

Another key to sustainability is to slow your metabolism once you no longer need to lose weight. Train your body to require less food. As good, non-toxic food becomes more expensive, rather than eating cheap carbs or toxic produce, simply eat less of the good stuff. If you eat mostly raw organic or sustainable food, you get more nutrients for the buck.

Don't compromise your health by filling your belly excessively with grains, starchy vegetables, or sweet hybrid fruits. Stay on a diet of greens, apples, berries, avocados, olives, nuts, seeds, eggs, fish, and small amounts of quality land meat. Just eat less. It is easier to eat less on a low-glycemic diet.

If Everyone Became Vegetarian, Most of the World Would Starve!

Few know better than I do about the agony of not being able to breathe. In the past, I have had asthma attacks that were so great I could not lie down and had to sit up all night gasping for air. Breathing became my full focus, both a meditation and exercise. So I feel the pain of a fish being caught even more than the average vegan. This doesn't take away the point that a large human population depends on fish for food. Three quarters of the earth is ocean, and this is where we get a huge chunk of our food.

If some vegan and vegetarian activists who exclude fish got their way, the world would stop eating fish. Don't they realize that the world's poorest people depend on fishing to survive? There is a reason that about 50 percent of the world's people live relatively close to the coastal regions — and it isn't for those nice walks on the beach at sunset (though that ranked high with me when I lived in San Diego). If everyone adopted this philosophy, billions would die of starvation.

It is true that many of the large fish are disappearing from being overfished and that they are toxic with mercury, PCBs, and other man-made pollutants. These facts do not negate the fact that we evolved eating seafood and need the nutrients seafood contains. I believe we have the technology to clean the ocean, and we have the ability to repopulate the fish. It is just a matter of politics. I hope this gets handled soon.

Some people, including John Robbins, author of several vegan books, think it is not so bad to eat wild fish, since after all, they were not factory farmed. This is true, and fish are one of the most healthful foods. But as the political situation stands today, if we were all to eat fish to the exclusion of land animals, we would find the already dwindling fish population disappearing faster than ever.

We cannot all depend on fish as some native people have done, because most of the world's fisheries are now depleted or in steep decline, and because our oceans and lakes are polluted and many of today's fish are high in mercury and other toxic contaminants.[17]

As for me, I am not going to let my brain rot while I wait for politicians and corporations to get their acts together in cleaning and replenishing the ocean. Pass the sardines, please!

Another important consideration is that only about 11 percent of the earth's land is arable. Large portions of our planet's land — deserts and mountainous areas — are not suitable for growing crops, but some of this land could be used to feed grazing animals. It would be ludicrous to waste that land. Nomads in the desert, where few edible plants can grow, depend largely on animal products from camels and goats. Note that some deserts were actually created by animal overgrazing, which is another reason crop rotation is so crucial.

In the UK, mountainous regions which cannot grow crops are able to sustain sheep, the UK's major livestock. If they gave up their sheep and fishing, huge portions of the population would starve to death or lead shortened lives in pseudo-health with a diet of grains.

If everyone decided it was morally wrong to eat animal foods, much of the world would starve. There simply isn't enough land for growing vegetarian food for everyone to be in peak health — especially the low-calorie, mineral-rich vegetables we would need more of to compensate for the lack of preformed vitamin A and other nutrients we depend on animal products for.[*]

There are ways to "green the desert" and improve our situation.[18] Nonetheless, most people still need to consume some animal products for peak health.

As indicated earlier in chapter 4, a vegan diet that ensures peak health is in many ways a luxury reserved for the middle and upper-middle classes. Many super foods imported from around the world and a variety of costly supplements are necessary to

---

[*]See chapter 15.

compensate for what is missing when you forgo nutrient-dense animal foods.

I once saw an episode of *Wife Swap*, a reality TV show that pits two very opposite families against each other. One family was raw vegan and they verbally duked it out with a lower-income family that hunted deer to eat. At the end of the two weeks, the vegan family finally got it that this family would not have very much food to eat if they didn't hunt deer.

Is there anyone out there who thinks billions of people should starve so that animals might live a slightly longer life?

In Vitro Meat

The evolution of our bodies is not likely to catch up with the evolution of our minds and spiritual awareness any time soon.

However, our technology has *almost caught up* with our spiritual/moral consciousness. In about 10 years, we should be able to buy *in vitro* meat — cultured meat that has never been part of an animal. Such meat doesn't impact the environment, since animals are not raised; neither does it involve slaughtering a sentient being. No nervous system is feeling pain. NASA and Dutch researchers have started working on it.

PETA has even offered one million dollars to the first company that could bring lab-grown chicken meat to consumers by 2012. They arrived at that figure by calculating that approximately a million chickens are killed every hour in the US.

In vitro meat is not synthetic and therefore should be safe, at least after the technique is perfected. The process involves taking a muscle cell from any animal through a biopsy and joining it with a protein that helps the cell grow into large portions of meat. It is cultivated similarly to the process of culturing yogurt. Once it grows, no more biopsies beyond the initial one are needed. For cells to mature, they must soak in a nutrient-rich soup, which is currently a costly fetal bovine serum but may soon be replaced by a plant-based substitute that will be more economical and will satisfy many vegetarians.

In a *Time* magazine article, journalist D.J. Siegelbaum explains the process.

Scientists biopsy stem or satellite muscle cells from a livestock animal, such as a chicken, cow, or pig. The cells are then placed in a nutrient-rich medium where they divide and multiply and are then attached to a scaffolding structure and put in a bioreactor to grow. In order to achieve the texture of natural muscle, the cells must be physically stretched and flexed, or exercised, regularly. After several weeks, voila, you have a thin layer of muscle tissue that can be harvested and processed into ground beef, chicken, or pork, depending on the origin of the cells. But don't expect to see big, juicy in vitro steaks anytime soon; the technology has not yet been able to synthesize blood vessels or grow large, three-dimensional pieces of meat.

Though it sounds a lot like Frankenfood, scientists note that in vitro tissue engineering is not the same as genetic engineering, a common misconception. "We use natural cells from natural animals," says Dr. Vladimir Mironov, a tissue engineer and assistant professor at the Medical University of South Carolina. "We don't change Mother Nature, we just try to imitate it." But there's always room for improvement — scientists can design meat, for example, that is high in healthy fats, such as omega-3s and -6s. Creating the meat in a lab also decreases its exposure to bacteria and disease, which have riddled the livestock industry, injuring consumers and causing extensive meat recalls.[19]

Again, the benefits are numerous: health and ethical considerations, environmental impact (no use of fresh water to raise cattle, no methane gas to add to global warming), reduced cost, and availability of meat for space explorations and natural disasters.

Nonetheless, as with many of man's experiments, we must be cautious. Until in vitro meat withstands the tests of time, anyone eating it long-term will be a guinea pig. I think I'll stick with Nature's methods until then.

In the Meantime...

If you are at less than peak health, forget about saving the *planet*; save *yourself*! Do the best you can by growing your own food if you can and getting in the best physical shape possible.

Saving the world is too big a task for a tired, malnourished, insulin-resistant body. You need to first work on yourself. Remember Linda Hamilton in the blockbuster movie *Terminator 2*? She was getting "buffed up" while in prison, making herself the best she could be, getting in gear to save the planet. Only when she was in great shape could she take on her destiny of saving the world.

So let's get in gear by eating the right diet!

Part 5

What's for Dinner?

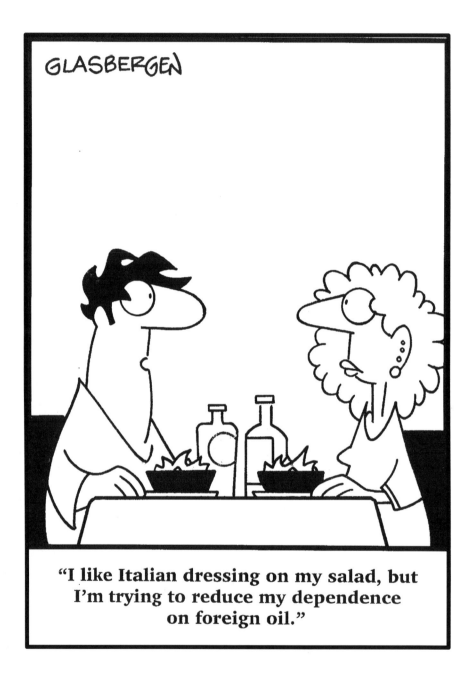

"I like Italian dressing on my salad, but
I'm trying to reduce my dependence
on foreign oil."

Chapter 23

Diet: It's All about Balance!

Diet is the essential key to all successful healing. Without a proper balanced diet, the effectiveness of herbal treatment is very limited.

—Michael Tierra, CA, ND, author of numerous books, including *The Way of Herbs* and *Planetary Herbology*

What your grandmother said was true: nutrition is all about *balance*! Our paleolithic ancestors ate a wide variety of foods — hundreds of plants and animals. Eating a varied diet not only helps you get all the obscure nutrients for optimal health, but it also prevents certain toxins from accumulating to the point that they can cause damage.

In *The Live Food Factor*, I cited scientific studies documenting that cooking food creates toxic by-products, chaotically produced chemicals that appear unpredictably and therefore impossible to fully adapt to.[1] However, many uncooked foods also contain toxins, even in their natural state.

If you consume more than about 5 percent of your calories in dairy products that contain the protein casein, even raw dairy, you may be exposing your cells to carcinogens and increasing your chances of getting cancer, according to the China Study.

If you overindulge in meat, especially cooked, your body tissues will become increasingly acidic, and your pancreas may even secrete excessive amounts of insulin. You might also lack enough antioxidants from fruits, berries especially, and sufficient plant fiber. With excessive intake of methionine, you may put yourself at risk for Alzheimer's, heart attacks, strokes, and depression. Americans eat an average of 9 ounces of meat a day; anything over 6 ounces is risky for some people.

One study found that meat eaters were about 20 percent more prone to dementia than vegetarians.[2] This is because cooked meat creates toxic by-products, such as heterocyclic amines. Many cured meats also contain nitrosamines, implicated in Alzheimer's.[3] Poultry and fish, however, have been found to deter Alzheimer's.[4]

Another study tested lab animals that ate the same percentage of saturated fats as the typical American: 10 percent. The animals developed severe brain and memory dysfunction![5]

If you overeat grains and lentils, to a much lesser degree sprouted, you will block mineral absorption because of their phytates.

If you overeat fruit, your blood insulin levels will swing alternately too high and too low due to the fruit's sugar content — unless you go on a very low-fat diet, in which case you may suffer deficiencies of essential minerals and fats. You could also gain too much weight from these high insulin levels, which tell the body to store fat. And don't forget the possible damage to your teeth!

If you overeat nuts and seeds, you will take in too much fat and may become overweight from all the calories. You may also experience fatigue, since nuts and seeds can be hard to digest. If you overeat any of them except walnuts, hemp seeds, flaxseeds, and chia seeds, your body's ratio of omega-6 to omega-3 fatty acids will become unbalanced, leading to disease and possible memory problems. If you overeat flaxseeds, you may damage your thyroid.

If you overeat green leaves and vegetables, you may become bloated from too much cellulose. Also, you will be spending a lot of money or a lot of effort in gardening, as these are low in calories. You would need to eat quite a lot to make them a huge part of your caloric intake. If you can afford the time and money, juicing them is a great option.

If you overindulge in wheatgrass juice, you may experience nausea. At the 2004 Portland, Oregon, raw food festival, there was a wheatgrass juice-drinking contest, and people who vomited were automatically eliminated.

This is why we need to eat in balance from a wide variety of foods. Your grandmother, or great-grandmother, was right. If you are over 50, it may even have been your mother.

Even if you eat a 100 percent raw, 100 percent

vegan, and 100 percent organic diet, your body is still battling exogenous toxins because nearly every food has its own inherent toxins. Plants often have naturally toxic compounds to guard against overeager predators. Or a toxin may be present to protect the plant from spoiling when damaged by weather, handling, UV light, or microbes.[6] When concentrated at high enough levels, phytotoxins can make a person sick.

Let's look at some specific plant toxins:

- The brassica species (cabbage, cauliflower, broccoli, rutabaga, kohlrabi, kale, collards, bok choy, rapeseed, and more) contain goitrogens, which bind iodine and inhibit thyroid gland function.[7] These goitrogens are destroyed by cooking, so one should never eat them excessively in raw form. However, cooking them also destroys many of their valuable nutrients, less so if lightly steamed.

- Potatoes have glycoalkaloids, especially solanine. These are not destroyed by cooking, but if you remove any green or damaged parts, you can minimize these toxins. Cut out the eyes if they are sprouting. Tomatoes and eggplants also contain glycoalkaloids in the green parts.

- Spinach and rhubarb contain oxalic acid, which is toxic in excess and also inhibits calcium absorption. Significant amounts of oxalates are also found in cabbage, beet greens, carrots, peas, mushrooms, tea, chard, and cacao.[8] Overdosing on this toxin can even lead to kidney stones.

- Zucchini has a group of natural toxins called *cucurbitacins*.

- Apple and pear seeds, as well as apricot pits, contain amygdalin, which can turn into cyanide in the stomach. Amygdalin is also known as vitamin B_{17}, or laetrile, which is said to protect against cancer, but no more than two apricot kernels a day should be consumed, unless they

are of the Hunza variety, which is not so toxic.

- Aflatoxin is a mold that is sometimes found growing on peanuts, grains, nuts, sunflower seeds, and certain spices, such as black pepper and coriander.[9] This mold is one of the most powerful liver carcinogens known!

- Lectins are found in seeds, grains, and legumes. They bind minerals, preventing them from being assimilated in the digestive process.

- Phytates are found in soybeans, whole wheat, and rye. These also bind minerals.

- Plantains are rich in indoles the body converts to a toxin known as *3-hydroxyanthranilic acid*. Africans who eat a lot of them have high rates of bladder cancer.

- Tannins are found in pomegranates, persimmons, berries, nuts, smoked foods, herbs, spices, tea, coffee, beer, wine, and legumes, including coffee beans and cocoa beans. Tannins impede the digestion of protein and the absorption of iron and zinc if taken at the same time.

These are just examples. A comprehensive list might be quite long. Probably every plant has some number and amount of toxins for self-protection. If you eat a wide variety of foods, you will be much less likely to be significantly affected by any of these toxins. If you eat foods natural to the human species, even less so.

☞ Balance is key: rotate your foods, eating them in moderation. Eat a wide variety of foods from the species-specific diet that we evolved eating.

Dr. Mark Berry, who is in charge of research at Unilever, agrees.

> The main hallmark of the palaeolithic diet was a huge diversity of plants. Nowadays we try our best to eat five portions of fruit and veg a day. They ate 20 to 25 plant-based foods a day.[10]

Chapter 24

Is Eating Raw Natural?

The raw food diet is a fad that has lasted millions of years. —Susan Schenck

Here is a simple test designed to see if you should be a raw fooder: Are you a living creature on this earth? If you answered yes to that question, you are genetically designed to eat a raw diet. Can you name any other creature that cooks its food? If cooking were necessary for health, how did our hominid ancestors thrive without it?

As I explain in my book *The Live Food Factor*, we were unquestionably designed to eat a diet of uncooked food containing lots of fruit, vegetables, nuts, and seeds, just as our primate cousins in the wild still eat. Now I am saying you may have to, like our primate cousins, add a bit of raw (or lightly heated) eggs and/or meat to your diet also.

Many anthropologists nonetheless applaud cooking as having enabled humans to eat foods that would otherwise be toxic in their natural state, like beans and grains. While it is true that grains and legumes, which have long shelf lives, enable humans to get by in sparse times, it is really clear they are neither our original nor our ideal foods. They are so full of antinutrients that one should question whether we should even be eating them outside of emergencies or insufficient funds. These foods have doubtless allowed humans to overpopulate the earth and destroy the balance of nature via chemical agriculture.

While researching the history of human diet, I found that numerous anthropologists felt cooking had some advantages that enhanced man's evolution. I got a copy of a cooking manifesto, *Catching Fire: How Cooking Made Us Human*, by Richard Wrangham, professor of biological anthropology at Harvard University.

Amusingly, my husband thought this was another book promoting the raw food diet. To him, being human is *not* a plus; we should instead identify with our divine natures!

In the first chapter, Professor Wrangham discusses studies showing that raw fooders do not get enough calories, claiming that this could not have sustained our ancestors; thus a raw food diet was not what we evolved on. Cooking increases the number of calories absorbed. This could be because cooking food increases both its glycemic index and its glycemic load, causing the body to secrete more insulin, thereby stimulating the body to store more fat.

However, the raw fooders from the studies he cites were mainly on low-fat, vegan diets, which tend to be lower in calories. Even for many raw vegan diets, what about the highly caloric nuts, seeds, olives, and avocados, which made some of us raw fooders (like me!) actually struggle with our weights? These, he insists, were only seasonally available before modern times.

OK, I get it. But that only proves we were not raw *vegans*. What about all the raw meat and eggs our ancestors ate? These were very nutrient dense. Wrangham goes on to argue that cooking meat and eggs has been shown in tests to enhance digestibility and absorption of calories. The argument that raw fooders use against cooking meat — that cooking denatures protein — is something that he views as an *advantage*. He claims that denaturing meat makes it easier to digest.

Wrangham cites a study in which physician Dr. William Beaumont, MD, observed the digestion of Alexis St. Martin, one of his patients. In 1822, St. Martin was accidentally shot in the stomach. A hole remained in his stomach that never fully healed. Beaumont convinced him to agree to be part of some studies on digestion. Beaumont performed experiments to observe how his digestion worked by looking through the window into his stomach. Wrangham insists cooked meat digests more easily than raw meat because it is more tender.

I bought the book by Dr. Beaumont to see for myself and noticed that in every case in which a food was eaten raw, it was digested *faster*! In other words, contrary to Wrangham's claims, raw or lightly cooked meat is faster and therefore *easier* to digest than more thoroughly cooked meat.

Wrangham argues that the advantage of obtaining more calories from cooked starches ensured that humans got enough energy for survival. Perhaps so, but given our obesity epidemic, eating cooked starches is hardly an advantage in modern times. Furthermore, cooked grains and legumes, according to experts on the paleo diet, were also not common in our diet until agriculture developed.

From an evolutionary perspective, if cooking causes a loss of vitamins or creates a few long-term toxic compounds, the effect is relatively unimportant compared to the impact of more calories.[1]

OK, so cooking allows us to get enough calories to overpopulate the planet. But evolution is not concerned about the longevity of the individual, only the survival of the species. For example, getting enough calories to remain fertile is great for the survival of the species, but studies abound showing that a calorie-restricted diet enables the individual to live longer. So if cooking otherwise toxic quantities of tubers, grains, and legumes helped us overpopulate the world, cooking did its job to ensure the survival of *Homo sapiens*. But for the individual, eating raw is conducive to superior health and longevity, as proven by all the studies described in *The Live Food Factor*.[2]

Dr. Wrangham argues that the studies which show cooking produces toxins need not alarm us, because these toxins will affect only animals, since humans have adapted to them. About half the studies summarized in my book are on humans. They show conclusively that eating raw, giving the body a break from these toxins, helps one to detox.

Wrangham correctly points out that some of our ancestors have been cooking for tens of thousands of years, which he considers enough time to adapt to the toxins. The problem is that the molecules created each time one cooks are so randomly and unpredictably formed that some experts believe we will *never* be able to adapt.[*]

Further, blood tests on people who eat cooked food show intestinal *leukocytosis* — an aggregation of white blood cells in that area. Such tests on people after they eat raw food do *not* demonstrate this increase in white blood cells! This increase of leukocytes is thought to be because they are needed for extra digestive support since cooked foods do not contain their own active enzymes that would otherwise assist in the digestive process. The pancreas thus becomes overburdened and needs the extra assistance of this emergency crew, even though the pancreas itself approximately triples in size in an attempt to keep up when cooked food is habitually eaten.[4]

Wrangham repeats the false assertion that it doesn't matter if we eat food with enzymes or not, because the stomach digests those food enzymes. However, Dr. Edward Howell showed more than half a century ago that during the first 30 to 60 minutes after a food is ingested, the naturally occurring digestive enzymes in all raw foods help to digest the food while it rests in the *cardiac* portion of the stomach, its upper section. It isn't until they reach the lower *pyloric* section that they become inactivated, where some, but not all, are destroyed by stomach acids. Those that survive reactivate in the small intestines and continue to aid in further digestion of the food.

I always tell people that if you don't believe it, just eat everything raw for a few days, and see how much more energy you have. So far, everyone I know who's tried it sees a huge difference. When we eat raw, we spare our pancreases much labor in cranking out digestive enzymes to compensate for food enzymes lost in the heat of cooking.

Wrangham argues that the human brain became larger not just from eating meat, but also from cooking. I wonder then, how does he explain the *11*

---

[*]"The substances generated are endless chains of new molecules that are variously toxic, aromatic, peroxidizing, antioxidizing, mutagenic, and carcinogenic. For example, in a broiled potato alone, Maillard identified 450 novel chemicals and tested them one by one for toxicity. Every one of the first 50 he tested was proven to be carcinogenic to laboratory animals. At that point, his employer terminated that line of research and *(continued in the next column)*

gave Maillard something else to work on before he could test the others."[3]

There were 450 novel chemicals isolated from a broiled potato. Consider what happens when other food items (cheese, salt, butter, oil) are added to the potato under various cooking methods (frying, microwaving, baking, et al.), and try to compute how many additional chemicals require genetic adaptation. It's impossible. Plus adaptation requires selective pressure. Where is the selective pressure?

percent shrinkage of the human brain that coincides with when we began to *cook much more*?

Furthermore, how does cooking food add brain nutrients like B_{12}, DHA, and EPA? If anything, it destroys some of them.

This book did make me realize that cooking began much earlier than I had thought. He cites evidence of cooking having occurred 2 million years ago and credits the reduction of our guts, teeth, and mouth sizes to eating cooked foods.

To the author's credit, I no longer feel so bad about steaming my turkey. At least I am not getting the whole toxic burden that comes with barbequing or grilling it. However, it remains clear to me, even with my occasional cheats, that *raw is law*.

Enzymes and Nutrients Destroyed by Cooking

Dr. Edward Howell devoted his entire career to studying enzymes and wrote a few books on the topic. To this day, ignorant doctors say it doesn't matter whether you eat raw or not because food enzymes are broken down in the stomach anyway, along with all other proteins. This is not true. As explained earlier, the food enzymes go to work for 30 to 60 minutes in the upper, cardiac section of the stomach before proceeding to the sections where pepsin and hydrochloric acid act.[5]

One interesting thought is that if food enzymes were destroyed in the stomach, then how is it that the stomach's own enzymes, those produced by the body, are *not* destroyed? Moreover, even mainstream nutritionists agree that mother's milk contributes hormones and antibodies, which are proteins, to the suckling infant. How is that possible if all proteins are destroyed by stomach acids?

Dr. Howell found that when we eat cooked food, our pancreases have to work overtime to crank out digestive enzymes, and this ages us. For the average food, heating it above 118° F for 30 minutes denatures nearly 100 percent of the food enzymes. Dr. Howell believed that our bodies inherit only so much enzyme production potential at birth. When this runs out, we die. Thus the more cooked food we eat, the *sooner* we die!

By age 40, the average person has only 30 percent of his lifetime enzyme production capacity left.[6] This a major reason for increasing tiredness with age.[*]

> The length of life is inversely proportional to the rate of exhaustion of the enzyme potential of an organism. ...
>
> It is shown that when the enzyme potential is exhausted beyond a particular point, it triggers the end of the life span.[8]

In other words, by incorporating more raw foods into your diet, you extend your life. You also have more energy freed up. Energy no longer needed for digestion often goes to the higher chakras, creating spiritual awakening, renewed creativity, mental alertness, enhanced optimism, and concentration.[†]

Cooking Just Allows You to Eat Toxic Food

Cooking allowed humans to expand their repertoire of plant food, since cooking destroys many toxins and antinutrients, as nutritional anthropologist Dr. Leon Abrams explains.

> Most plants eaten by humans today contain toxins, such as enzyme inhibitors, physiological irritants, allergens, favism substances, cholinesterase inhibitors, cyanogens, hemagglutinins, lathyrogens, goitrogens, vitamin and mineral antagonists, and poisonous alkaloids. Cooking neutralizes these toxins, rendering the foods that contain them safe for human consumption; therefore, there is a direct relationship between human consumption of most plant foods and cooking. When man developed the use of fire for cooking, he greatly expanded the number of plant foods that he could utilize.[9]

The problem is, cooking doesn't destroy *all* the antinutrients and toxins. It just disarms enough of them so a person doesn't get sick. Raw fooders claim that we are simply better off not eating any food that demands to be cooked. In that respect,

---

[*]Dr. Howell reviewed hundreds of studies, including one from Michael Reese Hospital in Chicago in which the enzymes found in the saliva of young adults were determined to be 30 times more concentrated than in people over 69.[7]

[†]The first chapter of *The Live Food Factor* presents a complete summary of all the benefits to "going raw."

they agree with those adhering to the paleodiet. If you want peak health, stick to man's original foods.

Cooking Adds New Toxins to Food

As detailed in *The Live Food Factor*, cooking creates toxic by-products, such as acrylamides, advanced glycation end products, lipid peroxides, and heterocyclic amines. The book summarizes dozens of studies showing the superiority of raw over cooked.

An additional study that was done after *The Live Food Factor* came out compared allergic reactions to raw vs. cooked or processed foods. The allergic reactions to the cooked and processed foods were by far more dramatic. The researchers concluded from the study that the formation of AGEs as a result of cooking contributes to inflammation, autoimmune reactions, aging, diabetes, and neuro-degeneration.[10]

I remarked earlier that the studies on macronutrients are enough to drive a health seeker crazy. There are studies and books showing that a diet high in protein leads to cancer and other diseases.[11] There are studies and books convincing us how dangerous insulin is. Hence a high-carb diet is to be avoided.[12] And there are studies and books showing that eating a high-fat diet is the recipe for early death.[13]

The dilemma is that when you reduce the percentage of one macronutrient, you must increase the percentage of another! Even if you cut back on calories, as beneficial to health and longevity as that is, those percentages will remain. We could consider the Zone Diet (30 percent fat, 30 percent protein, 40 percent carbs), but then the advocates of low-fat and low-protein diets would claim we were nonetheless in danger.

I asked Dr. Stanley Bass about this quandary in a phone conversation. His reply:

All these studies have been done on cooked foods. We don't know what the results would be on raw foods, but we do know that raw foods do not contain nearly as many toxins as cooked foods do. Eating a raw food diet, one doesn't have to be so overly concerned with getting the ratios so precise.

I know that was the case with me, except that I went way over my carb limits at the expense of pro-

tein needs.

Lots of Other Reasons to Eat Raw

There are many reasons to eat raw, because that is the way we evolved eating. Cooking food raises its glycemic index. Raw food is easier and faster to digest.[14] As I detailed in *The Live Food Factor*, cooking destroys, damages, or eliminates many valuable things in food, including phytochemicals, biophotons, oxygen, water, electrons, chlorophyll, friendly bacteria, minerals, vitamins, and probably many things we haven't even discovered yet![*]

Raw foods are also richer in vitamins. Viktoras Kulvinskas created a list of the various nutrients destroyed by cooking. He compiled this list from numerous scientific journals and detailed them on page 48 of his classic book *Survival into the 21st Century*. He discovered that about 45 to 55 percent of B vitamins are lost in heated foods, as well as 70 to 80 percent of vitamin C, and 50 percent of vitamin E, for example.

Cooking does not improve the nutritional value of food. It destroys or makes unavailable 85 percent of the original nutrients.

Raw Food Helps You Heal Not Just from Disease, but Also from Accidents

I know of people who even used raw foods as a main part of healing from accidents. Take Aajonus Vonderplanitz. Four MDs told him that his son, injured in a car accident, would be brain dead for life. Using raw foods, Aajonus got his son to emerge from his coma with full recovery of his brain and muscles. His son went on to graduate from a university.[†]

Then there is Dr. Joe Dispenza, who appears in the films *What the (Bleep) Do We Know?* and *What If?* He tells his story in his book *Evolve Your Brain*. Joe was injured in a car accident and was diagnosed

---

[*]Chapter 10 of *The Live Food Factor* goes into detail on the many food ingredients destroyed by cooking.

[†]His book *We Want to Live*, details the entire story.

with "multiple compression fractures of the thoracic spine with the T-8 vertebra more than 60 percent collapsed." The doctors recommended Harrington rod surgery (implanting a stainless steel surgical device), but Joe was haunted by the outcomes of all the patients he had seen that had had this surgery. They never really healed, never regained their spinal flexibility, and many lived the rest of their lives addicted to pain medications. Infused with conviction of the body's innate healing powers, he rejected surgery and used raw foods plus rest and visualization to recover.

Darrell Stoffels used raw foods and enzymes as a major part of his healing protocol. He was pronounced "dead on arrival" in a 1970 car accident, upgraded to "coma," and later graduated to a wheelchair. He attributes much of his recovery to enzymes and essential fatty-acid nutrition, along with a few other modalities.[15]

Finally, there is my husband, who injured his back from lifting weights at the gym. He was diagnosed with a herniated disc and told he needed surgery, but he continued with his raw diet, getting lots of rest, and doing plenty of stretching exercises. His MRI a year and a half later showed complete healing!

The Case for Raw or Rare Meat

The biggest problem I have in convincing people to go raw is that they think they have to become vegan, which most people believe is too nutritionally restrictive. By now you know our ancestors ate raw meat. However, meat was probably the first thing they cooked. During the Ice Age, if they didn't eat the kill immediately, it froze. So they had to heat it to some degree at least in order to thaw it out. The Eskimos, however, simply buried their meat so deep that it wouldn't freeze.

Raw meat sounds disgusting to civilized man, yet nearly every culture has a history of eating it. Consider sushi from Japan, seviche from Peru, steak tartare from France.

I told my friends I was writing about eating raw meat, and they were utterly disgusted. I then reminded them that we had just eaten at a restaurant at which we had all shared some lightly seared raw tuna. We had paid *two dollars* for each small strip of lightly seared meat.

I would never eat raw pork (too risky for parasites) or raw beef without knowing it is from pastured cows (too risky for sick tissues contaminated with harmful *E. coli* and other toxic waste matter).

Many Reasons for Eating Meat Raw or Rare

Most people won't like the idea of eating meat raw. If you don't, at least you can cook it very lightly to avoid adding more toxins to it. Organically raised meat should not have any harmful bacterial contamination. If it does by chance, due to bad handling procedures, the bacteria would be only on the surface. Bacteria would grow from the outside to the inside, so slightly searing the meat would kill any supposedly dangerous microbes, yet the meat would be raw at the core. Of course, if you had ground the meat, any bacteria in it would be dispersed all over, which is why hamburger gets contaminated so easily.

Later we will discuss how to eat raw or lightly cooked meat safely by freezing it first, as well as how to make it tasty.

Raw meat has many advantages over cooked. Below is a list of benefits from eating it, just as our hominid ancestors did.

Raw meat contains protease enzymes to help us digest it.

Even if it has been commercially frozen, about 70 to 75 percent of the enzymes are still viable. This makes it far easier to digest and doesn't give you that "heavy brick" feeling in the stomach that cooked meat does.

Its micronutrients (B_{12}, zinc, B_6, et al.) are not ruined if you don't cook the meat. One study found that cooking meat destroys around 33 percent of the B_{12}.[16]

In fact, some raw organs even contain vitamin C! The Eskimos traditionally lived on a diet of 100 percent raw meat at least six months out of the year, since there was no vegetation then. They displayed no evidence of scurvy, which arises when vitamin C is deficient.

Its protein is better digested.

Because it is raw, the protein is not coagulated and therefore better assimilated. Cooking destroys 20 to 50 percent of its amino acids.[17]

It doesn't get the toxic by-products of cooking.

Raw or rare meat doesn't have toxic lipid peroxides from the cooked fat in the meat. In addition, when fat drips onto the heat source and smokes, the smoke surrounds your food and can transfer cancer-causing polycyclic aromatic hydrocarbons (PAHs) to the meat. Eating a steak may be more dangerous than smoking, since a pound of charcoaled steak has as much benzopyrene as found in the smoke of 300 cigarettes.[18] Benzopyrene has led to leukemia and gastric tumors in mice.[19]

Raw or rare meat also doesn't contain heterocyclic amines, carcinogenic by-products produced in cooked meat, especially when cooked at high temperatures. HCAs are affected by four factors: the type of food, the cooking method, the cooking temperature, and the cooking time. The higher the temperature and the longer it is cooked, the more HCAs are produced. HCAs are found only in cooked muscle meats — very little or no HCAs are found in cooked organ meats, such as liver. Neither are they found in heated dairy and eggs.[20]

Frying, broiling, and barbequing produce the greatest amount of HCAs because of the high temperatures involved. Stewing, boiling, or poaching cooks at lower temperatures (212° F), so negligible amounts of these chemicals are produced. Oven roasting and baking produce moderate amounts. One study showed that when the cooking temperature was increased from 392° F to 482° F, the content of HCAs tripled.[21]

High heat also destroys the nutrient carnosine,* changing it into the toxic carcinogen acrylamide, which reacts with the creatine in meat, forming N-methyl-acrylamide.[22]

Raw meat is more alkaline than cooked meat.

Dr. Rosedale once mentioned that raw meat doesn't create the acidifying effect on the body that cooked meat does because the volatile ammonia contained in raw meat that could neutralize its acids is driven off almost immediately by heating it.

Dr. Timothy Brantley, PhD, ND, who turned supermodel Carol Alt on to a raw diet, points out that the more you cook meat, the more difficult it becomes to break it down and release its individual amino acids. When amino acids are not broken down properly, by enzymatic activity, bits of undigested protein can result in the body's production of excess uric acid, which acidifies the body, stressing the kidneys and other organs. An acidic environment lowers cellular oxygen levels, which enables cancer and microbes to grow. Parasites thrive on undigested protein and an acidic, low-oxygen environment.[23] The acidity and intestinal blockages resulting from eating cooked meat cause body odor.[24]

People historically ate raw meat before using fire.

Cro-Magnon man — living 35,000 years ago, a mere blink compared to our entire hominid existence — is believed to have eaten raw meat. Ever since that time, people have been eating raw meat in nearly every culture: steak tartare, seviche, sushi, et al.

S. Boyd Eaton and Melvyn Konner reviewed about 80 scientific papers, articles, and books on the paleolithic diet and wrote an article on paleolithic nutrition in 1985. They found that man depended on meat for high-energy food for over 2 million years, and at the beginning was eating the flesh raw, since fire was not widely used at first.

It may be argued that 1.4 million years of using fire is enough time to adapt to cooked food. However, as previously discussed, each time you cook, the chemical reactions are slightly different, making the foreign chemicals produced harder to adapt to. This is why, to this day, meat is associated with cancer: The studies use cooked meat. To my knowledge, no studies have been done using raw meat from wild, or at least free-range, properly fed animals. Even if we briefly cook our meat at low temperatures, we greatly minimize toxic by-products.

When properly marinated in lemon or lime juice, raw meat tastes and often looks similar to cooked meat.

---

*see chapter 17

Parasites may not pose a threat.

According to veteran raw meat eaters Dr. Stanley Bass and Aajonus Vonderplanitz, parasites do not flourish if one is on a raw diet, especially one that isn't high in carbs. As we will see, if the meat has been frozen at subzero temperatures for two weeks, the parasites are killed. Even if some survive, Aajonus claims that parasites are beneficial, at least in a person eating a healthful raw diet, as they can help eat up the toxins in the body.

Thousands of times, I ate raw meats and raw milk that were "microbe-infected" during my 32 years of experimentation and everyday life. According to the assumptions of the medical and scientific communities, I should have suffered bacterial or parasitic food poisoning thousands of times. I did not. Not once. Thousands of other "at-risk" individuals who switched to eating raw animal products to reverse their diseases and/or to improve their health also did not get sick.[25]

In fact, one man even recovered from ulcerative colitis by intentionally eating parasitic worms![26]

The important amino acid glutamine is heat sensitive.

Bodybuilders love glutamine because it aids in muscle growth and endurance. The body uses it to speed up healing after operations, and it is also useful in treatment of injury, trauma, serious illnesses, burns, and "side" effects of cancer treatment.[27] It can be destroyed by cooking.

Moreover, the toxic excitotoxin MSG forms when glutamine is heated in cooking.

Raw or rare meat digests much faster than cooked.

When Dr. Beaumont performed his experiments on St. Martin, he saw that raw pork digested in 3 hours, but it took the same pork 5¼ hours to digest when roasted, 4½ hours boiled, 4¼ hours fried, and 3¼ hours broiled. Raw oysters took 2 hours 55 minutes, but roasted ones took 3¼ hours, and stewed took 3½ hours. Raw beef digested in 3 hours, but boiled beef digested in 3 hours 36 minutes, and fried roast beef took 4 hours. Similarly raw eggs took 2 hours, but hard-boiled ones took 3½ hours.

The bottom line: The higher the temperature you cook something, and the longer you cook it, the longer it takes to digest.[28] These studies took place in the 1800s and should be common knowledge by now. Could it be that food processing companies and mainstream medicine, which are the media's major sources of funds through advertising, don't want this to be part of general public awareness?

It is easier to detect if meat has gone bad when it is raw.

Cooking is no guarantee of safety. The *E. coli* infections that have sickened or even killed people have almost always been from meat that was eaten cooked. If someone tries to eat that same meat raw, he will usually detect that it is spoiling: the foul odor and taste are very strong.

Doctors aware of these benefits often recommend raw meat.

Dr. Mercola touts the benefits of raw meat on his website, www.mercola.com. Dr. Stanley Bass also encourages his patients to eat raw meat.

Dr. Timothy Brantley conducted a two-year study in which his participants would eat meals from either food group A (standard American diet), food group B (transitional diet, which was a cooked whole-food diet, no processed foods or added sugars, coffee, or tea allowed) or food group C (a 75 to 80 percent raw diet of whole foods, including lightly cooked or raw meat and raw dairy, but no beverages except water and fresh juice). He found group C superior on all tests: food and blood sugar testing; electrodermal screening; live blood analysis; applied kinesiology; pH testing; client interviews, responses to foods, and feedback.

He had one group stay on foods from only food group C for a prolonged period. This group experienced a correction of all measurable imbalances. The stunning results included rehydration of every organ, gland, and tissue; more oxygenated, more vibrant, less toxic, healthier, and more balanced blood; more balanced body pH; more balanced and harmonious meridian systems; more balanced and unclogged organs, glands, and tissues.[29]

Dr. James Wilson, author of *Adrenal Fatigue*, explains.

Proteins have more food value and are easier to digest when eaten lightly cooked or raw. The amino acids are delivered intact (and therefore more usable) in uncooked or lightly cooked food rather than in the denatured (irreversibly changed) form produced by high heat or long cooking.

However, it is always necessary to fully cook poultry and pork to avoid potential microbial danger and to make sure that raw fish, shellfish, and beef are free from contamination. If you can be sure of the safety of the source, then sushi, sashimi, and seviche are excellent sources of protein, as is steak tartare and similar preparations from fresh, organically raised beef.[30]

Dr. Wilson warns that people with adrenal fatigue might not have enough hydrochloric acid (HCl) to properly break down protein food in the stomach and may therefore experience gas, bloating, and heaviness after eating a meal with proteins. Some people then eat more carbs, which only exacerbate the problem. Quality proteins are essential to adrenal recovery. The solution, he says, is to take HCl supplements with the meal.

The late Dr. Henry Bieler, MD, advocated raw meat.

[It] forms no putrefactive acids in the urine and (unlike cooked meat) is a hydrophilic (water soluble) protein similar to raw egg whites. Both cooked egg white and meat become hydrophobic (water insoluble) colloidal proteins.[31]

Bieler emphasized that cooked protein impairs the liver.

Some people may not be able to digest meat very easily, raw *or* cooked, after having been vegetarian awhile. They may have lost much of their hydrochloric acid production.

- Adding a few tablespoons of lemon juice will aid digestion until they are used to it.

- Adding green smoothies to their diets will also increase their bodies' hydrochloric acid output within in a few weeks, according to the Roseburg study detailed in Victoria Boutenko's book *Green for Life*.

- Taking HCl supplements is another option.

Dr. Beaumont's research showed that vinegar, also acidic, tenderizes the meat and can be added to it before it is eaten.[32] A couple of tablespoons of lemon or lime juice also does the trick with less toxicity, since vinegar is *acetic acid*, a toxic waste product of fermentative bacteria.

An interesting case of someone who thrived on raw meat was that of a certain Dr. F.L. Stone. Dr. Stone believed that eating the flesh of animals immediately after slaughter was the key to peak health. Using his own body as an experiment, he lived on fresh flesh for 25 years. In his later years, he lived in a jungle area of Kenya in Africa and lived on wild game.

Dr. Robert Gunther, his physician, declared that although Dr. Stone was nearly 70, he had "the youthful and robust health of a chap of 25 or 30." Dr. Stone's unique experiment came to an abrupt end in 1943 when he was fatally wounded by wild animals during a hunting expedition.[33]

Safety of Raw Meat

The most important thing to consider if you eat meat, raw *or* cooked, is to be sure it is from a healthy animal that was free range and fed its natural, organic, species-specific diet. Know the source of your meat. Factory-farmed, grain-fed, caged animals make for unhealthy animals that are unhealthful to eat. Spend more and compensate by eating less. For many people, eating three to six ounces of meat a day, five to seven days a week, is plenty. For some carb types, even this much may not be needed.

When people hear of eating raw meat, they first think of worms and parasites, and with good reason, since some are dangerous. But Joe Weinstock, MD, director of gastroenterology and hepatology at Tufts Medical Center in Boston, points out that there is an inverse relationship between worms and autoimmune diseases. Worms are very powerful inducers of immune regulation.

Dan Hurley interviewed Weinstock and wrote about it.

Intestinal worms, Weinstock told me, have co-evolved with humans, learning a neat trick along the way essential for their survival: turning down the molecular rheostat on our immune system, so that our white blood cells don't attack them. So reliant have we become on this process that without the worms, our immune systems, like a car engine idling too high, start going after our lungs (producing asthma), intestines (producing bowel disease), nerve linings (producing MS), pancreas (producing diabetes), or other organs.[34]

Note that even some fruits and vegetables may contain parasites. A friend of mine who has been a strict vegan for six years got roundworms from some fruit in Ecuador. A friend of mine from India says that some cabbages have to be cooked there because they contain parasites that can lead to blindness.

Does Freezing Destroy Bacteria and Parasites?

Sally Fallon, author of *Nourishing Traditions*, offers a solution to the parasite problem.

The problem of parasites in beef or lamb is easily solved. Simply freeze the meat for 14 days. According to the United States Department of Agriculture, this will kill off all parasites.[35]

Ask your grocer how long the meat has been frozen. Here is what the US Department of Agriculture's website says about freezing meat.

Freezing to 0º F inactivates any microbes — bacteria, yeasts and molds — present in food. Once thawed, however, these microbes can again become active, multiplying under the right conditions to levels that can lead to food borne illness. Since they will then grow at about the same rate as microorganisms on fresh food, you must handle thawed items as you would any perishable food.

Trichina and other parasites can be destroyed by sub-zero freezing temperatures. However, very strict government-supervised conditions must be met. It is not recommended to rely on home freezing to destroy trichina. Thorough cooking will destroy all parasites.

Note that they call for zero temperatures, well within the operating range of most home refrigerator freezers.

Raw Meat May Be Harder to Chew Unless Processed

People probably began cooking meat long before they began cooking plant food. Meat during the Ice Age sometimes had to be thawed out by heating. Unless eaten immediately, dead animals would freeze solid. Cooking of meat occurred in ovens that date back to over 200,000 years ago.[36]

No doubt cooked meat other than seafood is easier to chew. I choked on raw meat a couple of times until I realized this. I learned to marinate it overnight, cut it up into small pieces, and chew it thoroughly. I also sometimes dehydrate the meat, which makes it much, much easier to chew.

Traditional peoples have eaten raw meat after it is processed by the following methods: adding acidity (like marinating it in lemon or lime juice), drying it in the sun (like jerky), or adding salt (like jerky). Chimpanzees have been observed to process raw meat by chewing it together with tough, mature leaves, termed *wadging*.

Richard Wrangham made an experiment with his friends: They all chewed on raw goat meat with mature avocado leaves. They discovered that the leaves gave traction, and the bolus of chewed meat was reduced faster than when no leaves were used.[37]

Making the meat tender through whatever method makes it easier to digest.[38] You lose some of the enzymes from some of these methods, but it is a tradeoff, as it becomes easier to digest in other ways.

Another way to process raw meat is grinding. Just as green smoothies take advantage of high-tech blenders to make greens more digestible, we can use food processors to grind up meat before making dishes like steak tartare. Better yet, have the butcher grind it for you, but only if you plan to use it immediately or freeze it, as it oxidizes faster when chopped.

Raw Meat Preparation

I learned from Aajonus Vonderplanitz how to prepare raw meat to make it tasty, or at least tolerable. In my opinion, there is no tastier way to eat raw meat than to simply dehydrate it at 105° F for about 15 to 20 hours. As a scavenger, prehistoric man would find a dead animal dehydrated from the sun's heat. It was Nature's first jerky. I have found there is a reason you cannot buy chicken jerky: for some reason, dehydrating it makes it smell bad. Dehydration works best with red meat and fish and somewhat well with turkey.

Dr. Timothy Brantley has people sear meat on each side so that it looks (on the outside) and tastes cooked. I sometimes steam it so that it is cooked on the outside but raw inside. This tricks my brain into thinking it is cooked, and it even tastes cooked!

Raw meat can also be marinated in lemon or lime juice diluted with pure water, which makes it look and taste more like cooked meat. This also softens the meat. I like to thinly slice chicken and marinate it, adding curry powder and maybe some chopped onions, tomatoes, and cilantro.

Cutting or slicing meat always makes it digest faster, according to the experiments done by Dr. Beaumont. There are people who like to improve the digestibility of raw meat by letting it age.

> The digestibility of most meats is improved by incipient putrefaction, sufficient to render the muscular fibre slightly tender.[39]

The Eskimos were also in the habit of doing this, as is Aajonus Vonderplanitz.

If You Must Cook Your Meat

Most people can't stand the thought of eating raw meat, so they have to ease into it by lightly cooking it. If you feel you must cook it, doing so for shorter times and at lower temperatures will lessen the formation of toxic by-products, such as heterocyclic amines. For example, steam or sear the meat briefly so only the outside is cooked.

I found through experimentation that the more I cooked my meat, the longer it would take to digest, and the more it would putrefy in my intestines. The indisputable proof lies in the bathroom smells, which are especially strong after eating grilled or barbequed meat! Raw or rare meat doesn't have an odor going out.

Here are some low-temperature guidelines from Dr. Joseph Mercola.

> Use a glass casserole dish with a cover. (The cover is very important.) The tighter the cover fits, the better. The size of the casserole dish should be appro-
priate for the amount of food being cooked. In other words, the casserole dish should be about the same size as what you are cooking and should not be too big. Cook your food in the oven at 225º Fahrenheit, *no higher*! Allow for 12–15 minutes of cooking time per each 4 ounces of food being cooked, but decrease or increase the cooking time as needed. Other healthy methods of cooking that are acceptable to use with nutritional typing include crock-pot cooking, poaching, steaming your food lightly, or searing your food (on the outside, and leaving the inside very rare).[40]

Dr. Ron Schmid lists the ways he prepares raw or lightly cooked meat. He may braise it by melting raw butter and coconut oil in a pan on low heat, then heating for a minute only some cut-up, bite-sized strips. Or he will sear larger portions in a skillet for 30 seconds on each side using again raw butter or coconut oil. Sometimes he will put it in the oven several hours at low temperatures between 140° and 150° F.

His favorite way to prepare fish is "Eskimo style." He boils water and immerses chunks in the water for 45 to 90 seconds. Sometimes he will do this with beef or lamb as well. The meat is then cooked on the outside but pink inside. He pours off the water and places the chunks of meat in a bowl with seasonings of butter, Celtic salt, lemon, and pepper.

Dr. Timothy Brantley advises searing the meat so that on the inside it is raw, but on the outside it looks and tastes cooked. The same thing can be done with steaming. This way you get the "cooked" look but eat most of it raw. Note that this does not destroy all parasites, however.

Now that we've learned how to eat meat in a healthful manner, let's look at ways we can eat it consciously and make it a better world for the animals too.

Chapter 25

Increase the Demand for Clean Meat, and Eat It Consciously

Consuming unhealthy animals raised in suppressive environments results in the human nervous system recording all those negative qualities of those animals. Because factory-farmed chickens, loaded with antibiotics and suffering from numerous diseases, are among the most popularly and quantitatively consumed foods today, the effects of this 'food' on consumers are also among the most obvious.
—Steve Gagne, *Food Energetics*

It is very unlikely that vegetarians will convince the majority of the population to forgo meat, simply because most people feel better when they include it in their diets. Contrary to what many vegetarians claim, it is not about taste alone. It is not about being addicted to meat because of childhood conditioning or fast-food commercials or convenience or appetizing sauces. It is about eating the way we genetically evolved so that we can experience peak health.

Some of us can wean ourselves from meat, most notably the carb types. Some absolutely need at least a little meat to be healthy. Then there are those who can experience meso-, or medium, health without meat but prefer peak health. These need at least some meat to attain and maintain that.

Even famous vegetarians like Molly Katzen, author of several vegetarian cookbooks, have decided to resume eating meat a few times a week. Many do so for health reasons and to support those local farmers who raise animals compassionately.[1]

Healthy Animals Are Healthful to Eat

Many of us have been led to believe that eating animal products is a dangerous, unhealthful thing. We have been flat out lied to about cholesterol and saturated fats being dangerous, as they can be when cooked. Nonetheless, food products derived from factory-farmed animals do not support optimal health. Eating meat from a factory-farmed animal that is improperly fed is not good for you or for the livestock. All the dietary and medical toxins fed to the animals are passed on to you when you eat their flesh. The TV commercial that says "happy cows come from California" should instead say "happy cows come from free-range pastures."

All animals should be fed their proper foods in organic form. Beef from grass-fed cows is four times higher in vitamin E, contains less fat with higher quality (the proper ratio of fatty acids), has a negligible risk of mutant *E. coli* contamination, contains a negligible risk of mad cow disease, and is higher in beta-carotene.[2] Grass-fed meat also stays fresher longer.[3]

Studies show that cows which are free range and pastured have CLA levels 3 to 5 times higher than their grain-fed counterparts. Their milk also has higher levels of CLA. Bison that were grass fed had omega-6 to omega-3 ratios of 4 to 1, whereas the grain-fed bison had ratios of 21 to 1. The meat of pastured animals is also lower in fat.[4]

Meat from grass-fed animals has up to four times as much beta-carotene as that which is factory farmed. This increase in carotene creates a yellow rather than white color in the fat.[5] Grass-fed beef has the same low-fat profile as chicken breast but more of the good omega-3 fats.[6]

Factory Farms Hurt People Too

Many of us are familiar with the classic book *Slaughterhouse* and the movie *Meet Your Meat*, which reveal the injustices to animals meted out by conventional farming practices. Perhaps you have seen a few snippets on www.youtube.com or read reviews of books by concerned animal activists.

Factory farms hurt *people* too. The book *Animal Factory* by David Kirby reveals a number of troubling aspects to this form of animal rearing.

- Concentrated Animal Feeding Operations (CAFOs) are polluting local communities' air and adding to global warming.

- Manure, traditionally a source of fertilizer, pollutes rivers to the point that their fish die.
- Fishermen get sores and memory lapses from its toxins!
- Overuse of antibiotics creates harmful bacteria that don't respond to antibiotics.
- Novel viruses like the H1N1 swine flu proliferate.

The community loses jobs because illegal workers must be hired to keep costs competitive.

In addition, factory farms feed their animals rendered products. Rendering companies collect slaughterhouse waste (such as bones, heads, hooves, and blood), euthanized pets, road kill animals, and supermarket rejects for recycling. They also gather the used grill and deep fryer grease from fast food chains and other restaurants.

All of this grease and animal matter is then melted into a boiling acid bath which is later neutralized with lye. This soup may be contaminated with toxins from pesticides and antibiotics fed to the cattle, euthanasia drugs given to pets, and all of the carcinogenic chemicals that grilling and deep frying create. Worse, sometimes metal pet or cattle ID tags get into the soup, adding lead poisoning to the mix. Even plastic from Styrofoam trays from unsold packs of supermarket meats, chicken and fish can end up in the soup!

Any undissolved solids that float to the top, such as hooves and fur, are skimmed off and removed. This is dangerous work. The acid fumes can get into workers' lungs, and an unfortunate few have fallen into the boiling vats of sulfuric acid. Once the solids have been removed, the remaining mixture is then cooled and formed into bricks of grease that are later sold to farmers as supplemental livestock feed.[7]

When you eat the fatty flesh of animals fed this toxic mixture, *you* are consuming these carcinogenic chemicals also as they recycle through your own veins and arteries and end up in your fat tissues.

Animal factories are caught in the system, as they need to show profits for shareholders; yet a report demonstrated that the only reason these factory farms are profitable is that the externalized costs, like environmental cleanup, are borne not by the farm, but by the public tax payer. These corporations are taking advantage of the system and lax laws at the expense of the public. If they didn't get the free ride from tax payers, they might be motivated towards better ecology. They could actually profit by capturing and converting methane or manure into power-producing electricity.[8]

Americans demand cheap food. According to Kirby, people in the US spend about half the percentage of their incomes on food that they did in 1966. But cheap at the checkout doesn't translate into cheap in the long run, as farm activist Helen Reddout explains.

If you look at the actual cost of protein in the supermarket and then factor in the corporate welfare system and the cost of damaging the environment, creating antibiotic resistance and sickening people who live nearby; and then if you consider the inferior product we are getting as a result, then in that sense, we have the most expensive food in the world.[9]

Animal Factory takes us on a journey of activism, a very detailed journey starring ordinary people who were brave enough to fight back, get media attention, change some laws, and raise awareness in mass consciousness that this is not just a problem, but a major crisis. These activists, who include Rick Dove, Helen Reddout, and Karen Hudson as star reformers, bravely soldiered on despite death threats, drive-by obscenities, nasty comments from neighbors, and working long hours without pay.

> *CAFOs claim the animals need to be separated so that they don't establish a pecking order and fight each other, as well as compete for food. By such logic, perhaps all humans should be confined in prisons!*

CAFOs defend their cruel policy of keeping animals trapped in tiny spaces in which they often can't even turn around. They claim the animals need to be separated so that they don't establish a pecking order and fight each other, as well as compete for food. By such logic, perhaps all *humans* should be confined in prisons!

The best thing we can all do to help the situation is to boycott factory-farmed meat and buy it only from reputable sources, like small, local farmers. All meat should come from animals that are free range, antibiotic free, hormone free, and if possible, vaccination free. Pay double the price if need be for maximal quality; just eat less meat. If you need more protein, use hemp seeds and eggs to supplement your meat. Vote with your money! When this idea catches on, just as organic food caught on, big stores will start providing clean meat from compassionately raised animals. See the Resources section for where to get reputable meat.

Sustainable farmer Catherine Friend advises that we take baby steps toward compassionate carnivorism. Set goals like "I will buy three dozen eggs from uncaged hens this month," or "I will make five phone calls in search of happy meat."[10]

One such step to take is that when you go to a restaurant, order a vegetarian meal, since all meat from restaurants has been factory fed unless otherwise specified.

David Kirby gives us some tips to becoming a more sustainable shopper:

- Be aware of labels like "humane," "cage free," and the most stringent of all, "animal welfare approved" (AWA).

- Go red-tag shopping at the meat department. Find out what days of the week they get rid of their older, often deeply discounted meat. Buy it and freeze it if you don't use it right away.

- Seek out a local food co-op or local sustainable agriculture farm.

- Go online to Sustainable Table and its Eat Well Guide with a database searchable by zip code for farms, markets, and restaurants in your area that offer food that is friendly to humans, animals, and the environment.

Finally, eat less meat. Many Americans think they need to eat meat twice or even thrice a day,

and it just isn't so. You can supplement with hemp seeds and plant proteins. It is always better to have less with higher quality.[11]

Eating Consciously

Have you ever been guilty of eating while talking on the phone, driving, walking, reading, working, e-mailing, or watching TV? If so, you have probably noticed that the sandwich, protein bar — or whatever you were eating — vanished before you even realized you had begun eating it.

This makes you want to eat more so you can relish the taste, since you didn't savor what you ate unconsciously. This mindless eating is no doubt part of the cause of our obesity epidemic. Eating should be a sacred act, not part of our multi-tasking lifestyles.

In his book *Savor: Mindful Eating, Mindful Life*, Buddhist author and monk Thich Nhat Hanh lists seven practices for eating mindfully. I think the first one, *honor the food*, should especially apply to eating animal products.

Thich also says to start the meal with your traditional grace or gratitude, or with five contemplations that he provides. The first two of these contemplations are especially relevant if you are eating animal foods:

- This food is the gift of the whole universe: the earth, the sky, numerous living beings, and much hard, loving work.

- May we eat with mindfulness and gratitude so as to be worthy to receive it.

Practicing mindful eating, I now enjoy eating more than ever, despite eating less food than I ever have.

We also need to stop throwing meat away. An animal died for your nourishment, even if not willingly. As compassionate farmer Catherine Friend reminds us, "If we're going to kill millions of animals every year for food, the least we can do is respect those animals by actually eating them."

Chapter 26

If You Still Aspire to Remain Vegan or Vegetarian

Vegetarian — that's an old Indian word meaning "lousy hunter."
—Andy Rooney, American radio and television commentator

I hope that if you are vegan, you will now at least consider becoming vegetarian and adding eggs and/or some fermented dairy to your diet. Vegan diets are much more restrictive than vegetarian diets. There has never been a vegan tribe in "primitive" societies.

The best time to attempt veganism is in your 20s. When you are young and healthy, you can still make the conversions from plant nutrients to forms that are found only in animal foods: beta-carotene to vitamin A, omega-3s to DHA and EPA, vitamin K_1 to K_2, essential amino acids to nonessential ones, and vitamin D_2 to D_3.[*] On the other hand, if you start before your 20s, your brain and nervous system are still growing. You will want to maximize your full brain growth potential by eating brain foods like fish and eggs.

Raw or Nearly So Is Best

I will say this: if you are forced into a situation in which you must become vegetarian or vegan for religious or economic reasons, you will be *much better off* doing it raw. One problem with plant-based diets is that they tend to be very high in carbs. So it is best to eat them raw, as the carbs will not be absorbed as much. Cooking approximately doubles the glycemic index of a food. For low-glycemic raw vegan recipes, get Dr. Gabriel Cousens's *Rainbow Green Live-Food Cuisine* and *There Is a Cure for Diabetes.*

Raw fooders know how to soak, rinse, sprout, and ferment foods so that the mineral-binding phytates and lectins are largely removed. Most raw fooders avoid toxic soy, since it is edible only when cooked unless you eat it fresh off the plant. Raw

tempeh may be allowed, since the antinutrients have been mostly removed, and enzymes have been added back via fermentation.

Many people think it is easier to eat a cooked vegan diet because you can add soy and other proteins like cooked grains and beans, but these proteins are not healthful options! Instead, consume raw hemp seeds, chia seeds, and sprouted peas and/or lentils for protein. Supplement with other seeds and nuts, especially walnuts for omega-3 fats, and if you are not vegan, raw eggs. Some people can also tolerate raw goat dairy or raw kefir.

There is evidence that given the proper combinations and preparations, plant protein diets of root vegetables, leaves, fruits, and nuts can be adequate in amino acid content.[1] History shows that our bodies can survive on restricted diets. Our bodies were designed to live through famines, droughts, and food shortages. But to thrive a long time at peak health, the mostly raw, omnivorous paleodiet (as they ate it) is best for most people.

Keep Updated on Nutrition

If you wish to remain vegan, read some nutrition books and studies outside the vegetarian/vegan arena, which tends to be biased. I've read over 200 books through the years on those topics and found nothing that addressed the health issues I was experiencing with a deficiency of DHA, D_3, and K_2 in my diet and an excess of omega-6s from seeds. It wasn't until I did research outside the "veg" box that I found the solution.

You have to stay current with research and new discoveries. You need to be a virtual nutritionist if you want to stay healthy on such a highly restricted diet. Even then, it is easy to be deceived by propaganda, as it has been for many regarding the hype about soy being healthful. It is always safest to eat like our cavemen ancestors: a wide variety of

[*]See chapters 15 and 17.

organic vegetables, greens, nonsweet fruits, and meats — wild or free range when possible — supplemented with some nuts and seeds. Unless you are a carb type, go easy on the sweet fruits.

Forget Locavorism

In most places of the world, you will have to throw out the idea of being a locavore if you are a vegan. Super foods, which are those rare plant foods that contain nutrients found in animal foods, must be imported from around the world.

As we will see in the next section, super foods like Brazil nuts, coconuts, hemp seeds, shiitake or reiki mushrooms, and more are needed on a vegan diet. In most cases, these must be imported.

Even fruits, nuts, and seeds are usually seasonal and must be imported most of the year unless stored in the freezer or canned.

Because there are few regions that contain all of these foods, doesn't it seem *highly unlikely* that we could have evolved on vegan diets? Rather, it is the type of diet that some of us are trying to adapt to as long as we have sufficient fossil fuel to transport these foods around the planet.

For moral vegans, many deficiencies can theoretically be avoided with supplements, but even the best are not bioavailable for everyone. Supplements are unnatural and can be unbalancing, as well as toxic in many cases.[2]

Foods to Eat and Foods to Avoid

The two plant sources highest in zinc are wheat germ and pumpkin seeds, but the phytates in wheat germ make much of the zinc unavailable to the body. Since a plant diet is high in copper, you need a lot of zinc to balance out the copper. The catch is that if you eat a lot of pumpkin seeds or wheat germ, you may also be overdosing on omega-6 fatty acids, so you will also need to eat a lot of walnuts and chia seeds. Or take flax oil for balance.

Your brain needs DHA, which you can get from the purslane weed or from algal supplements — some of which can be neurotoxic, however. Blue-green algae are rich in DHA, but since they contain neurotoxins, this should be proof positive that that we didn't evolve as vegans, as algae are the only significant plant sources known to have this crucial brain nutrient fully formed.

If you are vegetarian, you can instead consume eggs labeled high omega-3 or DHA. Some vegans can synthesize enough DHA and EPA from omega-3 plant sources.

Brazil nuts are the most significant vegan source of selenium, unless the soil where your food grows happens to be high in selenium.

Hemp seeds (found online if not locally) have the most complete plant protein profile and one of the few plants with a proper omega-3 to omega-6 ratio.[3] Eat as much as half a cup (80 grams hulled) a day. They aren't cheap, but if you want to depend on plants to stay healthy, your diet should be composed of mostly super foods that are amino-acid balanced, omega-6:3 balanced, and mineral rich.

Be sure to eat nuts and seeds for methionine, an amino acid found primarily in flesh foods. Sesame seeds and Brazil nuts are adequate in methionine, as is soy protein.

A common mistake in raw veganism is assuming nuts and seeds have sufficient quantities of all the amino acids you need. The truth is that a *few* do, but since they are 70 to 90 percent fat, you would have to eat a great deal of them to get sufficient amino acids.

It might be wise to do what cooked vegetarians and vegans do — add legumes, which contain lysine. Nuts and seeds are relatively low in this essential amino acid. The two complementary proteins (legumes with nuts and/or seeds and/or sprouted grains) should be eaten.

Do some research, as certain legumes, such as red kidney beans, are considered to be toxic when eaten raw. But most legumes, such as peas, lentils, mung beans, and garbanzo beans, can be soaked, rinsed, and sprouted to get rid of antinutrients. It is hard to overeat them as much when raw as when cooked. Legume sprouts may be bloating for some people. For this reason, some raw fooders will steam the sprouted lentils just three to five minutes to break down their cellulose walls. This can make a huge difference in digestibility, even though many enzymes perish.

Your body needs saturated fat. Your liver makes it, but you may need to supplement that with dietary saturated fat as well. The chief plant sources with significant amounts are coconuts, palm nuts, and cacao butter, some of which should be staples in vegan diets. Vegetarians can get these fats from eggs and dairy.

Eat sea vegetables to get adequate iodine and some calcium.

Seek out natto, as it is the only known plant source of vitamin K_2.

Remember that Dr. Price found that people with truly robust health consumed *ten times* the amount of vitamins A and D eaten by Americans of his day. If you forgo the cod liver oil or other animal source rich in vitamin D (like liver), you would probably have to sunbathe for hours in a swimsuit, several times a week if not daily. I lived in sunny San Diego with year round temperatures of about 70° F, yet I knew no one who had time to do that.

I also know no one who has time to juice the amount of produce needed to get ten times the RDA of vitamin A. You need loads of beta-carotene, precursor to vitamin A. Remember that Dr. Price found we need much more for robust health. You may need to consume the equivalent of three pounds of carrots a day to get enough vitamin A for robust health. You can buy dehydrated carrot juice, however.

I highly recommend that your "cheat" be a tablespoon or two of cod liver oil. Be sure to compare brands to find one that contains a significant amount of D. Some people feel it's best to get the same ratios as those found naturally in the cod fish, as excesses can be toxic. Even raw vegan leader Rev. George Malkmus, founder of the raw vegan Hallelujah Acres program, recognizes the value of fish liver oil. He allows cod liver oil for those following his diet, although he himself takes a daily 5,000 IU vitamin D_3 supplement instead.

Sunflower seeds also have some vitamin D_2, though they are overloaded in omega-6 fats. The vitamin D_2 from plants is not efficiently converted to D_3 either.

Otherwise, try eating plenty of sundried shiitake or reiki mushrooms, which tend to be expensive, two of the only known plant sources of vitamin D. But you would have to eat about *13 ounces* (400 grams) a day to get just the *minimum* RDA of 400 IU.[*]

If vegan, you may need to take B_{12} sublingual lozenges or other B_{12} supplement, preferably in methylcobalamin form. You may need injections if the B_{12} doesn't absorb (determined with blood tests). The injections contain toxic preservatives, so they should be a last-ditch resort. I would advise giving up veganism if you get to that point; I did!

If vegetarian, simply eat three egg yolks a day to satisfy B_{12} requirements. Fortified yeast is another option, but be aware that it is not raw and not advisable for anyone fighting a candida overgrowth.

Avoid most grains, cereals, soy, and starchy vegetables. Eat legumes and a few nongluten grains, such as wild rice, corn, buckwheat, millet, and quinoa,[†] but only after soaking them overnight, rinsing them, and sprouting them. If you insist on eating cooked legumes, soak the beans two days like traditional Indians, or at least overnight. Then cook them in a pressure cooker to deactivate most of the remaining lectins. A study on Turkish beans found this helpful, but be aware that pressure cooking also destroys nutrients because of its high heat.[5]

Unless you are a carb type and you know you can get fruit that has been picked ripe, minimize fruit intake. Eat mainly apples, plums, and berries, which don't stimulate insulin secretion as much as sweeter fruits.

If Vegan, Consider Vegetarianism

In the raw food movement, people are mostly raw vegans. This is because many people who are already vegan naturally decide that eating raw is the next step to taking it further. Others come to the raw food movement directly from a standard American diet, and they become vegan because "everyone else is."

Another reason most raw fooders are vegan is that raw dairy is unavailable in most states, and the thought of eating raw meat or eggs can seem rather unappetizing. Why? Because we were not brought

---

[*]By some accounts, such as the USDA standards, you would need much more.[4]

[†]See chapter 28.

up eating it raw culturally, and our ancestors have likely been cooking animal foods longer than anything else.

Where in the raw food movement are the raw *vegetarians*? I think they are more than might be imagined. I know there are some out there. Three people — Frédéric Patenaude, Bob Avery, and Victoria Boutenko — who are even well known in the raw movement have been open about the fact that they sometimes eat raw eggs. David Jubb lists raw goat cheese in one of the recipes in his book. Kevin Gianni now eats krill oil. Brother Nazariah eats dairy and eggs. There are probably some who don't make it public or put it in their books because they don't want to be ostracized by zealots. I *know*; I was *one* of them!

Every time there is a raw food event, it nearly always has in the title *vegan* after *raw*. I would like sometime to see an event that says "raw vegetarian."

What would raw vegetarians eat that a raw vegan wouldn't? They could add eggs and some dairy (preferably fermented) to their diet to gain valuable nutrients. If they were sensitive to dairy, they could enjoy two or three raw egg yolks a day. This would give them vitamins A, D, and B_{12}, and brain-specific minerals. Providing the eggs come from chickens fed omega-3-rich feed, the eggs would also provide DHA and EPA.

Clean Yourself Out

Whenever someone fails at a vegan diet, other vegans rarely blame vegan diets per se for possible nutrient deficiencies. They speculate instead, "He wasn't eating the correct kind of vegan diet," or "Well, he just wasn't cleaned out enough."

Yet this certainly doesn't apply to everyone. There have been plenty of people who have tried every kind of vegan diet but failed. There are also those who practiced fasting and have gone 100 percent raw (which is a cleansing diet) for years but nonetheless found their vegan diets inadequate. Examples already mentioned include the Westbrook family, who were raw vegans for 6 years, and Aajonus Vonderplanitz, who was a raw vegan for 11 years.

Nonetheless, it *does* help to take purification

measures periodically. Toxic accumulations increase our need for various nutrients and also may inhibit absorption of new ones. So, if you fast periodically and eat at least 80 percent of your calories raw, it will indeed help with micronutrient absorption and lower your dietary need for large amounts of them. For example, vitamin D status improved after weight loss, which involves a loss of toxins, in one study.[6] Another example is that toxic antinutrients in some plant foods increase the need for iodine.[7]

Start Young but Not Too Young

It also helps to be young when you start, but not too young, as these diets are not best for all growing children. Those who start in their 20s or 30s seem to have, on the average, better success rates than those who start later in life. They haven't usually accumulated as many toxins. To be a successful vegan, your body must be good at nutrient conversions and synthesizing nutritional elements.[*] These conversions are often inefficient even in the healthiest person and are often impossible in the sick, elderly, toxic, or very young.

Cheat with Super Foods

Do as the Muslims advise: "Pray to Allah, but tie up your camel." Be 90 to 95 percent vegan, but take a few raw animal super foods for insurance: a tablespoon or two of cod liver oil, a couple of sardines, a few egg yolks, a tablespoon of powdered raw beef liver from Argentina. Peter Singer, author of *Animal Liberation*, said not to eat anything with a face. Even a "faceless" diet could include super foods like eggs, clams, and oysters.

Get Blood Tests

Finally: Always, always get that annual blood test done, including a check of all your vitamin and mineral levels. Be aware that it may take years for certain deficiencies to show up. Stay on top of it with periodic blood tests — at least yearly for vitamins B_{12} and D. Your body can store B_{12} and fat-

---

[*]See chapters 15 and 17.

soluble vitamins for many years.

If you can't afford a regular blood test, at least get a mineral analysis of your hair. It would be better to do both. If you can't or won't do any of that, then at least be aware of what symptoms can be caused by these various deficiencies, and keep paying attention to whether you are developing any of them so you can take appropriate remedial actions before the situation gets too serious.

Get tests for triglycerides and cholesterol. Make sure your triglycerides are low and your HDL is high.

My attitude as a raw vegan was that I felt so good, why get tested? But when I finally did, I realized I was on my way to osteoporosis and nervous system hell. The beauty of blood and hair tests is that they can give you previews of where you are headed if you don't change your diet, revealing subclinical deficiencies that may take years or even decades to show up in your state of health. Many people feel so confident in what they are doing that they shun such tests. When the deficiencies manifest overtly, it is sometimes too late to fully undo the damage.

If you find after a dozen years of veganism that you are in great health, *celebrate*! But don't judge others who have failed. It's not their fault. Because of our genetic diversity, there is no "one diet fits all."

Chapter 27

Pregnant, Lactating, or Feeding the Kids: Why Animal Products May Be Crucial

Veganism [is] a risky way to achieve normal brain development in animals as divergent as rats and humans. That is not to say it is impossible, just more difficult.

—Dr. Stephen C. Cunnane, *Survival of the Fattest*

As we will see in this chapter, certain brain foods from animal products are key factors in reaching a child's peak brain potential.

Pregnancy Increases Animal Product Needs

There are several nutrients that a pregnant woman needs that are hard to get on a vegetarian diet, let alone vegan: iron, vitamin D, and DHA are among them.

In *The Live Food Factor*, three women gave testimony to their successful raw vegan pregnancies. However, all three were very new to their diets when pregnant, so they would have undoubtedly held many nutritional reserves in their bodies.

Nonetheless, for assurance of a smart and healthy baby, I would never recommend that a woman remain vegan while pregnant. Raw *yes*, vegan *no*!

Becoming pregnant after years of veganism is even riskier, as stored nutrients needed by the developing fetus may be depleted. You can compensate somewhat by taking algae for DHA, but algae contain toxins. The fact is, we don't know enough about nutrition, a relatively new science. It is worth repeating: there could be some elements found only in animal foods that we have not yet discovered.

I am sure you may protest and say you know someone who had a successful child while vegan, but do you know for sure that the child developed his or her full brain possibilities? Defend your philosophy all you want, but is it really worth risking the greatest potential of your child's health and intelligence? As we've seen, fish, shellfish, and/or eggs play a critical role in brain development and maintenance. You definitely increase your child's odds of fulfilling his or her genetic potential with a nutrient-dense diet.

One study on rats showed that eating the long-chain omega-3 fats DHA and EPA caused their babies to have more brain cells than if they were to take those plant foods with precursors to these long-chain fats. You shouldn't count on your fat conversion rate being high enough if you want your children to have optimal intelligence.[1]

Another study on rats showed that those fed a diet high in choline (found chiefly in eggs, beef, organ meats, and fish) in utero did not experience the normally expected age-related decline.[2] The implication is that the pregnant mom's diet can help prevent dementia in her offspring.

Stephen Cunnane, author of a textbook on human brain evolution, warns us that "there is just one chance, one critical period, to get brain development correct."[3] Humans have big brains that need to develop in the womb and very quickly postnatally.

> *"There is just one chance, one critical period, to get brain development correct."*

Dr. John Fielder doesn't agree with veganism. He found that of his vegan patients, three percent had mentally retarded babies, and there was no environmental toxin exposure to explain this. Is it really worth the risk that your child would be mentally challenged just so that you can stick with your vegan diet while pregnant or lactating?

I had heard that low birth weights were bad, but I never knew why. Considering the obesity epidemic, I thought, wouldn't it benefit a baby to be born thin? Now I know why low birth weights, which are often found among vegans and smokers, can be dangerous. It has to do with the baby's brain. The baby has three ways to get DHA:

- It is stored in his or her baby fat. (This is for infants, not adults, so don't use that as an excuse to be overweight!)
- Another is to make it from omega-3s.
- The third is the DHA it gets from mom's milk or other foods.

Cunnane cites a study by researcher and medical doctor Maureen Hack that showed the importance of a baby's growing brain. She found that 12 percent of those with very low birth weights had abnormally small head sizes at birth. After 10 weeks, 24 percent had smaller head sizes than normal. After eight months, the figure was 13 percent. This shows how hard it is for the baby's brain size to catch up, even given proper medical care. The study found that those with a small head at eight months old were almost guaranteed to have poor school age performance.

Her conclusion:

Head circumference during the first year of life is a good measure of quantitative features of normal neurological development: i.e., the size, volume, cell density, and DNA and lipid content of the brain.[4]

> *One study found that infants born to vegetarian mothers, compared to those born to omnivores, had lower birth weights, head circumferences, and lengths, as well as less DHA in their plasma and cord artery phospholipids.*

One study found that infants born to vegetarian mothers, compared to those born to omnivores, had lower birth weights, head circumferences, and lengths, as well as less DHA in their plasma and cord artery phospholipids.[5]

Michael Crawford, an anthropological expert on the influence of omega-3s and DHA, claims that poor nutrition can even affect the fetus prior to con-

ception. Eating a poor diet reduces the size of follicle development in the mother's ovary and affects the earliest stages of reproduction.[6]

You also need adequate protein while pregnant, or you risk that your baby's brain will not reach its full potential. Protein restriction can decrease all the enzymes involved in producing DHA.[7]

> *Protein restriction can decrease all the enzymes involved in producing DHA.*

Risks of Raising Vegan Children

Malnutrition at birth reduces the number and size of an infant's brain cells. If malnutrition occurs before the critical period in early infancy when brain cell count is established, it is too late. Brain function will be permanently impaired. If the brain cell count is established as healthy but cell size is small due to malnutrition, proper nutrition can restore some normal brain development.[8]

While some babies can manufacture sufficient DHA from omega-3s in plants, you *don't* want to risk that your baby is not good at making those conversions. Besides, don't you want your kid to be as smart as possible and have an abundance of DHA? The way to ensure that is to give him or her food that has *fully formed* DHA in it. Furthermore, EPA, a fatty acid for the brain's well-being, is pretty much only in fish, fish oil, and shellfish, not algae.

Restrictive diets are not best for growing children, who need a very nutrient-dense diet for optimal health. Children cannot easily convert betacarotene into vitamin A, which is needed for sight.

If you wanted to give a child some soup, what would be the surest way he would get it, by giving him an already made soup, or giving him the ingredients and hoping he could make it successfully? What if you gave him only part of the ingredients, or insufficient amounts of some of the ingredients? Could he make it then? What if the child were sick? Or an infant? Would he be able to make that soup?

Do you see that it is always more efficient to

take the nutrient in its ready-made form instead of hoping your body can synthesize it?

While there are some children who grow up vegan and appear healthy, it is still a risk. There is no way we can determine whether they reached their highest health potential. Though this is true for everyone, we know we can increase the brain's potential with brain food. For one thing, DHA is needed for the brain. B_{12} is also needed for the nervous system and is found in significant quantities only in animal foods.

Furthermore, as we have seen, some plant protein sources (grains and legumes) have the potential to stunt a child's growth. Their phytates can bind with zinc, iron, and calcium if not removed by soaking/sprouting. Soy is one of the worst protein sources.

Obtaining sufficient zinc and iron can be hard for children, even when they eat beef.[9] This is probably due to cooking, which makes the minerals less assimilable. To get enough on a plant diet can really be a challenge.

Mom's Postnatal Diet Must Be Nutrient Dense

👉 DHA is actually extracted from the mother's brain when she is pregnant in order to form the baby's brain. If she eats a diet rich in DHA, the amount could take four years to replace! If she is not consuming adequate amounts of fats rich in DHA, each of her offspring becomes progressively less intelligent, according to Dr. Sears, who bases this on animal studies.[10] This forms the basis of the observation that the first born is often the most intelligent.

DHA is very important for preventing postpartum depression. Taking antidepressants for postpartum blues does not resolve the cause; replacing the mother's DHA and/or other depleted nutrients is what the brain needs. Some years ago, actor Tom Cruise criticized actress Brooke Shields for using drugs for postpartum depression, to which she took offense. He was right. Drugs don't get to the root of the problem. Nutrition does.

👉 Women lose 3 to 5 percent of brain volume during the last trimester of pregnancy. That volume is likely to consist largely of essential fatty acids.[11] Antidepressants don't replace the essential brain fat. Taking fish or fish oil does.

But drug companies can't patent fish oil. This is why the media, which depend on advertising revenue from drug companies, sided with Shields and made Cruise out to be a lunatic, citing his jumping for joy on *Oprah* as evidence that he was "crazy." The media witchhunt impacted Cruise's popularity, forcing him to publicly apologize for his comment in a later interview.

The mother's diet should be rich in nutrients not only for her own recovery from pregnancy's nutrient drain on the brain, but also for the quality of her breast milk. Vegan mother's milk was found to be nearly the lowest in the world in DHA. Mothers in the US in general have low DHA in their milk, but European vegans had the lowest of all except for the milk of mothers in Sudan, a poor African country.[12]

Studies show that vegan women often don't have adequate B_{12} in their breast milks.[13] This can be a huge problem and cause serious developmental regression in their infants, including smaller brains![14] Some vegan babies thrive, but others die.[15] Why take the risk?

Other crucial nutrients often low in vegetarian or vegan mothers' milk include vitamin D, taurine, and carnitine.[16]

If you are breastfeeding and do not produce enough milk, simply adding animal products to your diet will increase milk production. That is a widely known fact in Chinese medicine. If you do not want to do that, then at least feed your baby raw goat's milk. Goat's milk is more akin to human milk than cow's milk and is easier to digest.

On the other hand, if you feed your baby soy milk, you will be giving your baby the estrogen equivalent of five birth control pills a day. If the infant is a boy, the result can be so drastic that his testicles may not descend, and his sexual organs may not develop. Furthermore, the baby's brain can be damaged by manganese overdose.[17]

The child could have problems all his or her life from having been fed soy as a baby! She could develop breasts and menstrual cycles as early as age seven. He or she could have a damaged thyroid gland, reading disabilities, or various other complications.

If you feed the baby hemp seed, there will not likely be damage, but the amount of nutrients still won't be enough. I once met a vegan woman feeding her newborn hemp seed milk because she couldn't lactate enough. *Hemp seed!* She was feeding her baby hemp seed instead of milk! I guess that's better than soy, but how will her baby get vitamin K_2? How will she get vitamin A and DHA?

A growing baby needs lots of vitamins A, K_2, B_{12}, as well as DHA and the minerals zinc, iron, and calcium. At least with milk from a cow or goat, the basic components of proteins, fats, carbohydrates, vitamins, and minerals are very similar to those found in human breast milk. The milks of mammals evolved to enable the same functions of building bone, muscle, and nervous system.

Vegans say, "Man is the only species that drinks the milk of another species." That is true only for adults. I have seen numerous photos of dogs suckling kittens, cats suckling puppies, dogs or cats suckling baby squirrels, and even a dog suckling baby tigers and another a baby lion.

In one case, a zoo tiger grew depressed when her cubs died. After zookeepers gave her piglets to nurse, she became content again! Animals seem to be generous when it comes to babies that need to be fed, even when it is of a different species. In fact, early European explorers of North American observed that some Native American women loved their pets so much they even suckled the young animals at their breasts.[18] Women from New Guinea love piglets so much that they sometimes breastfeed them.

Crucial Nutrients Often Found Insufficient in Vegan Breast Milk

Numerous studies have found these nutrients to be frequently insufficient in the breast milk of vegan mothers.

- DHA
- Vitamin B_{12}
- Vitamin D
- Taurine
- Carnitine

Chapter 28

A Balanced, High-Raw, Near-Paleolithic Diet

Don't eat anything your great-great grandmother wouldn't recognize as food. ... There are a great many foodlike items in the supermarket your ancestors wouldn't recognize as food (Go-Gurt? Breakfast-cereal bars? Nondairy creamer?); stay away from these.

—Michael Pollan, author of several books about food

I recommend that you never blindly follow diet gurus, including me. Instead, experiment to find out what works for *you*. Nonetheless, there are a few universal principles:

- Eat whole foods, avoiding fractionated foods as much as possible.

- Eat mainly raw.

- Eat as closely as possible to what our paleo-ancestors would have eaten.

- Keep a food journal every day, noting how you felt later in the day and the next morning, so you can tweak your diet to suit your unique body metabolism.

If you want to get really proficient at finding out what diet suits you, you can write in your daily log easily tested baseline biomarkers upon waking in the morning: pulse rate, blood pressure, and temperature. For each of these markers, lower is better. Note your stool consistency and any gas you may have had. Note if you get constipated. If you eat beets, you can test how fast the food goes through your intestines, since your stools will be tinted red when beet residue comes out. (Sometimes a pink tint shows up in the urine as well.)

Also note how much exercise and sunshine you got that day and whether your sleep was adequate. All of these factors affect your state of health and will be reflected in your biomarkers.

As I said earlier, I was about 95 percent raw and 99 percent vegan for six years, but I ran into deficiencies over the long haul, as well as constant bloating. I now continue to eat about 85 to 95 percent raw, but only about 80 to 90 percent plant food. I have found what works for me: mostly raw, mostly plant, and mostly paleolithic: the diet of our ancestors.

I feel fantastic, and my blood work, which includes cholesterol, triglycerides, vitamins (especially D_3 and B_{12}), and inflammation, confirms I am on the right track. I am also no longer in denial about my body's design as a meat eater. I am no longer fighting nature, trying to adapt to a high-carb diet devoid of animal products, a diet which my ancestors didn't evolve eating.

What I found was that at first I craved animal foods and had three to six ounces of meat every day. Sometimes I had a few eggs or raw kefir in addition to that. I discovered raw beef liver for B_{12} and cod liver oil for vitamins A, D, DHA, and EPA. In other words, since I had been deficient for some time, I wanted to take several sources of animal foods a day until the stores were built up again.

Later I craved salads and smoothies again and needed less animal food. I nonetheless made the beef liver, eggs, small fish, and cod liver oil staples in my diet, since they represent a fast, convenient, and cost-effective way to get crucial nutrients.

This diet is quite simple: eat mostly like cavemen. They ate mainly raw, whole-food diets, although some of the meat may have been occasionally cooked. Everything was natural, unrefined, and organic. Don't overdo the complicated recipes, as this increases the chance of bad food combinations.[*]

Select animal protein from organically fed, free-range sources. Try to order wild meat as often as you can afford it, or even take up hunting. You don't need to eat as much meat as paleolithic man did, because you don't have to spend a lot of energy hunting for the meat. Usually about three to six ounces a day is enough, even less if you are a carb

---

[*]The importance of proper food combining and the rules pertaining to it are treated in depth in chapter 17 and Appendix F of *The Live Food Factor*.

type — and not even every day if you supplement with quality protein sources like eggs and hemp seeds. Eat meat rare, raw, dehydrated, or steamed.

Organ meats are the richest in nutrients that are scarce in plant-only diets. Liver is great for B_{12}, but be sure it is from a wild or free-range, organically fed animal so you don't get overdosed with toxins, since the liver is a storehouse of toxins as well as nutrients.

Eat red meats and organ meats in moderation, since they have the potential to create the inflammatory type of prostaglandins that can lead to gout. Eating eyeballs, full of vitamin A, benefits the eyes. Eating brains is good for the brain, but with such conditions as mad cow disease, this is no longer advisable unless the source is reliable. Eating adrenals is good for the adrenal glands, eating hearts is good for the heart, and so on.

I occasionally enjoy free-range turkey. It is about 97 percent protein and thus the cheapest source of protein next to eggs. I know that "free range" doesn't hold the same significance it did when I was a kid in the 1960s, but I do the best I can until I find a better source. Poultry is also easier on the environment than mammals are. In addition, their slaughter is not performed at a slaughterhouse and is usually very quick, with the animals experiencing minimal fear because of the swiftness of execution. This is not always the case with mammals.

The best plant protein comes from hemp seeds, chia seeds, walnuts, macadamia nuts, and flaxseeds — all organic, fresh, and raw. These all have the best ratios of omega-3 to omega-6s fats. Enjoy small amounts of Brazil nuts for selenium, as well as other nuts and seeds.

Overeating protein can increase insulin secretion, though not as easily as carbs can. Overeating protein foods, especially those high in the amino acid methionine, which is found mainly in flesh foods, is also not good if your goal is longevity.[1] This is a good reason not to *overdo* meat, as is so customary in developed countries.

Legumes are low in methionine, but one should soak them overnight, rinse them, and sprout them to get rid of their lectins, which inhibit mineral absorption, as well as enzyme inhibitors, which make digestion more difficult. So an additional source of protein can be sprouted lentils or other small legumes, which are very inexpensive. If you find their cellulose too bloating, you can lightly steam them, which breaks the down cellulose walls.

Cavemen probably didn't eat legumes, but if you don't overdo them, you can enjoy these foods as long as their antinutrients are taken out as much as possible. Beans are not a source of complete amino acids and are thus often partnered with grains in the diet. But best is to avoid most grains and instead eat animal products for your main protein sources.

You need plenty of plant food for antioxidants, minerals, and phytochemicals. Oh yes, and although the need for fiber has been exaggerated, you still need the fiber from greens, fruits, and vegetables — just not from the grains.

Eat unrestricted amounts of nonstarchy vegetables. These are the above-ground vegetables. They are mineral rich and low in calories.

Indulge in nonsweet fruits, usually classified as vegetables, as much as you like: bell peppers, cucumbers, tomatoes, zucchini, summer squash. Avocados, another nonsweet fruit, are high in calories, so eat in moderation if you are concerned with overweight.

You may use olive oil or hemp seed oil in moderation and just squeeze some lemon or lime juice on salads for dressing. If you don't have those on hand, use raw apple cider vinegar. Each of those options has been found to help prevent Alzheimer's.[2]

Enjoy olives and avocados with your salads.

Consume raw cream in moderation. A pint of it makes great ice cream when blended with a few raw egg yolks, a bit of raw honey, and a few tablespoons of raw coconut butter.

Enjoy raw or lightly steamed winter squash or yams just once in a while. Unless you know you are a carb type, starchy vegetables like these should be considered treats, not staples. Ironically, sweet potatoes have a lower glycemic index than do white potatoes, even though they are sweeter tasting.

Eat as many greens as you like, as they are very low in calories and therefore carbs. Their alkaline minerals are important. I like to make green smoothies, but instead of using fruit, I often use stevia, lemon juice, and ginger to mask any bitterness of the greens. Greens are full of chlorophyll, which gives you a huge energy boost.

Raw food leader Victoria Boutenko has written a couple of books on the benefits of green smoothies.[3]

Nutritionist Natalia Rose concurs.

Drinking the juice of green plants ... infuses the body with the sun's energy, renewing every cell it reaches. It cleans the blood through its rich alkalinity [and] near bio-identical makeup to hemoglobin, delivers the most absorbable form of minerals, floods the body with fresh Life Force Energy, and makes you feel absolutely fresh and energetic.[3]

Supa Nova Slom, medicine man to hip-hop musicians, claims he has surpassed veganism to become a "chlorophyllian," living largely on greens.

What Toxitarians and Starchitarians and the majority of Americans ignore is the cleansing and nutritive power of greens. Carnivore or vegan, overweight or underweight, the secret to cleansing and detoxifying and reenergizing your life is the same: eat green.[4]

Though cavemen didn't have blenders, I still like to drink my smoothies. I blend greens in a heavy duty blender with hemp seeds and other super foods for a nutrient-rich drink. Super foods include mineral-rich foods like goji berries, maca, spirulina, blue-green algae, chlorella, alfalfa, bee pollen, royal jelly, acai berry, and more. This is where we can improve on the caveman diet, at least if we are not concerned with using fossil fuels to import foods from all over.

Of course, if you grow much of your own food in high-quality soil that increases the food's mineral content, you won't need many of these super foods.

Avoid dairy unless you have the gene mutation that keeps lactase in the intestine into adulthood. Some people, especially of Northern Europe descent, have the capacity to digest dairy. Even then, it's very questionable how well. The late Finnish health guru Paavo Airola experienced heart disease and allergies from excess dairy consumption, dying of a stroke at 64. For most of us, it is mucus forming and constipating, even leading to asthma in some of us.

This warning doesn't apply to the pure dairy *fat*. Cream and butter don't contain the protein casein that makes dairy so hard to digest. Most people are also lactose intolerant and need to supplement

with the enzyme lactase. This doesn't apply if the dairy is fermented. Goat dairy is also easier to digest than cow dairy, since its composition is closer to human milk.

Avoid most processed foods. However, by experimenting throughout generations, traditional cultures found that some forms of processing actually increase nutrients and/or decrease antinutrients. These include culturing of dairy products. By fermenting or souring milk and making yogurt, kefir, and clabber, the milk's lactose is broken down and the casein predigested.

Eat fermented foods like sauerkraut for extra enzymes and probiotics.

Soaking, rinsing, sprouting, and fermenting grains and legumes are other aids to digestion and get rid of many antinutrients. Sprouting increases certain nutrients. Fermenting, pickling, and leavening can increase available nutrients.[5]

Try to avoid most grains at all costs. The exceptions might be some soaked or sprouted buckwheat, quinoa, brown rice, or spelt on occasion. If you crave noodles, seek out kelp noodles at your local health store, found in the refrigerated section, or order them online at www.kelpnoodles.com. These are very low in carbs and calories. When soaked, they can take the place of pasta, absorbing the flavor of any sauce.

Experiment to see what ratio of macronutrients is optimal for you. What works best for me is a ballpark caloric ratio of 40 to 50 percent carbs, 15 to 20 percent protein, and the rest fat.

Good, healthful fats increase leptin sensitivity. I don't experience fatigue eating lots of fat so long as I stay low carb, and so long as I don't overdo nuts and seeds, which I find hard to digest even when soaked and rinsed.

If you cheat with a high-carb treat, immediately take a brisk walk or do some exercise to burn off the sugar to avoid an insulin spike. Carbs are great for "turbocharged energy," which is why athletes and laborers can get away with eating a lot more of them.

Avoid soy except for natto and moderate amounts of tempeh and miso.

For sweets, you can enjoy low-glycemic fruits like berries, plums, and apples, especially green apples. Unless you are a carb type, eat sweet, sugary fruits in moderation, more often if you buy them locally at a farmers' market so you know they were picked ripe.

Dates, raisins, and other dried fruit are high on the glycemic index scale.

Remember, the Eskimos thrived without fruit other than some berries in the summer. Dr. Richard Bernstein explains why fruit can be so bad.

Fruits still cause an unacceptably large blood sugar rise. Some people fear that they will lose important nutrients by eliminating fruit, but that shouldn't be a worry. I haven't eaten fruit in more than thirty years, and I haven't suffered in any respect. Nutrients found in fruits are also present in the vegetables you can safely eat.[6]

He notes that non-sweet fruits like avocados, bell peppers, cucumbers, and summer squash are just fine.

Avoid refined sugar and minimize the use of honey and raw agave. Use stevia as a sweetener instead. For some people, the brain is tricked even by stevia, a low-glycemic and very low- or no-calorie sweetener, into stimulating the pancreas to release insulin. For most people, insulin levels are not influenced by this sweetener.

I have found yacon root syrup from Peru to be the best tasting low-glycemic sweetener. It is only 16 calories per tablespoon, but its sugar consists of fructooligosaccharides (FOS) that pass right through the body mostly unmetabolized, since the body has no enzyme to hydrolyze FOS. These undigested sugars serve as food for friendly bacteria in the small intestines and colon.[7] In the US, it is possible to get a raw version of this super food.

When you first try yacon syrup, it will not seem as sweet as honey, sugar, or agave, but after you have gone low glycemic awhile and made your taste buds more sensitive, yacon tastes every bit as divine as high-glycemic sugars. The only drawback is that it is extremely expensive, which is why I buy it in bulk. Yacon has made this diet so easy for me; I feel like I have given nothing up, even when I am hovering around or in ketosis!

Be sure to get a couple of servings a day of monounsaturated fats, the secret behind the Mediterranean diet and a key in keeping a flat belly as well as preventing Alzheimer's. Sources include avocados, olives, olive oil, nuts, and seeds.

Oils are often badmouthed in the raw food community, since they are a fractionated food, but extra virgin olive oil has been found in studies to keep a strong heart, dense bones, low blood pressure, better blood cholesterol and coagulation, and a better brain.[8]

Unless you are a carb type, start out the day with a high-protein breakfast. I discovered this by accident. The idea of eating meat for breakfast sounded disgusting to me, but one night I dehydrated some wild buffalo. The next morning I just couldn't wait to try this highly acclaimed super food. I had been keeping a food journal and noticed that I felt great all day long. I observed afterwards that when I had meat or eggs at breakfast, meat especially, I was not hungry all day. I ate less overall on those days and was most productive.

According to Dr. Adrienne Denese, this is because it is critical to start out the day without carbs. Insulin responds more briskly in the morning than at any other time of the day. Furthermore, if you start out the day with insulin levels boosted, you will be hungry all day. Dr. Denese also recommends eating meat for breakfast.[9]

In fact, once in a while I eat "dinner" for breakfast: lightly steamed turkey or chicken with lightly steamed vegetables! The only "problem" with eating meat for breakfast is that you feel so good all day, with such stable blood sugar, that you often forget to eat lunch. After a high-protein breakfast, you will be so satisfied that you won't feel the need to make fancy recipes anymore. Just graze on nuts, salad, olives, avocados, vegetables, berries, and a green apple.

When it comes to vegetables, I steam some and I eat some raw. According to studies, if you steam them, you make the beta-carotene more bioavailable. Yet you obtain fewer vitamins and no enzymes.

> *It is critical to start the day without carbs. Insulin responds more briskly in the morning than at any other time of day.*

So it is best to alternate. Or you can juice or blend the produce to break down the cellulose walls to get the beta-carotene and the benefits of eating the vegetables raw.

Dr. Bernstein also discusses other tradeoffs when you cook vegetables.

Cooked vegetables tend to raise blood sugar more rapidly than raw vegetables because cooking makes them more digestible and converts some of the cellulose to glucose.[10]

Of course, converting the cellulose to glucose would also increase the calories absorbed, though nonstarchy vegetables are so low in calories that this shouldn't be a problem.

You may wish to go on a periodic fast from animal products. You may do this for weeks or even for a couple of months once a year. It is good to also do regular juice cleanses or water-only fasting as outlined in *The Live Food Factor*.

You might also find times in your life that you don't feel the need to eat much meat, just eggs, a bit of dairy, and fish for the brain, but no land animals. I found this to be the case for me after about a year into my return to flesh eating.

You could find yourself being "flexitarian" at times, just eating meat on occasion. An example might be when you are relaxing thoroughly in a pristine environment, as found in areas like certain parts of Costa Rica. In general, reducing pollution and stress decreases the body's needs for nutrients.

On the other hand, there may be times you crave more meat, such as when pregnant, lactating, or involved in extra muscle-building physical activity.

Remember to always, always *get that annual blood test done*, checking all of your vitamin and mineral levels, especially those listed in chapter 17. Blood tests give you previews of what your health will be like years later if you keep on doing what you're doing. Hair tests for minerals are relatively inexpensive if you can't afford blood tests.

Visit an alternative doctor once in a while. Even though there are many webinar and online nutrition classes, nothing replaces seeing a local health practitioner who can actually see you in person.

Finally, listen to the final authority on your health status: your own body. *The body never lies!*

Epilogue: Thoughts about the Future

There are known knowns. There are things we know we know. We also know there are known unknowns. That is to say, we know there are some things we do not know. But there are also unknown unknowns, the ones we don't know we don't know.
    —Donald Rumsfeld, United States Secretary of Defense, February 12, 2002.

The stimulus for writing this book was this question: are we genetically meant to be vegan, or is veganism something we are evolving into?

I am convinced that someday we will have our vegan paradise. As it says in the Bible, "The wolf also shall dwell with the lamb. … The lion shall eat straw like the ox."[*] But the vegan paradise isn't happening in my body. If it ever does happen globally in some sort of quantum leap, I want to be alive and in robust health to witness it.

My metaphysically minded friends keep me informed on the latest theories of how it is all going to play out. For example, "We are now carbon-based but will soon be shifting to a silicon base, and for some reason, none of us will need to eat meat then."

How things turn out may not be exactly as the vegans have envisioned: that we will all be eating luscious, sweet fruit or living off air and solar energy, bypassing the mitochondria altogether. The vegan paradise may come via technology before our bodies catch up with our evolution in consciousness. Perhaps when we perfect the science of in vitro meat culturing, the entire planet — domestic animals included! — can become vegans in the sense that no animal need die for our food.

On the other hand, I will not rule out the possibility that the spiritual paradigm plays out with a quantum leap in human consciousness and physical evolution. Who knows?

It could also be that we as a species are being forced to evolve into vegetarian diets, if not vegan ones, due to overpopulation and destruction of our ocean life. Those who are able to adapt to vegan diets may survive and pass on this genetic heritage. Maybe our genes might alter at a much more accelerated pace if all the metaphysical (including some scientific!) ways of thinking are true about the future.

After I wrote the fifth draft of this book, I joined the world in watching the devastation of history's largest oil spill. I pondered, "What will this mean down the road for the average person's brain? Will only the rich be able to afford the best sources of brain food?"

In the end, it may be those who adapt best to vegan or at least vegetarian diets who survive. If the population explodes to 11 billion by 2050 as some predict, we may all be living on beans and rice. (Hopefully by then, hemp seed will also be legal and widely available.) This may accelerate if the bees continue to die out. Only those who are good at making nutrient conversions will thrive. It might even get to the point when only those who adapt to plant diets will be able to reproduce.

Another possible scenario: We take all the energy and monetary investments that we currently use for war and focus on cleaning the oceans and environmental pollution. We replenish the soil. We perfect in vitro meat, making it compatible with our genes, and make it within reach of everyone's budget. We educate the masses and give them all sustainable jobs. The entire planet will be fed according to genetic needs. Who knows?

This may not be going to happen anytime soon, so meanwhile *be true to what your body needs*. Give your body the nutrients it requires so you can be healthy when that time comes. Don't resist nature. Even if others may be making the necessary genetic mutations, this doesn't mean you necessarily are — *yet*.

---

[*]Isaiah 11:6–7

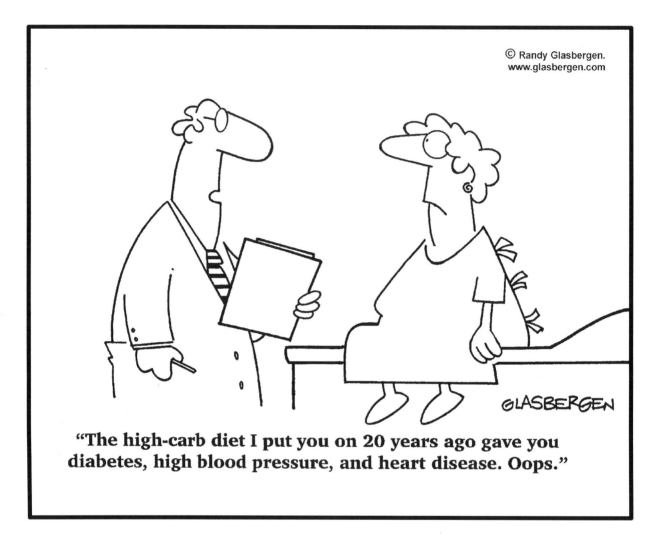

"The high-carb diet I put you on 20 years ago gave you diabetes, high blood pressure, and heart disease. Oops."

Notes

Chapter 1 (page 5)

1. Craig and Mangels, "Position of the American Dietetic Association: Vegetarian Diets," *J Am Diet Assoc*, 2009, 109 (7):1266–82

2. Corwin, "Forgotten Food Factors," *P-P Jnl of Hlth & Healng*, 1979, 4 (1)

3. Schenck, *Live Food Factor*, ch. 8, App. D

4. For more information about man's longevity potential, see the *Holy Bible*; Hilton Hotema, *Man's Higher Consciousness*; and De Vries, *Primitive Man*.

5. McDonald, *Perfect Gene Diet*, 22

Chapter 2 (page 11)

1. Billings, "Correcting the Vegetarian Myths about Ape Diets," www.beyondveg.com, accessed 1-21-10

2. Abrams, Jr., "Vegetarianism: Another View," www.biblelife.org/abrams2.htm, accessed 1-24-10

3. Abrams, Jr., "What We Can Learn from the Diet of Monkeys and Apes in Their Natural Habitat about Human Nutritional Needs," *P-P Jnl of Hlth & Healng,* 1979, 4 (2)

4. De Vries, *Primitive Man*, 19

5. Liebenberg, "Persistence Hunting by Modern Hunter-Gatherers," Wenner-Gren Foundation for Anthropological Research, *Current Anthropology*, Dec 2006, 47 (6):1017–25

6. Lieberman and Bramble, "The Evolution of Marathon Running Capabilities in Humans, *Sports Med*, 2007, 37 (4–5), 288–90

7. Bramble and Siegel, University of Utah, "How Running Made Us Human," *University of Utah News Release*, 17 Nov 2004

8. Lindeberg, *Food and Western Disease*, 56

9. For more information, read Cohen, *Health and the Rise of Civilization*; Steckel, *Backbone of History*.

10. Norat et al., "Meat, fish, and colorectal cancer risk: the European Prospective Investigation into cancer and nutrition," *J Natl Cancer Inst*, 15 Jun 2005, 97 (12):906–16

11. Sinha et al., "Meat intake and mortality" *Arch Intern Med*, 2009, 169 (6): 562–71

12. Mills et al., "Cancer incidence among California Seventh-Day Adventists, 1976–1982," *Am J Clin Nutr*, 1994, 59 (5 Suppl):1136s–42s

13. Key et al., "Health effects of vegetarian and vegan diets," *Proc Nutr Soc*, Feb 2006, 65 (1):35–41

14. Jönsson et al., "A paleolithic diet confers higher insulin sensitivity, lower C-reactive protein and lower blood pressure than a cereal-based diet in domestic pigs," *Nutrition & Metabolism*, Nov 2006, 3:39

15. Rosevear, "The Lesson of Price's Disappointment, Should We Be Strict Vegetarians?" *P-P Jnl of Hlth & Healng*, 1991, 15 (1–2)

16. Schenck, *Live Food Factor*, 188

17. Cordain and Campbell, "The Protein Debate," www.cathletics.com/articles/proteinDebate.pdf, accessed 9-14-10

18. Rose, *Detox for Women*, 22

19. Taubes, *Why We Get Fat*, 192, cites "The Battle of Weight Loss Diets: Is Anyone Winning (at Losing)?" Christopher Gardner, director of Nutrition Studies at Stanford Prevention Research Center, www.you tube.com/watch?v=eREuZEdMAVo.

20. Krajcovicova-Kudlackova et al., "Advanced glycation end products and nutrition," Physiological Research, 2002, 51:313–16

21. Hipkiss, "Would carnosine or a carnivorous diet help suppress aging and associated pathologies?" *Ann N Y Acad Sci*, May 2006, 1067:369–74

22. Fraser and Shavlik, "Ten years of life: is it a matter of choice?" *Arch Intern Med*, 2001, 161:1645–52

23. Colpo, *Great Cholesterol Con*, 299–302

24. Key et al., "Health effects of vegetarian and vegan diets," *Proc Nutr Soc*, Feb 2006, 65 (1):35–41

25. Chang-Claude et al., "Lifestyle determinants and mortality in German vegetarians and health-conscious persons: results of a 21-year follow up study," *Cancer Epidemiology, Biomarkers & Prevention*, 14 Apr 2005, 963

26. Ginter, "Vegetarian diets, chronic diseases, and longevity," *Bratisl Lek Listy*, 2008, 109 (10):463–66

27. Willett, "Convergence of philosophy and science: the Third International Congress on vegetarian nutrition," Am J Clin Nutr, 70 (suppl):434s–38s; 1999

28. Key et al., "Mortality in vegetarians and nonvegetarians: detailed finding from a collaborative analysis of 5 prospective studies," *Am J Clin Nutr*, 1999, 70 (suppl):516s–25s

29. Shibata, "Nutrition for the Japanese elderly," *Nutr Health*, 1992, 8 (2–3): 165–75

30. Ibid.

31. Smith, *Diet, Blood Cholesterol, and Coronary Heart Disease: A Critical Review of the Literature*, Vol 2, Vector Enterprises, Nov 1991; Russell Smith, "Vegetarian Studies — A Summary" P-P Jnl of Hlth & Healng, 1998 (4)

32. Smith and Pinckney, *Diet, Blood Cholesterol, and Coronary Heart Disease: A Critical Review of the Literature, vol. 2*, Vector Enterprises, CA, 1991. A shortened adaptation of Smith's section on vegetarianism and longevity was published in *P-P Jnl of Hlth & Healng,* 1998, 22 (4), 27–29. See also Fallon and Enig, *Wise Choices, Healthy Bodies*, Wise Traditions, Winter 2000, 15–21, www.westonaprice.org/womens-health/641-wise-choices-healthy-bodies.html, accessed 1-15-11; Burr and Sweetnam, "Vegetarianism, dietary fiber, and mortality," *Amer J Clin Nutr*, 1982, 36:873.

33. Schenck, *Live Food Factor*, App. C

34. Weaver, *Butcher and Vegetarian*, 68

Chapter 3 (page 19)

1. http://naturalhygienesociety.org/articl es/paleo2.html, accessed 4-22-10
2. Ibid.
3. Harris, *Food and Evolution*, 449
4. Harris, *Cows, Pigs, Wars*, 30
5. Abrams, Jr., "An Anthropological Observation: Vegetarianism," *P-P Jnl of Hlth & Healng,* 1978, 3 (1)
6. Malhotra, *Indian Journal of Industrial Medicine*, 1968, 14:219; Malhotra, "Epidemiology of ischaemic heart disease in India with special reference to causation," *British Heart Journal*, 1967, 29:895–905
7. www.vegetariantimes.com/features/a rchive_of_editorial/667, accessed 3-25-10
8. *New York Times*, 22 Nov 2009
9. De Vries, *Elixir of Life,* ch. 8
10. Crayhon, *Carnitine Miracle*, 46
11. Marcus et al., "Strict vegan, low-calorie diet administered by care giving daughter to elderly mother — is this elder abuse?" *Med Law* 2005 Jun, 24 (2):279–96
12. http://naturalhygienesociety.org/diet -nazariah.html, accessed 1-31-10
13. Ibid., accessed 1-29-10
14. Robbins, *Healthy at 100,* 142–43
15. Boutenko, *12 Steps to Raw* (2007), ch. 11
16. Donaldson, "Omega-3 vs. Omega-6 Fats, How to Maintain Proper Balance," *Hallelujah Acres Health News,* Nov/Dec 2010, 64
17. www.drbenkim.com, accessed 1-25-10
18. According to Geary, "Former Vegan Confesses All," www.truthaboutabs .com/vegan-confesses-health-problems .html, accessed 12-11-10. Natasha's website is www.voraciouseats.com, accessed 2-14-11.

Chapter 4 (page 25)

1. Key et al., "Raised thyroid stimulating hormone associated with kelp intake in British vegan men," *J Hum Nutr Diet*, 1992, 5:323–26
2. Anon., www.foxnews.com/story/0,29 33,422767,00.html, accessed 4-17-10; Vogiatzoglou et al., "Vitamin B_{12} status and rate of brain volume loss in community-dwelling elderly," *Neurology*, 2008, 71:826–32
3. Price, *Nutrition and Physical Degeneration*, 109
4. Private e-mail correspondence, Dec 2008
5. Gedgaudas, *Primal Body, Primal Mind,* 235
6. "Nutritional pros and cons of meat-based and vegetarian diets," www.ac u-cell.com/veg.html, accessed 1-25-10
7. Schenck, *Live Food Factor*, 151–53.
8. www.johnfielder.com.au/interview.ht ml, accessed 1-29-10
9. "Eating for Optimum Health," *East West Journal*, 22, 1992, http://natura lhygienesociety.org/articles/paleo2.ht ml, accessed 2-1-10
10. Wilson, *Adrenal Fatigue*, 140
11. Schmid, *Traditional Foods*, 18–19
12. Fallon, *Nourishing Traditions*, 24
13. http://naturalhygienesociety.org/diet3 .html#8, accessed 1-29-10
14. Vance, "Raw Foodist Celebrates his 109th Birthday," www.myfoxphoenix .com/dpp/morning_show/bernando-la pallo-celebrates-birthday-08172010?C MP=201009_emailshare, accessed 11-30-10.
15. He is "only" 101 according to Intelius: http://tinyurl.com/2e4dxdh, accessed 8-1-11.
16. Private telephone conversation, 2010
17. Schenck, *Live Food Factor*, ch. 2, presents testimonials and photos.
18. Winnicki et al., "Fish-rich diet, leptin, and body mass," *Circulation,* 2002, 106:289
19. Lindeberg, *Food and Western Disease*, 136–38
20. Gittleman, *Beyond Pritikin*, 6
21. Córdova-Fraga et al., "The colon transit time in different phases of the menstrual cycle: assessed with biomagnetic technique," *Neurology and Clinical Neurophysiology*, 30 Nov 2004, 31
22. Westbrook, *What Happened*, 27
23. George, "Discrimination and bias in the vegan ideal," *Journal of Agricultural and Environmental Ethics*, Mar 1994, 7:1, 19–28
24. Sapontzis, *Food for Thought*, 59, 261
25. Ibid., 266
26. Ibid., 268

Chapter 5 (page 35)

1. Hobbs and Haas, "Methionine: Amino Acid Support for Your Liver," www.dummies.com/how-to/content/ methionine-amino-acid-support-for-y our-liver.html, accessed 12-3-10; Maroufyan et al., "The effect of methionine and threonine supplementations on immune responses of broiler chickens challenged with infectious bursal disease," *American Journal of Applied Sciences*, 2010, 7 (1):44–50, www.scipub.org/fulltext/ajas/ajas714 -50.pdf; van Brummelen and du Toit, "L-methionine as immune supportive supplement: a clinical evaluation," Tshwane University of Technology, Gezina, South Africa, *Amino Acids*, 29 Sep 2006, www.biomox.com/res ources/publication%20amino%20acid %20journal.pdf
2. Gittleman, *Eat Fat, Lose Weight*, 63
3. Robb, *Fat Burning Diet*, 194
4. Fallon, "Twenty-Two Reason Not to Go Vegetarian," www.westonaprice .org/twenty-two-reasons-not-to-go-ve getarian.html, accessed 1-26-10
5. Private e-mail, Sep 2010
6. According to "Former Vegan Confesses All," www.truthaboutabs.com /vegan-confesses-health-problems.html, accessed 12-11-10. Natasha's website is www.voraciouseats.com, accessed 2-14-11
7. Ibid.

Chapter 6 (page 43)

1. Keith, *Vegetarian Myth*, 147
2. Lindeberg, *Food and Western Disease*, 4
3. Ibid., 56
4. Ibid., 62
5. For more information: Eaton, *Paleolithic Prescription*; Crawford, *Driving Force*
6. Finch, *Biology of Longevity*, 391–402
7. Ungar, *Evolution of Human Diet*, 4
8. Seinandre, *Los Orígenes del Hombre*, (Spanish Edition), Larousse: Paris, France, 2005; Klein, *Cambridge Encyclopedia of Human Evolution*, 1994 ed., 25; Klein, *Human Career*, University of Chicago Press, 1999, 93; Campbell et al., *Primates in Perspective*, Oxford University Press, 2007, 11
9. Humphries, "The Diet of Early Humans: What did our ancestors eat?" www.ivu.org/history/early/ancestors.html, accessed 1-12-10
10. Gathered from various anthropological texts, including those by Eaton et al. and Cunnane
11. Bunn, ed., *Meat-Eating and Evolution*, 318
12. Leakey, *Origin of Humankind*, 55–57
13. Leakey, *Origins*, 148
14. Leakey, *Origin of Humankind*, 39–40
15. Abrams, Jr., "Vegetarianism: Another View," www.biblelife.org/abrams2.htm, accessed 1-24-10
16. http://en.wikipedia.org/wiki/Mitochondrial_Eve, accessed 4-18-11
17. Sears, *Omega Rx Zone*, 17; for more information about how seafood saved humanity, see www.scientificamerican.com/article.cfm?id=interactive-seas-saved-humanity, accessed 11-15-10.
18. Bunn, ed., *Meat-Eating and Evolution*, 214
19. Aiello and Wheeler, "The expensive-tissue hypothesis: the brain and the digestive system in human and primate evolution," *Curr Anthropol*, 1995, 36:199–221, quote on 208
20. Ungar, *Evolution of Human Diet*, 349
21. Ibid., 349
22. Bunn, ed., *Meat-Eating and Evolution*, 312
23. Ungar, *Evolution of Human Diet*, 350
24. Ibid., 351
25. Ibid., 6
26. Finch, *Biology of Longevity*, 385–86
27. Wrangham, *Catching Fire*, 139
28. Corliss et al., "Should We All Be Vegetarians?" www.time.com/time/magazine/article/0,9171,1002888-8,00.html, 15 Jul 2002
29. Leakey, *Origins*, 11
30. Leakey, *Origin of Humankind*, 43
31. Ungar, *Evolution of Human Diet*, 354
32. Cunnane, *Survival of Fattest*, 220
33. Fallon and Enig, "The Cave Man Diet," *P-P Jnl of Hlth & Healng*, 1997, 21 (2)
34. Groves, "The Naïve Vegetarian," www.second-opinions.co.uk/vegetarian.html, accessed 1-11-10
35. Ungar, *Evolution of Human Diet*, 192
36. Ibid., 194
37. Ibid., 199
38. Bunn, ed., *Meat-Eating and Evolution*, 28
39. Ungar, *Evolution of Human Diet*, 205
40. Roxby, "Recreating the caveman diet," www.bbc.co.uk/news/health-11075437, accessed 11-25-10
41. De Vries, *Primitive Man*, 12
42. Ibid., 19
43. Ibid., 132–33
44. Eades, *Protein Power Life Plan*, 2
45. Coleman, "Comparative Anatomy and Taxonomy vs. Opportunistic Feeding," http://home.earthlink.net/~mr.kerchak/VEGAN.html, accessed 4-13-11
46. Fallon and Enig, "The Cave Man Diet," *P-P Jnl of Hlth & Healng*, 1997, 21 (2)

Chapter 7 (page 55)

1. Wadley and Martin, "The Origins of Agriculture: A Biological Perspective and a New Hypothesis," *Australian Biologist*, Jun 1993, 96–105, http://iheartfruit.com/index.php?topic=134.0;wap2
2. Lindeberg, *Food and Western Disease*, 195
3. Crawford, *Driving Force*, 194
4. Ibid., 205, cites *Everyman Encyclopædia*, 1913, 6:384
5. Cochran, *10,000 Year Explosion*, 111–12
6. Ibid., 114–17
7. Hartmann, *Last Hours*, 17–19

Chapter 8 (page 57)

1. Several sources indicate this, including Cunnane, *Survival of Fattest*, 21
2. Holford, *Optimum Nutrition*, 35
3. Crawford, *Driving Force*, 221
4. This calculation is based on 100 billion in total, from Chudler, "Brain Facts and Figures," http://faculty.washington.edu/chudler/facts.html, accessed 11-9-10
5. www.inner.org/audio/aid/E_013.htm, accessed 1-5-10
6. Crawford, *Driving Force*, 189
7. Carper, *100 Simple Things*, 225
8. Kang et al., "Docosahexaenoic acid induces apoptosis in MCF-7 cells in vitro and in vivo via reactive oxygen species formation and caspase 8 activation," *PLoS ONE*, Apr 2010, 5:4, e10296
9. Sears, *Omega Rx Zone*, 108–11
10. Albanese et al., "Dietary fish and meat intake and dementia in Latin America, China, and India: a 10/66 Dementia Research Group population-based study," *Am J Clin Nutr*, 2009, 90:392–400
11. Carper, *100 Simple Things*, 124
12. Ibid., 125
13. Ibid., 171–73

14. Miller, "Fewer months 'R' safe for eating raw gulf oysters," http://findarticles.com/p/articles/mi_m1370/is_n5_v22/ai_6495708/, accessed 4-15-11

15. Williams and Burdge, "Long-chain n-3 PUFA: plant v. marine sources," *Proc Nutr Soc*, Feb 2006, 65 (1):42-50

16. Fallon, *Nourishing Traditions*, 10

17. Ibid.

18. Sears, *Omega Rx Zone*, 96

19. Ibid., 192

20. Ibid., 95

21. Eades, *Protein Power LifePlan*, 75

22. Vogiatzoglou et al., "Dietary sources of vitamin B_{12} and their association with plasma vitamin B_{12} concentrations in the general population: the Hordaland homocysteine study," *Am J Clin Nutr*, 2009, 89:1078–87

23. Henslin, *Your Brain on Joy*, 56

24. Fallon, *Nourishing Traditions*, 32

25. Turunen et al., "Mortality in a cohort with high fish consumption," *Int J Epidemiol*, 25 Jun 2008

26. Carr, *Shallows*, 115–116, 119, 126–127

27. Schoenthaler et al., "Controlled vial of vitamin-mineral supplementation: effects on intelligence and performance," *Person Individ Diff*, 1991, 12 (4):351–52, cited by Holford, *Optimum Nutrition*, 122.

28. Sears, *Omega Rx Zone*, 194–96

29. Raji et al., "Brain structure and obesity," *Human Brain Mapping*, Mar 2010, 31 (3): 353–64

30. Cournot et al., "Relation between body mass index and cognitive function in healthy middle-aged men and women," *Neurology*, 2006, 67:1208–14

31. Holford, *Optimum Nutrition*, 79

32. Ibid., 42

Chapter 9 (page 65)

1. Day, "Strict Vegan Diets May Be Dangerous, Especially for Expectant Mothers and Children ," http://chetday.com/vegandietdangers.htm, accessed 1-29-10

2. Billings, "Essential Fatty Acids (EFAs)," www.beyondveg.com/billings-t/comp-anat/comp-anat-7h.shtml, accessed 4-15-11, cites numerous sources.

3. Holford, *Optimum Nutrition*, 40

4. Crawford and Sinclair, "Nutritional influences in the evolution of the mammalian brain," *Ciba Found Symp*, 1971, 267–92

5. Crawford, *Driving Force*, 182

6. Sears, *Omega Rx Zone*, 78

7. Sears, "Fish Oil and Hexane," http://drsears.com/tabId/399/itemId/10846/Fish-oil-and-hexane.aspx, accessed 1-28-10

8. Holford, *Optimum Nutrition*, 40

9. File et al., "Soya phytoestrogens change cortical and hippocampal expression of BDNF mRNA in male rats," *Neurosci Lett*, 27 Feb 2003, 338 (2):135–38

10. Hales and Hales, "The Brain's Power to Heal," *Washington Post*, 21 Nov 1999, Parade Section, 10

11. Goddard, "Soy-Dementia in Men," http://iangoddard.com/soy.htm, accessed 1-17-10

12. Keith, *Vegetarian Myth*, 193

13. Ibid.

14. Ibid., 194

15. Groves, "The Naïve Vegetarian," www.second-opinions.co.uk/vegetarian.html, accessed 1-16-10

16. Gagne, *Food Energetics*, 160

17. www.beyondveg.com

18. See "A Former Vegan Confesses All" on www.truthaboutabs.com/vegan-confesses-health-problems.html, accessed 12-11-10. Natasha's website is www.voraciouseats.com, accessed 2-14-11.

19. Zavasta, *Raw Food Hot Yoga*, 241

20. Weaver, *Butcher and Vegetarian*, 78

21. Ibid., 171

22. Billings, "Comparative Anatomy and Physiology Brought Up to Date," www.beyondveg.com/billingst/comp-anat/comp-anat-9d.shtml, accessed 12-30-09

23. According to Natasha. See note 18 above.

24. White et al., "Association of mid-life consumption of tofu with late life cognitive impairment and dementia. The Honolulu-Asia Aging Study," *Neurobiol Aging*, 1996, 7 (suppl 4): 121; White et al., "Prevalence of dementia in older Japanese-American men in Hawaii," *JAMA*, 1996, 276: 955–60; White et al., "Brain aging and midlife tofu consumption," *J Am Coll Nutr*, 2000, 19:207–9, 242–55; Goddard, "Tofu study update," 9 Dec 1999, http://iangoddard.com/soy.htm

25. Wang et al. "Vitamin B_{12} and folate in relation to the development of Alzheimer's disease," *Neurology*, 8 May 2001, 56 (9):1188–94

26. Chang-Claude et al., "Lifestyle Determinants and Mortality in German Vegetarians and health-conscious persons: results of a 21-year follow-up study," *Cancer Epidemiology, Biomarkers, and Prevention*, Apr 2005 14:963

Chapter 10 (page 73)

1. Campbell, *China Study*, 104

2. Fallon and Enig, "Adventures in Macro-Nutrient Land," 2003, www.westonaprice.org/adventures-in-macro-nutrient-land.html, accessed 3-24-10

3. Wharton, *Metabolic Man*, 183

4. Ibid., 184

5. Ibid.

6. Ibid., 212

7. Ibid., 273

8. Mercola, *P-P Jnl of Hlth & Healng*, 2009, 33 (4)

9. Wharton, *Metabolic Man*, 183

10. Campbell, *China Study*, 99–101

11. Hyman, *Ultimate Metabolism*, 51

12. Cousens, *Conscious Eating*, 56–57

13. DeCava, "Food Fights (Part 2)," *P-P Jnl of Hlth & Healng*, 2001, 25 (4)

14. Melvin, *Paleolithic Prescription*, 74

15. McDonald, *Perfect Gene Diet*, 58

16. *Findings and Recommendations on the*

Insulin Resistance Syndrome, American Association of Clinical Endocrinologists, Washington, DC, 25–26 Aug 2002

17. For more information, see Pidcock, "High-Altitude Eating," www.pppon line.co.uk/encyc/0319.htm, accessed 11-10-10.

18. "Food Fight (Part 2)," *P-P Jnl of Hlth & Healng*, 2001, 25 (4)

19. Eades, *Protein Power LifePlan*, 30

20. http://en.wikipedia.org/wiki/Great_Fa mine_(Ireland)#Emigration, accessed 1-13-11

Chapter 11 (page 81)

1. McNamara, "The impact of egg limitations on coronary heart disease risk: do the numbers add up?" *Journal of the American College of Nutrition*, 2000, 19 (90005):540s–548s; McNamara, "The impact of egg limitations on coronary heart disease risk: do the numbers add up?" *Journal of the American College of Nutrition*, 2000, 19 (90005):540s–548s

2. Knopp and Retzlaff, "Saturated fat prevents coronary artery disease: an American paradox," *Am J Clin Nutr*, Nov 2004, 80:5, 1102–3

3. Keys, "Letter: normal plasma cholesterol in a man who eats 25 eggs a day," *New England Journal of Medicine*, 1991, 325:584

4. Mann et al., "Atherosclerosis in the Masai," *Am J Epidemiol*, 95 (1), 26–37

5. Mann et al., "Cardiovascular disease in African Pygmies: a survey of the health status, serum lipids, and diet of Pygmies in Congo," Apr 1962, *Journal of Chronic Diseases*, 15 (4), 341–71

6. DeBakey, *JAMA*, 1964, 189:655–59

7. Murray, *Drug Companies Won't Tell*, 127

8. Engelberg, "Low serum cholesterol and suicide," *Lancet*, 21 Mar 1992, 339 (8795):727–9; "Cholesterol and violence: is there a connection?" *Annals of Internal Medicine*, 15 Mar 1998, 128 (6), 478–87; Ellison and Morri-

son, "Low serum cholesterol concentration and risk of suicide," *Epidemiology*, 2001 Mar, 12 (2):168–72; Muldoon et al., "Lowering cholesterol concentrations and mortality: a quantitative review of primary prevention trials," *British Medical Journal*, 1990, 301:309–14; Hawthon et al., "Low serum cholesterol and suicide," *Br J Psychiatry*, Jun 1993, 162:818–25

9. Fallon, *Nourishing Traditions*, 11, cites Felton et al., *Lancet*, 1994, 344:1195.

10. Lindeberg, *Food and Western Disease*, 96, cites Mozaffarian et al., "Dietary fats, carbohydrate, and progression of coronary atherosclerosis in postmenopausal women," *Am J Clin Nutr*, 80:1175–84.

11. Fallon, *Nourishing Traditions*, 11, cites Watkins and Seifert, "Food lipids and bone health," *Food Lipids and Health*, 101, Marcel Dekker, Inc.: New York, NY, 1996.

12. Gittleman, *Eat Fat, Lose Weight*, 45

13. Berglund et al., "HDL-subpopulation patterns in response to reductions in dietary total and saturated fat intakes in healthy subjects," *Am J Clin Nutr*, Dec 1999, 70 (6), 992–1000

14. Mensink and Katan, "Effect of dietary fatty acids on serum lipids and lipoproteins: a meta-analysis of 27 trials," *Arterioscler Thromb*, Aug 1992, 12 (8):911–19

15. Colpo, *Great Cholesterol Con*, 257–59

16. Bowden, *Living Low Carb*, 67–68

17. Lindeberg, *Food and Western Disease*, 75

18. Eades, *Protein Power LifePlan*, 109

19. Ibid., 93

20. Wolf, *Paleo Solution*, 75.

21. Taubes, *Why We Get Fat*, 193

22. Ibid., 193

23. Key, Appleby, and Rosell, "Health effects of vegetarian and vegan diets," *Proc Nutr Soc*, Feb 2006, 65 (1):35–41; Lindeberg, *Food and Western Disease*, 82, cites 3 studies:

Bissoli et al., "Effect of vegetarian diet on homocysteine levels," *Ann Nutr Metab*, 2002, 46:73–9; Majchrzak et al., "B-vitamin status and concentrations of homocysteine in Austrian omnivores, vegetarians, and vegans," *Ann Nutr Metab*, 2006, 50:485–91; Mann et al., "The effect of diet on plasma homocysteine concentrations in healthy male subjects," *Eur J Clin Nutr*, 1999, 53:895–59.

24. Howard and Wylie-Rosett, "Sugar and cardiovascular disease: a statement for healthcare professionals from the Committee on Nutrition of the Council on Nutrition, Physical Activity, and Metabolism of the American Heart Association," *Circulation*, 2002, 106:523

25. Eades, *Protein Power LifePlan*, 95

26. Bowden, *Living Low Carb*, 42, cites Gaziano, "Fasting triglycerides, high-density lipoprotein, and risk of myocardial infarction," *Circulation*, 1997, 96:2520–25.

27. Taubes, *Why We Get Fat*, 188

28. Bowden, *Living Low Carb*, 73

29. Enig, *Know Your Fats*, 85–86

30. Liu et al., "Relation between a diet with a high glycemic load and plasma concentrations of high-sensitivity C-reactive protein in middle-aged women," *Am J Clin Nutr*, Mar 2002, 75:3, 492–98

Chapter 12 (page 89)

1. Hyman, *Ultra-Metabolism*, 46

2. Eades, *Protein Power*, 108

3. Abrams, H. Leon, Jr., "What is nutritional anthropology?" *P-P Jnl of Hlth & Healng*, 1982, 7 (1)

4. Graham, *80/10/10 Diet*, 132

5. Sharifi et al., "Effects of caloric restriction and the role of nitric oxide [NO] on hemodynamic condition of nondiabetic and stz-induced diabetics rats," *Iranian Journal of Diabetes and Lipid Disorders*, 2006, 6:177

6. Brodsky et al., "Glucose Scavenging of nitric oxide," *American Journal of Physiology, Renal Physiology*, 1 Mar

2001, 280 (3):F480–86; James et al., "Vasorelaxation by red blood cells and impairment in diabetes; reduced nitric oxide and oxygen delivery by glycated hemoglobin," *Circulation Research*, 16 Apr 2004, 94 (7): 976–83

7. Northrup, *Secret Pleasures of Menopause*, 28

8. Ibid., 34

9. Bowden, *Living Low Carb*, 14; Eades, *Protein Power Life Plan*, 50

10. Bowden, *Living Low Carb*, 14, cites Kekwick and Pawan, "Metabolic study in human obesity with isocaloric diets high in fat, protein, or carbohydrate," *Metabolism*, Sep 1957, 6 (5):447–60.

11. Layman et al., "A reduced ratio of dietary carbohydrate to protein improves body composition and blood lipid profiles during weight loss in adult women," *J Nutr*, Feb 2003, 133 (2):411–17

12. Bowden, *Living Low Carb*, 85

13. Ibid., 41

14. Rosedale, "Insulin Resistance: The Real Culprit," www.drrosedale.com /resources/pdf/Insulin%20Resistance.p df, accessed 11-10-10

15. Lindeberg, *Food and Western Disease*, 151, 189–90

16. Bowden, *Living Low Carb*, 44

17. Denese, *Ageless Skin*, 19–20

18. Lindeberg, *Food and Western Disease*, 151–52

19. Bernstein, *Diabetes Diet*, 21

20. Ibid., 23

21. Monastyrsky, *Fiber Menace*, 69

22. Wolf, *Paleo Solution*, 76–77

23. Monastyrsky, *Fiber Menace*, 16

24. Hyman, *UltraMind Solution*, 154

25. Alzheimer Research Forum live discussion transcript, 2006: Kinoshita, "Insulin resistance: a common axis linking Alzheimer's, depression, and metabolism?" *J ALzheimers Dis*, 9 (1):89–93

26. Hyman, *UltraMind Solution*, 155

27. Manninen, "Very-low-carbohydrate diets and preservation of muscle mass," *Nutr Metab* (Lond), Jan 2006 31, 3:9; Rosedale et al. "Clinical experience in a diet designed to reduce aging," *Jnl App Res*, 1 Jan 2009, 9 (4):159–165.

Chapter 13 (page 95)

1. Rosedale, *Rosedale Diet*, 16–17

2. Gittleman, *Beyond Pritikin*, 4

3. Sears, *Toxic Fat*, 29–34

4. Schwarzbein, *Schwarzbein Principle*, 91

5. Eades, *Protein Power LifePlan*, 53, 96; Bowden, *Living Low Carb*, 53. Both cite Marigliano et al., "Normal values in extreme old age," *Ann N Y Acad Sci*, Dec 1992, 26, 673:23–8, the last paragraph being a direct quote from the study.

6. Bowden, *Living Low Carb*, 103–5

7. http://en.wikipedia.org/wiki/Ketoacid osis, accessed 11-11-10

8. Kashiwaya et al., "D-beta-hydroxy-butyrate protects neurons in models of Alzheimer's and Parkinson's disease," *Proc Natl Acad Sci USA*, 9 May 2000, 97 (10):5440–44

9. Sharman et al., "A ketogenic diet favorably affects serum biomarkers for cardiovascular disease in normal-weight men," *J Nutr*, Jul 2002, 132, 7:1879–85

10. Freeman, *Ketogenic Diet*, 246–49

11. Atkins, *New Diet Revolution*, 60–61, cites Benoit, et al., "Changes in Body Composition During Weight Reduction in Obesity: Balance Studies Comparing Effects of Fasting and a Ketogenic Diet," *Annals of Internal Medicine*, 63, 1965, 604–12.

12. Bowden, *Living Low Carb*, 103

13. Cunnane, *Survival of Fattest*, 208

14. Beisswenger et al., "Ketosis leads to increased methylglyoxal production on the Atkins diet," *Ann N Y Acad Sci*, 2005 Jun, 1043:201–10

15. Cunnane, *Survival of Fattest*, 207

16. Taubes, *Why We Get Fat*, 211

17. Bowden, *Living Low Carb*, 105

18. Veech et al., "Ketone Bodies: Potential Therapeutic Uses," *IUBMB Life*, 2001, 51:241–47, www.niaaa.nih.gov /NR/rdonlyres/8334AC75-0432-4758 -BEA4-5571F4A00BC4/0/VeechIUB MBLife2001_241.pdf, accessed 2-10-10

19. Atkins, *New Diet Revolution*, 52

20. Yudkoff et al., "Response of brain amino acid metabolism to ketosis," *Neurochem Int*, Jul 2005, 47 (1–2): 119–28

21. El Mallakh and Paskitti, "The ketogenic diet may have mood stabilizing properties," *Med Hypotheses*, Dec 2001, 57 (6):724–26

Chapter 14 (page 101)

1. Crayhon, *Carnitine Miracle*, 43

2. Eades, *Protein Power*, 39

3. Wolf, *Paleo Solution*, 109

4. Gedgaudas, *Primal Body, Primal Mind*, 242

5. Ibid., 187

6. Eades, *Protein Power LifePlan*, 160

7. Gedgaudas, *Primal Body, Primal Mind*, 165

8. Eades, *Protein Power*, 102

9. Lindeberg, *Food and Western Disease*, 189

10. Smith-Warner and Stampfer, "Fat intake and breast cancer revisited," *J Natl Cancer Inst*, 2007, 99:418–19

11. Gittleman, *Beyond Pritikin*, 28

12. Muldoon et al., "Lowering cholesterol concentrations and mortality: a quantitative review of primary prevention trials," *British Medical Journal*, 1990, 301:309–14

13. Vonderplanitz, *Living without Disease*, 210

14. Baroody, *Alkalize or Die*, 58–61

15. Gedgaudas, *Primal Body, Primal Mind*, 225

16. Lindeberg, *Food and Western Disease*, 90

17. Harris, *Food and Evolution*, 216, an

anthology to which H. Leon Abrams, Jr. contributed

18. Bernstein, *Diabetes Diet*, 42

19. Eades, *Protein Power*, 37

20. Bowden, *Living Low Carb*, 36

21. Lindeberg, *Food and Western Disease*, 152

22. Bowden, *Living Low Carb*, 97

23. Westman, "Is dietary carbohydrate essential for human nutrition?" *Am J Clin Nutr*, May 2002, 75 (5):951–53

24. Lieb, "The effects of an exclusive long-continued meat diet," *JAMA*, 3 Jul 1926, 87 (1):25–26; Stefansson, "Adventures in Diet," *Harper's Monthly Magazine*, Nov 1935, Dec 1935, and Jan 1936, www.biblelife.org/stefansson1.htm, accessed 1-16-11

25. Stefansson, "Food of the ancient and modern Stone Age man," *J Amer Diet Assoc*, 1937, 13:2

26. Holford, *Optimum Nutrition*, 18. Raw fats are also "smokeless," while complex carbs may not always be.

27. Ibid., 151

Chapter 15 (page 107)

1. Cited by: Schmidt, *Dynamics of Nutrition*; Cousens, *Spiritual Nutrition*

2. Cheraskin et al., "The 'ideal' daily intake of threonine, valine, phenylalanine, leucine, isoleucine, and methionine," *Orthomolecular Psychiatry*, 1978, 7 (3):150–55

3. Gedgaudas, *Primal Body, Primal Mind*, 156

4. Lindeberg, *Food and Western Disease*, 54

5. Ibid., 218

6. Ibid., 54

7. Ibid., 199

8. Ibid., 209, cites Brune et al., "Iron absorption: no intestinal adaptation to a high-phytate diet," 1989, *Am J Clin Nutr*, 49:542–45.

9. Nutritional data in this chapter obtained from www.nutritiondata.com, accessed 11-18-10, unless otherwise specified

10. Brazil nut data obtained from http://nat.illinois.edu/mainnat.html, accessed 11-18-10

11. Simopoulos, "The importance of the ratio of omega-6/omega-3 essential fatty acids," *Biomed Pharmacother*, Oct 2002, 56 (8):365–79

12. www.phyticacidresearch.com, accessed 2-15-10

13. Cordain, *Paleo Diet*, 50

14. Ayerza and Coates, *Chia*, 121

15. Gittleman, *Fat Flush Plan*, 167

16. Ayerza and Coates, *Chia*, 121, cites Muis and Wes.

17. "Organic Shelled Hempseed," http://nutiva.com/nutrition/charts/organic-shelled-hempseed, accessed 11-18-10

18. Murdock, "Why Hemp Could Save the World," www.examiner.com/freethought-in-national/why-hemp-could-save-the-world, accessed 11-12-10

19. Lindeberg, *Food and Western Disease*, 202, cites Liesegang et al., "Influence of a vegetarian diet versus a diet with fishmeal on bone in growing pigs," *J Vet Med A*, 2002, 49:230–38.

20. White et al., "Association of midlife consumption of tofu with late life cognitive impairment and dementia: the Honolulu-Asia aging study," *Neurobiol Aging*, 1996, 7 (4):121; White et al., "Prevalence of dementia in older Japanese-American men in Hawaii," *JAMA*, 1996, 276:955–60; White et al., "Brain aging and midlife tofu consumption," *J Am Coll Nutr*, 2000, 19:207–9, 242–55; Goddard, "Tofu study update," 9 Dec 1999

21. Daniel, *Whole Soy Story*, 299

22. Key et al., "Raised thyroid stimulating hormone associated with kelp intake in British vegan men," *J Hum Nutr Diet*, 1992, 5:323–26

23. Daniel, *Whole Soy Story*, 376–77

24. Ibid., 373

25. Ibid., 374

26. Daniel, *Whole Soy Story*, quotes Professor Ieuan Hughes from a discussion forum on birth-defect links to vegetarian mothers at www.animalrig-hts.net.

27. Daniel, *Whole Soy Story*, 347

28. Ibid., 159

29. Ibid., 353

30. Cordain, *Paleo Diet*, 92

31. Carper, *100 Simple Things*, 61, 95–96

32. Bernstein, *Diabetes Diet*, 49

33. Lindeberg, *Food and Western Disease*, 100

34. Bond, *Natural Eating*, 62

35. Ibid., 61

36. Ibid., 63

37. Eades, *Protein Power LifePlan*, 136–51

38. Lindeberg, *Food and Western Disease*, 131

39. Ibid.

40. Wadley and Martin, "The origins of agriculture: a biological perspective and a new hypothesis," *Australian Biologist*, Jun 1993, 96–105, http://iheartfruit.com/index.php?topic=134.0;wap2

41. Lindeberg, *Food and Western Disease*, 211

42. Ibid., 214

43. Ibid., 110

44. Ibid., 155

45. Pfeiffer, *Nutrition and Mental Illness*, 26–32

46. Weaver, *Butcher and Vegetarian*, 106

47. Corwin, "Forgotten Food Factors," *P-P Jnl of Hlth & Healng*, 1979, 4 (1)

48. www.bryannaclarkgrogan.com/board/board_topic/580578/117826.htm, accessed 2-26-11, references studies on spirulina and blue green algae toxicity in footnotes.

49. Colpo, *Great Cholesterol Con*, 242

50. Monastyrsky, *Fiber Menace*, 61

51. Schmid, "Recovering from Vegetarianism," *P-P Jnl of Hlth & Healng*, 2006, 30 (3)

52. Lindeberg, *Food and Western Disease*, 19

53. Ibid., 189–90

54. Ibid., 110

55. Ibid., 80

56. "Vegetarian Myths and Facts," http://thehealthadvantage.com/vegetarians.html, accessed 1-17-10

57. Fallon, *Nourishing Traditions*, 37

58. www.salem-news.com/articles/april26 2010/gm-food-as.php, accessed 5-5-10

59. Engdahl, *Seeds of Destruction*, 272–73

60. Campbell, *China Study,* 30–31

61. Troen et al., "The atherogenic effect of excess methionine intake," *Proc Natl Acad Sci USA*, 9 Dec 2003, 100 (25):15089–94, www.ncbi.nlm.nih.gov/pmc/articles/PMC299913, accessed 11-28-10

62. Carper, *100 Simple Things*, 239

63. Ibid., 215

Chapter 16 (page 121)

1. Croveti et al., "The influence of thermic effect of food on satiety," *Eur J Clin Nutr*, 1998, 52:482–88

2. Batterham, et al., "Critical role of peptide YY in protein-mediated satiation and body-weight regulaton," *Cell Metab*, Sep 2006, 4 (3):223–33

3. Gittleman, *Beyond Pritikin*, 7

4. Johnston et al., "Postprandial thermogenesis is increased 100 percent on a high-protein, low-fat diet versus a high-carbohydrate, low-fat diet in healthy, young women," *J Am Coll Nutr*, Feb 2002, 21 (1):55–61

5. Gittleman, *Beyond Pritikin*, p 7

6. Lindeberg, *Food and Western Disease*, 223

7. Sears, *Toxic Fat*, 28

8. Ross, *Mood Cure*, 112

9. Fallon, *Nourishing Traditions*, 26

10. Fallon and Enig, "Adventures in Macro-Nutrient Land," www.westonaprice.org/adventures-in-macro-nutrient-land.html, 2003, accessed 3-25-10

11. Rosedale, *Rosedale Diet*, 22–23

12. Cousens, *Spiritual Nutrition*, 273

13. See note 10 above.

14. Knight et al., "The impact of protein intake on renal function decline in women with normal renal function or mild renal insufficiency," *Annals of Internal Medicine*, 2003, 138:460–67

15. Skov et al., "Changes in renal function during weight loss induced by high- vs. low-protein, low-fat diets in overweight subjects," *International Journal of Obesity and Related Metabolic Disorders*, Nov 1999, 23, 11:1170–77

16. Hannan et al., "Effect of dietary protein on bone loss in elderly men and women: the Framingham osteoporosis study," *Journal of Bone and Mineral Research*, 2000, 15 (12):2504–12

17. Devine et al., "Protein consumption is an important predictor of lower limb bone mass in elderly women," *Am J Clin Nutr* 2005, 81:1423–28

18. Bowden, *Living Low Carb*, 111, cites Heaney, "Editorial: protein and calcium: antagonists or synergists?" *Am J Clin Nutr*, Apr 2002, 75 (4):609–10

19. Atkins, *New Diet Revolution*, 87

20. Bilsborough S, Mann N, "A review of issues of dietary protein intake in humans," *Int J Sport Nutr Exerc Metab*, Apr 2006, 16 (2):129–52

21. Wolf, *Paleo Solution*, 67

22. Lindeberg, *Food and Western Disease*, 201

23. Spencer and Kramer, "Factors contributing to osteoporosis," *J Nutr*, 1986, 116:316–19

24. Spencer and Kramer, "Further studies of the effect of a high-protein diet as meat on calcium metabolism," *Am J Clin Nutr*, Jun 1983, 37 (6):924–29

25. Mazess and Mather, "Bone mineral content of North Alaskan Eskimos," *Am J Clin Nutr*, Sep 1974, 2:916–25

26. Price, *Nutrition and Physical Degeneration*, 59

27. Hu et al., "Dietary Protein and Risk of Ischemic Heart Disease in Women," *Am J Clin Nutr*, 1999, 81 (4A): 221–27

Chapter 17 (page 125)

1. Schenck, *Live Food Factor*, 521

2. Price, *Nutrition and Physical Degeneration*, 282

3. Craig and Mangels, "Position of the American Dietetic Association: vegetarian diets," *J Am Diet Assoc*, Jul 2009, 109 (7):1266–82

4. Fallon and Enig, "Vitamin Primer," www.westonaprice.org/vitamin–primer.html, accessed 3-23-10

5. West et al., "Consequences of revised estimates of carotenoid bioefficacy for dietary control of vitamin A deficiency in developing countries," *J Nutr*, 2002 suppl, 132:2920s–26s

6. Chris Masterjohn, "Vitamin A on trial: does vitamin A cause osteoporosis?" www.westonaprice.org/vitamin-a-on-trial-does-vitamin-a-cause-osteoporosis.html, 2006, accessed 3-24-10

7. Johansson and Melhus, "Vitamin A antagonizes calcium response to vitamin D in man," *Journal of Bone and Mineral Research*, 2001, 16 (10): 1899–1905

8. "Vegetarianism and Nutrient Deficiencies," www.westonaprice.org, accessed 12-24-09

9. Fallon and Enig, "Cod Liver Oil Basics and Recommendations," www.westonaprice.org/cod-liver-oil-basics-and-recommendations.html

10. Masterjohn, "Vegetarianism and Nutrient Deficiencies," www.westonaprice.org/abcs-of-nutrition/1640-vegetarianism-and-nutrient-deficiencies.html, accessed 11-9-10, who references West et al., "Consequences of revised estimates of carotenoid bioefficacy for dietary control of vitamin A deficiency in developing countries," *J Nutr.* 2002, 132 (9):2920s–26s.

11. Russell, "The enigma of beta-carotene in carcinogenesis: what can be learned from animal studies," *J Nutr*, 2004, 134:262s–268s

12. Fallon and Enig, "Vitamin A Saga," www.westonaprice.org/abcs-of-nutrition/167-vitamin-a-saga.html, accessed

11-27-10

13. Jones et al., "Choline availability to the developing rat fetus alters adult hippocampal long-term potentiation," *Brain Res Dev Brain Res*, 10 Dec 1999, 118 (1–2):159–67

14. Cousens, *Live-Food Cuisine*, 25

15. Cousens, *Spiritual Nutrition*, 283

16. Mozafar, "Enrichment of some B-vitamins in plants with application of organic fertilizers," *Plant and Soil*, 1994, 167 (2):305–11

17. Halstead, Carroll, and Rubert, "Serum and tissue concentration of vitamin B_{12} in certain pathological states," *N Eng J Med*, 1959, 260:575

18. *Nature's Way*, 1979, 10:20–30, cited by "Vitamin B_{12}: Vital Nutrient for Good," www.westonaprice.org/abcs-of-nutrition/174-vitamin-b12.html, accessed 11-27-10

19. Milea, "Blindness in a strict vegan," *N Engl J Med*, 2000, 342:897–98; Brocadello et al., "Irreversible subacute sclerotic combined degeneration of the spinal cord in a vegan subject," *Nutrition*, Jul–Aug 2007, 23 (7–8):622–24

20. Zhuo and Praticò, "Acceleration of brain amyloidosis in an Alzheimer's disease mouse model by a folate, vitamin B_6 and B_{12}, deficient diet," *Exp Gerontol*, Mar 2010, 45 (3):195–201, E-pub 11 Dec 2009

21. Carper, *100 Simple Things*, 271

22. Fallon and Enig, "Cod Liver Oil Basics and Recommendations," www.westonaprice.org/cod-liver-oil-basics-and-recommendations.html, accessed 1-25-10

23. Mercola, "Vitamin D Resource Page," www.mercola.com/article/vitamin-d-resources.htm, accessed 1-25-10

24. Weaver, *Butcher and Vegetarian*, 125

25. "Light-zapped mushrooms filled with vitamin D," www.msnbc.msn.com/id/12370708, *Associated Press*, 18 Apr 2006, accessed 1-30-10; Armas et al., "Vitamin D_2 is much less effective than vitamin D_3 in humans," *Journal of Clinical Endocrinology and Metabolism*, 2004, 89 (11):5387–91

26. Masterjohn, "On the Trail of the Elusive X-Factor," www.westonaprice.org/abcs-of-nutrition/175-x-factor-is-vitamin-k2.html, accessed 11-20-10, who references McKeown et al., "Dietary and nondietary determinants of vitamin K biochemical measures in men and women," *J Nutr*, 2002, 132 (6): 1329–34

27. www.westonaprice.org/on-the-trail-of-the-elusive-x-factor-a-sixty-two-year-old-mystery-finally-solved.html, accessed 1-21-10

28. Cockayne et al., "Vitamin K and the prevention of fractures: systematic review and meta-analysis of randomized controlled trials," *Arch Intern Med*, Jun 2006, 26, 166 (12):1256–61

29. www.smartbodyz.com/Vitamin-K1-K2-K-1-supplements-foods-source-information-Dose.htm, accessed 11-19-10

30. Craig, "Health effects of vegan diets," *Am J Clin Nutr*, May 2009, 89 (5):1627s–1633s, E-pub 11 Mar 2009

31. See the article "Spinach — how a data quality mistake created a myth and a cartoon character," http://it.toolbox.com/blogs/infosphere/spinach-how-a-data-quality-mistake-created-a-myth-and-a-cartoon-character-10166, accessed 11-14-10

32. From http://nutritiondata.self.com unless otherwise specified

33. *Soil Science Society of America Proceedings 1948*, vol. 13, 380–84 (The Soil Science Society of America, Madison, Wisconsin, 1949), also http://njaes.rutgers.edu/pubs/bearreport

34. Lindeberg, *Food and Western Disease*, 209, cites Rossander-Hulthen and Hallberb, "Dietary factors influencing iron absorption: an overview," *Iron Nutrition in Health and Disease*, Hallberb and Asp eds., 1996, John Libbey: London, 105–15.

35. Hunt and Roughhead, "Nonheme-iron absorption, fecal ferritin excretion, and blood indexes of iron status in women consuming controlled lactoovovegetarian diets for 8 weeks," *Am J Clin Nutr*, 1999, 69:944–52

36. Cunnane, *Survival of Fattest*, 134

37. Robbins, *Healthy at 100*, 151

38. Carper, *100 Simple Things*, 82–84, 179

39. www.frot.co.nz/dietnet/basics/copper.htm, accessed 11-14-10; "Introduction to Copper Toxicity," www.arltma.com/CuIntroDoc.htm, accessed 11-14-10

40. Gittleman, *Why So Tired*, 35

41. Ibid., 27

42. Gittleman, *Fat Flush Plan*, 170

43. Fallon, *Nourishing Traditions*, 26

44. Ibid.

45. Eades, *Protein Power LifePlan*, 9

46. Daniel, *Whole Soy Story*, 154, who cites four studies in support, including: Jackson, "Amino acids: essential and nonessential?" *Lancet*, 1983, 1: 1034–37; Irwin and Hegstead, "A conspectus of research on amino requirements of man," *J Nutr*, 1971, 101:387–429

47. Lindeberg, *Food and Western Disease*, 41

48. Crayhon, *The Carnitine Miracle*, 17; http://en.wikipedia.org/wiki/Carnitine#Food

49. Crayhon, *The Carnitine Miracle*, 58

50. Ibid.

51. Colpo, *Cholesterol Con*, 154

52. Hipkiss, "On the enigma of carnosine's anti-ageing actions," *Exp Gerontol*, Apr 2009, 44 (4):237–42. E-pub 11 Nov 2008

53. Hipkiss, "Could carnosine or related structures suppress Alzheimer's disease?" *J Alzheimer's Dis*, May 2007, 11 (2):229–40

54. Hipkiss, "Glycation, ageing, and carnosine: are carnivorous diets beneficial?" *Mech Ageing Dev*, Oct 2005, 126 (10):1034–39; Hipkiss et al., "Carnosine, the anti-ageing, antioxidant dipeptide, may react with protein carbonyl groups," *Mech Ageing Dev*, 15 Sep 2001, 122 (13):1431–45

55. Rashid, van Reyk, Davies, "Carnosine and its constituents inhibit glycation of low-density lipoproteins that

promotes foam cell formation in vitro," *FEBS Letters*, 2007, 581:1067–70

56. Andrews et al., "The effect of dietary creatine supplementation on skeletal muscle metabolism in congestive heart failure." *European Heart Journal*, Apr 1998, 19 (4):617–22; Gordon et al. "Creatine supplementation in chronic heart failure increases skeletal muscle creatine phosphate and muscle performance," *Cardiovascular Research*, Sep 1995, 30 (3):413–18

57. Laidlaw et al. "Plasma and urine taurine levels in vegans," *Am J Clin Nutr*, Apr 1988, 47 (4):660–63

58. Sturman et al., 1984, and Laidlaw et al., 1988

59. Lindeberg, *Food and Western Disease*, 177

60. Anon., "Beef Facts," *Nutrition*, Series No. FS/N 023, www.nebeef.org/post/lfu/MeatContaining_vs_VegDiets.pdf, accessed 2-25-11

61. Aro et al., "Inverse association between dietary and serum conjugated linoleic acid and risk of breast cancer in postmenopausal women," *Nutr Cancer*, 2000, 38 (2):151–57

62. Holford, *Optimum Nutrition*, 46

63. Cunnane, *Survival of Fattest*, 115–50

64. Vogiatzoglou et al., "Dietary sources of vitamin B_{12} and their association with plasma vitamin B_{12} concentrations in the general population: the Hordaland homocysteine study," *Am J Clin Nutr*, 2009, 89:1078–87, www.ajcn.org/cgi/content/full/89/4/1078, accessed 11-14-10

65. Holford, *Optimum Nutrition*, 46

66. Ibid., 36

67. Keith, *Vegetarian Myth*, 191–92

68. Daniel, *Whole Soy Story*, 213–14

69. Campbell et al., "Effects of an omnivorous diet compared with a lactoovovegetarian diet on resistance-training-induced changes in body composition and skeletal muscle in older men," *Am J Clin Nutr*, 1999, 70: 1032–39

70. Dreyer et al., "Role of protein and amino acids in the pathophysiology and treatment of sarcopenia," *Journal of the American College of Nutrition*, 2005, 24 (2):140s–45s; Paddon-Jones et al., "Role of dietary protein in the sarcopenia of aging," *Am J Clin Nutr*, May 2008, 87 (5):1562s–66s

71. Aubertin-Leheudre and Adlercreutz, "Relationship between animal protein intake and muscle mass index in healthy women," *Br J Nutr*, Dec 2009, 102 (12):1803–10

72. Thalacker-Mercer et al., "Inadequate protein intake affects skeletal muscle transcript profiles in older humans," *Am J Clin Nutr* 2007, 85:1344–52

73. Fallon and Enig, "It's the Beef," www.westonaprice.org/food-features/268-its-the-beef.html, accessed 1-14-11

74. Purdey, *J Nutr Med*, 1994, 4:43–82

75. See note 72 above.

76. Tappel, "Heme of consumed red meat can act as a catalyst of oxidative damage and could initiate colon, breast, and prostate cancers; heart disease; and other diseases," *Med Hypotheses*, 2007, 68 (3):562–64, E-pub 11 Oct 2006

77. Carper, *100 Simple Things*, 178–79

78. Ibid., 124–26, 180

Chapter 18 (page 139)

1. Vogiatzoglou et al., "Dietary sources of vitamin B_{12} and their association with plasma vitamin B_{12} concentrations in the general population: the Hordaland homocysteine study," *Am J Clin Nutr*, 2009, 89:1078–87

2. Cochran, *10,000 Year Explosion*, 77

3. Ibid., 97, cites Kritchevsky, et al., "Influence of type of carbohydrate on atherosclerosis in baboons fed semipurified diets plus 0.1 percent cholesterol," *Am J Clin Nutr*, 1980, 33l: 1869–87.

4. Ibid., 98

5. Harris and Ross, *Food and Evolution*, 236

6. Grant, "An ecologic study of dietary links to prostate cancer," *Altern Med Rev*, 1999, 4:162–69

7. Lindeberg, *Food and Western Disease*, 154

8. Ibid., 41

9. Mann et al., "Atherosclerosis in the Masai," *Am J Epidemiol*, 95:26–37

10. Lindeberg, *Food and Western Disease*, 223

11. Ibid., 213

12. Ibid., 154

13. Ibid., 153

14. Ibid., 130

15. Ibid., 214

16. Masterjohn, "Dioxins in Animal Foods: A Case for Vegetarianism?" www.westonaprice.org/dioxins-in-animal-foods-a-case-for-vegetarianism.html, accessed 1-26-10

17. Gumpert, *Raw Milk Revolution*, 100

18. Cowan, "Raw Milk," *P-P Jnl of Hlth & Healng*, 1997, 21 (2)

19. Gumpert, *Raw Milk Revolution*, xxviii

20. For more information, see Masterjohn, "The Biochemical Magic of Raw Milk and Other Raw Foods: Glutathione" www.westonaprice.org/blogs/printblog.html?index_php?view=article&id=2009&tmpl=component&print=1, accessed 11-15-10.

21. www.organicpastures.com/faq.html, accessed 1-27-10

22. Gumpert, *Raw Milk Revolution*, 123

23. Ibid., 115

24. Schenck, *Live Food Factor*, 160

25. Ibid.

26. De Vries, *Elixir of Life*, ch. 2

27. Ayerza and Coates, *Chia*, 127

28. Vishwanathan et al., "Consumption of 2 and 4 egg yolks/d for 5 wk increases macular pigment concentrations in older adults with low macular pigment taking cholesterol-lowering statins," *Am J Clin Nutr* 2009, 90: 1272–79

29. Hyman, *Ultra-Metabolism*, 37

30. Kern, Jr., "Normal plasma cholesterol in an 88-year-old man who eats 25

eggs a day. Mechanisms of adaptation," *N Engl J Med*, 28 Mar 1991, 324 (13):896–99

31. Mutungi et al., "Dietary cholesterol from eggs increases plasma HDL cholesterol in overweight men consuming a carbohydrate-restricted diet," *J Nutr*, Feb 2008, 138 (2):272–76

32. Eades, *Protein Power*, 97

Chapter 19 (page 145)

1. Schenck, *Live Food Factor*, App. D, cites several studies.

2. Crawford, *Driving Force*, 227

3. Eades, *Protein Power LifePlan*, 73

4. Taubes, *Good Calories, Bad Calories*, 94–95

5. http://paleosister.wordpress.com/20 10/10/18/130, accessed 12-11-10

6. According to "Former Vegan Confesses All," www.truthaboutabs.com/ vegan-confesses-health-problems.html, accessed 12-11-10. Natasha's website is www.voraciouseats.com.

7. Campbell, *China Study*, 76

8. Ibid., 78

9. Maroufyan et al., "The effect of methionine and threonine supplementations on immune responses of broiler chickens challenged with infectious bursal disease," *American Journal of Applied Sciences*, 2010, 7 (1): 44–50, www.scipub.org/fulltext/ajas/ajas7144– 50.pdf, accessed 12-3-10; Van Brummelen and du Toit, "L-methionine as immune supportive supplement: a clinical evaluation," Tshwane University of Technology, Gezina, South Africa, *Amino Acids*, 29 Sep 2006, 10:1007s, www.biomox.com/resources/publicat ion%20amino%20acid%20journal.pd f, accessed 12-3-10; Hobbs and Haas, "Methionine: Amino Acid Support for Your Liver," www.dummies.com /how-to/content/methionine-amino-ac id-support-for-your-liver.html, accessed 12-3-10

10. De Vries, *Primitive Man*, 55

11. Wharton, *Metabolic Man*, 185, 216, 275

12. Campbell, *China Study*, 242–43

13. Ibid., 358

14. Ibid., 230

15. Chen, Diet, *Life-Style, and Mortality in China: A Study of the Characteristics of 65 Chinese Counties*, Cornell University Press: Ithaca, NY, 1991, cited by Fallon, *Nourishing Traditions*, 7

16. Dr. Eades, "The China Study vs. the China Study," www.proteinpower.co m/drmike/cancer/the-china-study-vs-th e-china-study/#more-4213, accessed 9-10-10

17. Masterjohn, "The Truth about the China Study," www.cholesterol-and-health.com/China-Study.html, accessed 9-10-10; Colpo, "The China Study, More Vegan Nonsense!" http://antho nycolpo.com/?p=129, accessed 9-10-10

18. www.cholesterol-and-health.com/Cam pbell-Masterjohn.html#Figure1, accessed 11-15-10: scroll down to see figure 2 also.

19. McDougall et al., "Effects of a Very Low-Fat, Vegan Diet in Subjects with Rheumatoid Arthritis," *J Altern Complement Med.*, 2002, 8 (1):71–75; Esselstyn et al., "A strategy to arrest and reverse coronary artery disease: a 5-year longitudinal study of a single physician's practice," *J Fam Pract*, 1995, 41 (6):560–66

20. Campbell, *China Study*, 104

21. Schulsinger et al., "Effect of dietary protein quality on development of aflatoxin B$_1$-induced hepatic preneoplastic lesions," *J Natl Cancer Inst.*, 16 Aug 1989, 81 (16):1241–45

22. Mainigi and Campbell, "Subcellular distribution and covalent binding of aflatoxins as functions of dietary manipulation," J Toxicol Environ Health, May 1980, 6 (3):659–71

23. Appleton and Campbell, "Effect of high and low dietary protein on the dosing and postdosing periods of aflatoxin B$_1$-induced hepatic preneoplastic lesion development in the rat," *Cancer Res.*, May 1983, 43 (5):2150–54

24. Mercola, "The Dark Side of the China Study Supporting Vegetarianism," http://articles.mercola.com/sites/articl es/archive/2010/09/08/china-study.asp x, accessed 9-10-10

25. Cordain and Campbell, "The Protein Debate," www.cathletics.com/articles /proteinDebate.pdf, accessed 9-14-10

Chapter 20 (page 157)

1. Sapontzis, *Food for Thought*, 315

2. Friend, *Compassionate Carnivore*, 184

3. Pollan, *Omnivore's Dilemma*, 312

4. Sally Fallon, "Twenty-Two Reasons Not to Go Vegetarian," www.weston aprice.org/abcs-of-nutrition/1555-not-t o-go-vegetarian.html, accessed 1-13-11

5. Pollan, *Omnivore's Dilemma*, 326

6. Lanza, "Does Death Exist? New Theory Says 'No,' " www.huffington post.com/robert-lanza/does-death-exi st-new-theo_b_384515.html, accessed 1-28-10

7. Sapontzis, *Food for Thought*, 239

8. One example is Sheridan, *Animals and the Afterlife: True Stories of Our Best Friends' Journey Beyond Death*, Hay House: Carlsbad, CA, 2003

9. Shroder, *Old Souls*, 26

10. Here is a list of books on scientific proof of afterlife. I have read all of these: Tom Shroder, *Old Souls*; Kubis and Macy, *Conversations Beyond the Light with Departed Friends & Colleagues by Electronic Means*; Locher and Harsch-Fischbach, *Breakthroughs in Technical Spirit Communication*; Macy, *Miracles in the Storm: Talking to the Other Side with the New Technology of Spiritual Contact*; Martin, *Science of Life after Death: New Research Shows Human Consciousness Lives On*; Schwartz, *Afterlife Experiments: Breakthrough Scientific Evidence of Life after Death*.

11. Thompkins and Bird, *Secret Life of Plants*, 59, 145–62, ch. 10

12. Ibid., 1–32

13. Prechtel, *Long Life*, 347

14. Ibid., 349

15. Vonderplanitz, *We Want to Live*, 293

16. Budiansky, *Covenant of the Wild*, 45

17. Pollan, *Omnivore's Dilemma*, 322

18. Ibid., 325

19. Budiansky, *Covenant of the Wild*, 24

20. Ibid., 14

21. Ibid., 34

22. Ibid., 13

23. Sapontzis, *Food for Thought*, 156

24. Weaver, *Butcher and Vegetarian*, 169

25. Pollan, *Omnivore's Dilemma*, 330

26. Friend, *Compassionate Carnivore*, 151

27. Ibid., 164–65

28. Sapontzis, *Food for Thought*, 88

29. Ibid., 322

30. Weaver, *Butcher and Vegetarian*, 140

31. Sapontzis, *Food for Thought*, 120

32. DeVore, "Hog Heaven," www.yesmagazine.org/issues/food-for-life/339, accessed 4-11-10

33. Friend, *Compassionate Carnivore*, 132

Chapter 21 (page 167)

1. Billings, "30 years of transitions: from fruitarian to living foods to lacto-vegetarian," www.beyondveg.com/billings-t/bio/billings-t-bio-1b.shtml, accessed 11-20-10

2. Pfeiffer, *Mental and Elemental Nutrients: A Physician's Guide to Nutrition and Health Care*, 103

3. Rose, *New Energy Body*, 81

4. Ibid., 86

5. E-mail correspondence, Oct 2010

6. Narayanananda, *Secrets of Mind-Control*, 41

7. Ibid., 43–44

8. Zephyr, *Instinctive Eating*, 49–50

9. Ibid., 54

Chapter 22 (page 173)

1. Abend, "How Cows (Grass-Fed Only) Could Save the Planet," *Time*, 25 Jan 2010, www.time.com/time/magazine/article/0,9171,1953692,00.html, accessed 11-23-10

2. Coleman, *New Organic Grower*, cites *Light Connection*, San Diego, CA, Apr 2010, 15.

3. Clancy, "Greener Pastures: how grass-fed beef and milk contribute to healthy eating," www.ucsusa.org/assets/documents/food_and_agriculture/greener-pastures-exec-sum.pdf, accessed 4-3-10

4. Than, "Sun Blamed for Warming of Earth and Other Worlds," www.livescience.com/environment/070312_solarsys_warming.html; Ravilious, "Mars Melt Hints at Solar, Not Human, Cause for Warming, Scientist Says," http://news.nationalgeographic.com/news/2007/02/070228-mars-warming.html, accessed 1-26-10

5. Fallon, "Twenty-Two Reasons Not to Go Vegetarian," www.westonaprice.org/abcs-of-nutrition/1555-not-to-go-vegetarian.html, accessed 1-13-11

6. Figures obtained from www.goats4h.com/Sheep.html, accessed 11-23-10

7. According to "Former Vegan Confesses All," www.truthaboutabs.com/vegan-confesses-health-problems.html, accessed 12-11-10. Natasha's website is www.voraciouseats.com.

8. Or use rock powders, worm castings, and other high-brix tools and methods, as explained at www.highbrixgardens.com.

9. Purdey, "The (Vegan Ecological) Wasteland," www.westonaprice.org/farm-a-ranch/446-the-vegan-ecological-wasteland, accessed 9-18-10

10. Radhika et al., "Refined grain consumption and the metabolic syndrome in urban Asian Indians (Chennai Urban Rural Epidemiology Study 57)," *Metabolism*, May 2009, 58 (5): 675–81, www.ncbi.nlm.nih.gov/pubmed/19375591, accessed 11-23-10

11. Bond, *Natural Eating*, 35

12. Cordain, *Paleo Diet*, 29

13. Brittman, "Rethinking the Meat Guzzler," www.nytimes.com/2008/01/27/weekinreview/27bittman.html, accessed 4-7-10

14. Friend, *Compassionate Carnivore*, 45,

cites USDA figures.

15. Ibid., 48

16. Shapin, "Vegetable Love: The History of Vegetarianism," *New Yorker*, www.newyorker.com/arts/critics/books/2007/01/22/070122crbo_books_shapin, accessed 1-22-10

17. Robbins, *Healthy at 100*, 121

18. Gilman and Gilman, "Greening the Desert: Applying natural farming techniques in Africa," an interview with Masanobu Fukuoka, www.context.org/ICLIB/IC14/Fukuoka.htm, accessed 11-23-10

19. Siegelbaum, "In Search of a Test Tube Hamburger," *Time*, Apr 2008, www.time.com/time/health/article/0,8599,1734630,00.html, accessed 11-23-10

Chapter 23 (page 183)

1. Schenck, *Live Food Factor*, 147–72

2. Carper, *100 Simple Things*, 178

3. Ibid., 179

4. Ibid., 124–26, 180

5. Ibid., 37

6. Anon., "Natural Toxins in Fruits and Vegetables," www.foodsafetynetwork.ca/aspx/public/publication_detail_global.aspx?languageid=1&contenttypeid=5&id=83, accessed 12-1-10

7. For more information, see http://en.wikipedia.org/wiki/Cruciferous_vegetables and www.iodine4health.com/special/goitrogens/foods/goitrogenic_foods.htm, accessed 11-21-10.

8. Harris, *Food and Evolution*, 249

9. Anon., "Aflatoxin & Liver Cancer," www.niehs.nih.gov/health/impacts/aflatoxin.cfm, accessed 11-21-10

10. Roxby, "Creating the caveman diet," www.bbc.co.uk/news/health-11075437, accessed 11-25-10

Chapter 24 (page 185)

1. Wrangham, *Catching Fire*, 81

2. Schenck, *Live Food Factor*, ch. 8, App. D

3. Ibid., 175

4. Ibid., 153–54, summarizes Dr. Howell's findings, and 188–91 has more information on enzymes.

5. Howell, *Enzyme Nutrition*, 52–53

6. Boutenko, *12 Steps to Raw Food* (2001), 5

7. Ibid. cites Howell, *Enzyme Nutrition*, (1985), 25–29.

8. Howell, *Enzyme Nutrition*, 25

9. Abrams, Jr., "What IS Nutritional Anthropology?" *P-P Jnl of Hlth & Healng*, 1982, 7 (1)

10. Vojdani, "Detection of IgE, IgG, IgA, and IgM antibodies against raw and processed food antigens," *Nutrition & Metabolism*, 2 May 2009, 6:22, www.nutritionandmetabolism.com/content/6/1/22, accessed 11-27-10

11. Campbell, *China Study*, and Autio, *Digital Mantrap*, cite some of these studies.

12. Rosedale, *Rosedale Diet*; Melvin, *Paleolithic Prescription*; and Bowden, *Living Low Carb*, are a few.

13. Graham, *80/10/10 Diet*, is one such book.

14. Beaumont, *Physiology of Digestion*, 269–72

15. Stoffels, "Optimum Health: Leaving No Stone Unturned," *P-P Jnl of Hlth & Healng*, 1993, 17 (3–4)

16. Vogiatzoglou et al., "Dietary sources of vitamin B_{12} and their association with plasma vitamin B_{12} concentrations in the general population: the Hordaland homocysteine study," *Am J Clin Nutr*, 2009, 89:1078–87

17. Cheraskin et al., "The 'ideal' daily intake of threonine, valine, phenylalanine, leucine, isoleucine, and methionine," *Orthomolecular Psychiatry*, 1978, 7 (3):150–55

18. Brantley, *Cure*, 96, cites Kulvinskas, *Survival into the 21st Century*.

19. Neal and Rigdon, "Gastric tumours in mice fed benzo[a]pyrene: a quantitative study," *Tex. Rep. Biol. Med.*, 1967, 25:553; www.ncbi.nlm.nih.gov/pubmed/6082228, accessed 11-21-10; www.ncbi.nlm.nih.gov/pubmed/7589

05, accessed 11-21-10

20. http://en.wikipedia.org/wiki/Heterocyclic_amine, accessed 11-21-10

21. National Cancer Institute, "Heterocyclic Amines in Cooked Meats," www.cancer.gov/cancertopics/factsheet/risk/heterocyclic-amines, accessed 1-3-10

22. Yaylayan et al., "The role of creatine in the generation of N-methylacrylamide: a new toxicant in cooked meat," *J Agric Food Chem.* 2004, 52: 5559–65

23. Brantley, *Cure*, 91

24. Ibid., 96

25. Vonderplanitz, *Living without Disease*, 19

26. Cohen, "Man finds extreme healing eating parasitic worms," CNN, 8 Dec 2010, www.cnn.com/2010/HEALTH/12/09/worms.health/?hpt=T2, accessed 12-11-10

27. Anon., "Glutamine for muscle growth and fat loss," www.warriorfx.com/2008/06/glutamine-for-muscle-growth-and-fat-loss, accessed 5-2-10

28. Beaumont, *Physiology of Digestion*, 269–72

29. Brantley, *Cure*, 131–32

30. Wilson, *Adrenal Fatigue*, 139

31. Wharton, *Metabolic Man*, 193

32. Beaumont, *Physiology of Digestion*, 49; also his chart showing how it aided the digestion of cabbage, 272

33. De Vries, *Elixir of Life*, 48

34. Hurley, *Diabetes Rising*, 169

35. Fallon, *Nourishing Traditions*, 231

36. Wrangham, *Catching Fire*, 83

37. Ibid., 118

38. Beaumont, *Physiology of Digestion*, 127

39. Ibid., 46

40. Mercola, *Discover the Magic of Nutritional Typing: Nature's Best-Kept Secret for Optimizing Your Health and Weight*, E-book, 26

Chapter 25 (page 195)

1. Yabroff, "No More Sacred Cows," *Newsweek*, 31 Dec 2009, www.newsweek.com/2009/12/30/no-more-sacred-cows.html

2. Grinzi, "Grass-Fed Beef: There Is a Difference," *P-P Jnl of Hlth & Healng*, 2005, 29 (3)

3. Scollan, "Control of beef meat quality," *Annual Report and Accounts 2001*, Institute of Grassland and Environmental Research (IGER), Jan 2002; for a photo comparison of grass- vs. grain-fed beef after two weeks of refrigeration, see www.westwindfarm.biz/grassfedbenefits/freshness.html, accessed 12-3-10.

4. Mercola, "The Ominous Beef Cover Up: The Hidden Truth Behind the Meat on Your Plate," 23 Mar 2010, http://articles.mercola.com/sites/articles/archive/2010/03/23/how-grassfed-cows-could-save-the-planet.aspx, accessed 3-25-10

5. Friend, *Compassionate Carnivore*, 137

6. Ibid., 138

7. "Rendering Plants, Recycling of Dead Animals and Slaughterhouse Wastes," www.jivdaya.org/rendering_plants.htm, accessed 12-3-10

8. Friend, *Compassionate Carnivore*, 93

9. Kirby, *Animal Factory*, 444

10. Friend, *Compassionate Carnivore*, 199

11. Kirby, "6 Baby Steps toward a More Sustainable Animal Diet," www.huffingtonpost.com/david-kirby/6-baby-steps-toward-a-mor_b_481624.html, accessed 3-6-10

Chapter 26 (page 199)

1. Young and Pellet, "Plant proteins in relation to human protein and amino acid nutrition," *Am J Clin Nutr*, 1994, 59:1203s–12s

2. More in Clement, *Supplements Exposed*

3. More on hemp at www.innvista.com/health/foods/hemp/seedprot.htm and http://en.wikipedia.org/wiki/Hemp, both

accessed 11-23-10

4. www.nal.usda.gov/fnic/foodcomp/cgi-b in/list_nut_edit.pl, accessed 11-23-10

5. Lindeberg, *Food and Western Disease*, 53, cites Grant et al., "The effect of heating on the haemagglutinating activity and nutritional properties of bean (*Phaseolus vulgaris*) seeds," *J Sci Food Agri*, 1982, 33:1324–26.

6. Ibid., 196

7. Ibid., 218

Chapter 27 (page 205)

1. Destaillats et al., "Differential effect of maternal diet supplementation with α-Linolenic acid or n-3 long-chain polyunsaturated fatty acids on glial cell phosphatidylethanolamine and phosphatidylserine fatty acid profile in neonate rat brains," *Nutrition & Metabolism*, 2010, 7:2, www.nutritionandmetabolism.com/content/7/1/2, accessed 1-15-11

2. Carper, *100 Simple Things*, 68–69

3. Cunnane, *Survival of Fattest*, 168

4. Ibid., 105

5. Reddy et al., "The influence of maternal vegetarian diet on essential fatty acid status of the newborn," *Eur J Clin Nutr*, May 1994, 48 (5):358–68

6. Cunnane, *Survival of Fattest*, 106

7. Torres et al., "Protein restriction during pregnancy affects maternal liver lipid metabolism and fetal brain lipid composition in the rat," *Am J Physiol Endocrinol Metab*, Feb 2010, 298 (2): E270–77

8. Cunnane, *Survival of Fattest*, 107

9. Waylett et al., "The role of beef as a source of vital nutrients in healthy diets," *Environ*, Jul 1999; Anon., "Beef Facts: Beef/Meat-Containing vs. Vegetarian Diets and Health," www.beefnutrition.org/uDocs/ACF3A.pdf, accessed 1-25-10

10. Sears, *Omega Rx Zone*, 194

11. Bunn, ed., *Meat-Eating and Evolution*, 341

12. Sears, *Omega Rx Zone*, 195

13. Wagnon et al., "Breastfeeding and vegan diet," *J Gynecol Obstet Biol Reprod (Paris)*, Oct 2005, 34 (6): 610–12

14. Casella et al., "Vitamin B_{12} deficiency in infancy as a cause of developmental regression," *Brain Dev*, Dec 2005, 27 (8):592–94

15. Cundiff and Harris, "Case report of 5 siblings: malnutrition? Rickets? DiGeorge syndrome? Developmental delay?" *Nutr J*, 16 Jan 2006, 5:1; Day, "Strict Vegan Diets May Be Dangerous, Especially for Expectant Mothers and Children," www.chetday.com/vegandietdangers.htm, accessed 1-15-11

16. Sapontzis, *Food for Thought*, 60–61

17. Daniel, *Whole Soy Story*, 143, 251–58

18. Budiansky, *Covenant of the Wild*, 23

Chapter 28 (page 209)

1. Henderson, "The secret of a healthy old age may lie in right balance of proteins," www.timesonline.co.uk/tol/life_and_style/health/article6941392.ece, *Times*, accessed 1-13-10

2. Carper, *100 Simple Things*, 269–70

3. Rose, *Detox for Women*, 27

4. Slom, *Remedy*, xv

5. Fallon, *Nourishing Traditions*, 37

6. Bernstein, *Diabetes Diet*, 65

7. Wolfe, *Superfoods*, 245

8. Carper, *100 Simple Things*, 222

9. Denese, *Ageless Skin*, 31–32

10. Bernstein, *Diabetes Diet*, 76

Resources

Related Websites

Beyond Vegetarianism: www.beyondveg.com

The Paleolithic Diet Page: www.paleodiet.com

Dr. Joseph Mercola: www.mercola.com

Dr. Stanley Bass: 718-648-1500, www.drbass.com

The Price-Pottenger Nutrition Foundation: www.ppnf.org

The Weston A. Price Foundation: www.westonaprice.org

The International Natural Hygiene Society: naturalhygienesociety.org

Aajonus Vonderplanitz and the Raw Animal Food Diet: www.wewant2live.com

The International Network of Cholesterol Skeptics: www.thincs.org

Victoria Boutenko: www.rawfamily.com

Ursula Horaitis: www.vitalgourmet.eu and www.thehealthspeaker.com

Dr. Steve Monkiewicz, host of Real Health: www.healthylife.net

Susan Schenck: www.livefoodfactor.com
    Available for raw food coaching at livefoodfactor@yahoo.com

Doctors

Dr. Stanley Bass: 718-648-1500, www.drbass.com

Dr. John Fielder: (07) 4093 7989 (within Australia) and (61) 7 4093 7989 (international), www.johnfielder.com.au

Dr. Jeff Hazim: 954-640-4040, info@WellWithU.com, www.WellWithU.com and www.NutritionCrafters.com

Dr. Ben Kim: 415-578-4628, http://drbenkim.com

Dr. Ron Strauss: Natural Healing Educator and coach: rstrauss@mchsi.com

Clean Meat and Animal Foods from Healthy Animals

Pranther Ranch Meat Company: 415-391-0420, www.prmeatco.com

Sustainable Table: 212-991-1930, www.sustainabletable.org
    Sustainable Table has an Eat Well Guide with a database searchable by zip-code for farms, markets, and restaurants in your area that offer food that is friendly to humans, animals, and the environment.

American Grassfed Association: 877-774-7277, www.americangrassfed.org

American Pastured Poultry Producers Association: www.apppa.org

Eat Wild: 253-759-2318, www.eatwild.com
    A directory of pasture-based farms.

List of online nutrient data bases: www.ars.usda.gov/aboutus/docs.htm?docid=6300

Community Alliance with Family Farmer: 530-756-8518, www.caff.org

Eat Well Guide: 212-991-1858, www.eatwellguide.org

Selected Bibliography

Adams, Robert. *Silence of the Heart: Dialogues with Robert Adams*, Acropolis Books, Inc.: Atlanta, GA, 1999.

Atkins, Robert C., MD. *Dr. Atkins' New Diet Revolution*, M. Evan and Company, Inc.: New York, NY, 2002.

Autio, James. *The Digital Mantrap: A Training Program for Business Professionals*, Ebola Communications: Del Mar, CA, 2000.

Ayerza, Ricardo, Jr., and Wayne Coates. *Chia: Rediscovering a Forgotten Crop of the Aztecs*, University of Arizona Press: AZ, 2005.

Barnard, Neal D., MD. *Foods that Cause You to Lose Weight: The Negative Calorie Effect*, Avon Books: New York, NY, 1992.

Baroody, Theodore A., DC, ND, LMT, PhD (Nutr), Dipl. Acup. (IAMA). *Alkalize or Die: Superior Health through Proper Alkaline-Acid Balance*, Holographic Health, Inc.: Waynesville, NC, 1991.

Bass, Stanley S., ND, DC, PhC, PhD, DO, DSc, DD, *Discovery of the Ultimate (Vegetarian) Diet: Testing Nutritional Theories on Mice*, Volume II, Life Science Publishing: New York, NY, 1996.

Bass, Stanley S., ND, DC, PhC, PhD, DO, DSc, DD, *In Search of the Ultimate (Vegetarian) Diet: Testing Nutritional Theories on Mice*, Volume I, Life Science Publishing: New York, NY, 1994.

Bass, Stanley S., ND, DC, PhC, PhD, DO, DSc, DD, *With 3 Generations of Vegetarian Hygienists*, Life Science Publishing: New York, NY, 1994.

Bass, Stanley S., ND, DC, PhC, PhD, DO, DSc, DD, *Ideal Health through Sequential Eating: Perfection in Food Combining*, Life Science Publishing: New York, NY, 1996 (orig. 1993).

Bass, Stanley S., ND, DC, PhC, PhD, DO, DSc, DD, *Overcoming Compulsive Habits*, Life Science Publishing: New York, NY, 1980.

Bass, Stanley S., ND, DC, PhC, PhD, DO, DSc, DD, *Natural Health and Nutrition: Condensed Natural Hygiene Course*, Life Science Publishing: New York, NY, 1977.

Bass, Stanley S., ND, DC, PhC, PhD, DO, DSc, DD, *The Laws of Life*, Life Science Publishing: New York, NY, 1976.

Bass, Stanley S., ND, DC, PhC, PhD, DO, DSc, DD, *From the Average Diet to Superior Nutrition in 7 Weekly Programs*, Life Science Publishing: New York, NY, 1972.

Beale, Lucy and Joan Clark-Warner, MS, RD, CDE. *The Complete Idiot's Guide to Glycemic Index Weight Loss*, Alpha Books: New York, NY, 2010.

Beaumont, William, MD. *Experiments and Observations on the Gastric Juice and the Physiology of Digestion*, Kessinger Publishing Co., LLC, 2003. Orig. pub. F. P. Allen: Plattsburgh, NY, 1833.

Bernstein, Richard K., MD. *The Diabetes Diet: Dr. Bernstein's Low-Carbohydrate Solution*, Little, Brown, and Company: New York, NY, 2005.

Bird, Christopher and Peter Tompkins. *The Secret Life of Plants*, Harper and Row Publishers, Inc.: New York, NY, 1973.

Bond, Geoff. *Natural Eating, Nutritional Anthropology: Eating in Harmony with Our Genetic Programming*, Griffin Publishing Group: Torrance, CA, 2000.

Boutenko, Victoria. *Green for Life: The Updated Classic on Green Smoothie Nutrition*, North Atlantic Books: Berkeley, CA, 2010.

Boutenko, Victoria. *12 Steps to Raw Foods: How to End Your Dependency on Cooked Food*, North Atlantic Books: Berkeley, CA, 2007.

Bowden, Jonny, PhD, CNS. *Living Low Carb: How to Choose the Diet That's Right for You*, Sterling: New York, NY: 2010.

Brantley, Timothy, PhD, ND. *The Cure: Heal Your Body, Save Your Life*, John Wiley & Sons, Inc.: Hoboken, NJ, 2007.

Budiansky, Stephen. *The Covenant of the Wild: Why Animals Chose Domestication*, Yale University Press: New Haven, CT, 1999.

Bunn, Henry and Craig Stanford, eds. *Meat-Eating and Human Evolution*, Oxford University Press: New York, NY, 2001.

Campbell, T. Colin, PhD. *The China Study: Startling Implications for Diet, Weight Loss, and Long-Term Health*, BenBella Books: Dallas, TX, 2004.

Carper, Jean. *100 Simple Things You Can Do to Prevent Alzheimer's: And Age-Related Memory Loss*, Little, Brown, and Company Hachette Book Group: New York, NY, 2010.

Carr, Nicholas. *Shallows: What the Internet Is Doing to Our Brains*, W.W. Norton & Company, Inc.: New York, NY, 2010.

Carrington, Hereward. *Vitality, Fasting, and Nutrition: A Physiological Study of the Curative Power of Fasting, together with a New Theory of the Relation of Food to Human Vitality*, Rebman Co.: New York, MT, 1908.

Clement, Brian, PhD. *Supplements Exposed: The Truth They Don't Want You to Know about Vitamins, Minerals, and Their Effects on Your Health*, New Page Books: Franklin Lakes, NJ, 2010.

Cochran, Gregory and Henry Harpending. *The 10,000 Year Explosion: How Civilization Accelerated Human Evolution*, Basic Books: New York, NY, 2009.

Cohen, Mark Nathan, PhD. *Health and the Rise of Civilization*, Yale University: New Haven, CT, 1989.

Colpo, Anthony. *The Great Cholesterol Con: Why Everything You've Been Told about Cholesterol, Diet, and Heart Disease Is Wrong*, LuLu.com, 2006.

Cordain, Loren, PhD. *The Paleo Diet: Lose Weight and Get Healthy by Eating the Food You Were Designed to Eat*, John Wiley & Sons, Inc.: Hoboken, NJ, 2002.

Cousens, Gabriel, MD. *Spiritual Nutrition: Six Foundations for Spiritual Life and the Awakening of Kundalini*, North Atlantic Books: Berkeley, CA, 2005.

Cousens, Gabriel, MD. *Rainbow Green Live-Food Cuisine*, North Atlantic Books: Berkeley, CA, 2003.

Crawford, Michael and David Marsh. *The Driving Force: Food, Evolution, and the Future*, Harper & Row: New York, NY, 1989.

Crayhon, Robert. *The Carnitine Miracle: The Supernutrient Program that Promotes High Energy, Fat Burning, Heart Health, Brain Wellness, and Longevity*, M. Evans and Company, Inc.: New York, NY, 1998.

Cunnane, Stephen C. *Survival of the Fattest: The Key to Human Brain Evolution*, World Scientific Publishing Company: Hackensack, NJ, 2005.

D'Adamo, Peter, ND, and Catherine Whitney. *Eat Right for Your Blood Type: The Individualized Diet Solution to Staying Healthy, Living Longer, & Achieving Your Ideal Weight*, G.P. Putnam's Sons: New York, NY, 1996.

Daniel, Kaayla T., PhD, CCN. *The Whole Soy Story: The Dark Side of America's Favorite Health Food*, NewTrends Publishing, Washington, DC, 2005.

Denese, Adrienne, MD, PhD. *Dr. Denese's Secrets for Ageless Skin: Younger Skin in 8 Weeks*, The Berkley Publishing Group: New York, NY, 2005.

De Vany, Arthur, PhD. *The New Evolution Diet: What Our Paleolithic Ancestors Can Teach Us about Weight Loss, Fitness, and Aging*, Special Markets Department, Rodale, Inc: New York, NY, 2011.

De Vries, Arnold. *The Elixir of Life*, Chandler Book Company: Chicago, IL, 1958.

De Vries, Arnold. *Primitive Man and His Food*, Chandler Book Company: Chicago, IL, 1952.

Eades, Michael R., MD, and Mary Dan Eades, MD. *The Protein Power Lifeplan*, Warner Books: New York, NY, 2000.

Eades, Michael R., MD, and Mary Dan Eades, MD. *Protein Power: The High-Protein/Low-Carbohydrate Way to Lose Weight, Feel Fit, and Boost Your Health — in Just Weeks*, Bantam Books: New York, NY, 1996.

Eaton, S. Boyd, MD; Marjorie Shostak; and Melvin Konner, MD, PhD. *The Paleolithic Prescription: A Program of Diet and Exercise and a Design for Living*, Harper & Row Publishers: New York, NY, 1988.

Engdahl, F. William. *Seeds of Destruction: The Hidden Agenda of Genetic Manipulation*, Global Research: Montreal, Quebec, Canada, 2007.

Enig, Mary G., PhD. *Know Your Fats: The Complete Primer for Understanding the Nutrition of Fats, Oils, and Cholesterol*, Bethesda Press: Silver Spring, MD, 2008.

Enig, Mary G., PhD, and Sally Fallon. *Eat Fat, Lose Fat: The Healthy Alternative to Trans Fats*, Plume: New York, NY, 2005.

Fahey, Trish and William Wolcott. *The Metabolic Typing Diet: Customize Your Diet to Your Own Unique Body Chemistry*, Random House, Inc.: New York, NY, 2000.

Fallon, Sally, with Mary Enig, PhD. *Nourishing Traditions: The Cookbook That Challenges Politically Correct Nutrition and the Diet Dictocrats*, NewTrends Pub: Washington, DC, 2001.

Finch, Caleb, PhD. *The Biology of Human Longevity: Inflammation, Nutrition, and Aging in the Evolution of Lifespans*, Elsevier Inc.: New York, NY, 2007.

Freeman, John, MD; Eric H. Kossoff; Jennifer B. Freeman; and Millicent T. Kelly, RD. *The Ketogenic Diet: A Treatment for Children and Others with Epilepsy*, Demos Health: New York, NY, 2007.

Friend, Catherine. *The Compassionate Carnivore: Or How to Keep Animals Happy, Save Old MacDonald's Farm, Reduce Your Hoofprint, and Still Eat Meat*, Da Capo Press: Philadelphia, PA, 2008.

Gagne, Steve. *Food Energetics: The Spiritual, Emotional, and Nutritional Power of What We Eat*, Healing Arts Press: Rochester, VT, 2008.

Galland, Leo, MD. *The Fat Resistance Diet: Unlock the Secret of the Hormone Leptin*, Broadway Books: New York, NY, 2005.

Gedgaudas, Nora, CNS, CNT. *Primal Body, Primal Mind: Empower Your Total Health the Way Evolution Intended (...and Didn't)*, Primal Body-Primal Mind Publishing: Portland, OR, 2009.

Gittleman, Ann Louise, PhD, CNS. *The Fat Flush Plan: The Breakthrough Weight-Loss System*, McGraw-Hill: New York, NY, 2002.

Gittleman, Ann Louise, CNS, with Melissa Diane Smith. *Why Am I Always So Tired? Discover How Correcting Your Body's Copper Imbalance Can...*, Harper Collins: New York, NY, 1999.

Gittleman, Ann Louise, CNS. *Eat Fat, Lose Weight: How the Right Fats Can Make You Thin for Life*, Keats Publishing: Lincolnwood, IL, 1999.

Gittleman, Ann Louise, CNS. *Beyond Pritikin: A Total Nutrition Program for Weight Loss, Longevity, and Good Health*, Bantam Books: New York, NY, 1996.

Graham, Douglas N., DC. *The 80/10/10 Diet*, FoodnSport Press: Key Largo, FL, 2006.

Gumpert, David E. *The Raw Milk Revolution: Behind America's Emerging Battle over Food Rights*, Chelsea Green Publishing: White River Junction, VT, 2009.

Hanh, Thich Nhat and Lilian Cheung, DSc, RD. *Savor: Mindful Eating, Mindful Life*, HarperOne: New York, NY, 2010.

Harris, Marvin. *Cows, Pigs, Wars, and Witches: The Riddles of Culture*, Vintage Books: New York, NY, 1974.

Harris, Marvin and Eric B. Ross, eds. *Food and Evolution: Toward a Theory of Human Food Habits*, Temple University Press: Philadelphia, PA, 1987.

Hart, Cheryle R., MD, and Mary Kay Grossman, RD. *The Insulin-Resistance Diet: How to Turn Off Your Body's Fat-Making Machine*, Contemporary Books: Chicago, IL, 2001.

Hartmann, Thom. *The Last Hours of Ancient Sunlight: Waking Up to Personal and Global Transformation*, Three Rivers Press: New York, NY, 1999.

Henslin, Earl. *This is Your Brain on Joy: A Revolutionary Program for Balancing Mood, Restoring Brain Health, and Nurturing Spiritual Growth*, Thomas Nelson, Inc.: Highlands Ranch, CO, 2008.

Holford, Patrick. *New Optimum Nutrition for the Mind*, Basic Health Publications, Inc.: Laguna Beach, CA, 2009.

Howell, Edward. *Enzyme Nutrition: The Food Enzyme Concept*, Avery Publishing Group, Inc.: Wayne, NJ, 1985.

Hurley, Dan. *Diabetes Rising: How a Rare Disease Became a Modern Pandemic, and What to Do about It*, Kaplan Publishing: New York, NY, 2010.

Hyman, Mark, MD. *The UltraMind Solution: Fix Your Broken Brain by Healing Your Body First*, Scribner: New York, NY, 2009.

Hyman, Mark, MD. *Ultra-Metabolism: The Simple Plan for Automatic Weight Loss*, Atria Books: New York, NY, 2006.

Iserbyt, Charlotte Thomson. *The Deliberate Dumbing Down of America: A Chronological Paper Trail*, Conscience Press: Ravenna, OH, 1999.

Katz, David L., MD, MPH, FACPM, FACP. *Nutrition in Clinical Practice: A Comprehensive, Evidence-Based Manual for the Practitioner*, Lippincott, Williams & Wilkins: Philadelphia, PA, 2008.

Keith, Lierre. *The Vegetarian Myth: Food, Justice, and Sustainability*, Flashpoint Press: Crescent City, CA, 2009.

Kendrick, Malcom, MD. *The Great Cholesterol Con: The Truth about What Really Causes Heart Disease and How to Avoid It*, John Blake Publishing Ltd: London, England, 2008.

Kirby, David. *Animal Factory: The Looming Threat of Industrial Pig, Dairy, and Poultry Farms to Humans and the Environment*, St. Martin's Press: New York, NY, 2010.

Kulvinskas, Viktoras. *Survival into the 21st Century: Planetary Healers Manual*, 21st Century Publications: Fairfield, IA, 1981.

Leakey, Richard and Roger Lewin. *Origins: What New Discoveries Reveal about the Emergence of Our Species and Its Possible Future*, EP Dutton: New York, NY, 1977.

Leakey, Richard. *The Origin of Humankind*, BasicBooks: New York, NY, 1994.

Lindeberg, Staffan, MD, PhD. *Food and Western Disease: Health and Nutrition from an Evolutionary Perspective*, Wiley-Blackwell: Chichester, West Sussex, UK, 2010.

McCully, Kilmer S., MD, and Martha McCully. *The Heart Revolution: The Extraordinary Discovery That Finally Laid the Cholesterol Myth to Rest*, Harper/Perennial: New York, NY. 2000.

McDonald, Pamela, NP. *The Perfect Gene Diet: Use Your Body's Own APO E Gene to Treat High Cholesterol, Weight Problems, Heart Disease, Alzheimer's...and More!* Hay House, Inc: Carlsbad, CA, 2010.

Monastyrsky, Konstantin, CNC. *Fiber Menace: The Truth about Fiber's Role in Diet Failure, Constipation, Hemorrhoids, Irritable Bowel Syndrome, Ulcerative Colitis, Crohn's Disease, and Colon Cancer*, Ageless Press: Lyndhurst, NJ, 2008.

Morgan, Dan. *Merchants of Grain: The Incredible Story of the Power, Profits, and Politics behind the International Grain Trade*, Penguin Books: New York, NY, 1980.

Morse, Joseph S.B. *The Evolution Diet: What and How We Were Designed to Eat*, Amelior Publishing Co: San Diego, CA, 2008.

Murray, Michael T., ND. *What the Drug Companies Won't Tell You and Your Doctor Doesn't Know: The Alternative Treatments That May Change Your Life — and the Prescriptions That Could Harm You*, Atria Books: New York, NY, 2009.

Narayanananda, Swami. *The Secrets of Mind-Control*, Yoga Trust: Rishikesh, U.P., India, 1979 (orig. 1959).

Northrup, Christiane, MD. *The Secret Pleasures of Menopause*, Hay House, Inc.: Carlsbad, CA, 2008.

Perricone, Nicholas, MD. *Ageless Face, Ageless Mind: Erase Wrinkles and Rejuvenate the Brain*, Ballantine Books: New York, NY, 2007.

Pfeiffer, Carl C., PhD, MD. *Nutrition and Mental Illness: An Orthomolecular Approach to Balancing Body Chemistry*, Healing Arts Press: Rochester, VT, 1987.

Pollan, Michael. *The Omnivore's Dilemma: A Natural History of Four Meals*, The Penguin Press: New York, NY, 2006.

Prechtel, Martin. *Long Life: Honey in the Heart*, North Atlantic Books: Berkley, CA, 2004.

Price, Weston A., DDS. *Nutrition and Physical Degeneration: The Enduring Classic Work on How What We Eat Shapes Us...for Better and Worse*, The Price-Pottenger Nutrition Foundation, Inc.: La Mesa, CA, 1945.

Reaven, Gerald, MD. *Syndrome X: Overcoming the Silent Killer That Can Give You a Heart Attack*, Simon & Schuster: New York, NY, 2000.

Richards, Byron J., CCN, with Mary G. Richards. *Mastering Leptin: The Leptin Diet, Solving Obesity and Preventing Disease*, Wellness Resources Books: Minneapolis, MN, 2005.

Rigden, Scott, MD. *The Ultimate Metabolism Diet: Eat Right for Your Metabolic Type*, Hunter House, Inc.: Alameda, CA, 2009.

Robb, Jay. *The Fat Burning Diet: Accessing Unlimited Energy for a Lifetime*, Loving Health Publications: Encinitas, CA: 1999.

Robbins, John. *Healthy at 100: How You Can — at Any Age — Dramatically Increase Your Life Span and Your Health Span*, Ballantine Books: New York, NY, 2007.

Rose, Natalia. *Detox for Women: An All New Approach for a Sleek Body and Radiant Health*, William Morrow: New York, NY, 2009.

Rose, Natalia. *The New Energy Body: Discover a New Source of Energy That Will Amaze You*, Rose Program, 2007.

Rosedale, Ron, MD. *The Rosedale Diet: Turn Off Your Hunger Switch!* HarperCollins, New York, NY, 2004.

Ross, Julia, MA. *The Mood Cure: The 4-Step Program to Take Charge of Your Emotions — Today*, Penguin Group: New York, NY, 2002.

Sapontzis, Steve F., ed. *Food for Thought: The Debate over Eating Meat*, Prometheus Books: Amherst, NY, 2004.

Schenck, Susan, LAc, MTOM. *The Live Food Factor: The Comprehensive Guide to the Ultimate Diet for Body, Mind, Spirit, and Planet*, 2nd ed., Awakenings Publications: San Diego, CA, 2008.

Schmid, Ronald, ND. *Traditional Foods Are Your Best Medicine: An Eminent Naturopathic Physician Shares His Nutritional Techniques for Treating Modern Life's Maladies*, Ballantine Books: New York, NY, 1987.

Schmidt, Gerhard. *The Dynamics of Nutrition*, Biodynamic Farming & Gardening Association: Junction City, OR, 1982.

Schwarzbein, Diana, MD, and Nancy Deville. *The Schwarzbein Principle: The Truth about Losing Weight, Being Healthy, and Feeling Younger*, Health Communications, Inc.: Deerfield Beach, FL, 1999.

Sears, Barry, PhD. *Toxic Fat: When Good Fat Turns Bad*, Thomas Nelson, Inc.: Nashville, TN, 2008.

Sears, Barry, PhD. *The Omega Rx Zone: The Miracle of the New High-Dose Fish Oil*, HarperCollins Books: New York, NY, 2002.

Shroder, Tom. *Old Souls: Compelling Evidence from Children Who Remember Past Lives*, Rockefeller Center, New York, NY, 1999.

Slom, Supa Nova. *The Remedy: The Five-Week Power Plan to Detox Your System: Combat the Fat, and Rebuild Your Mind and Body*, Wellness Central: New York, NY, 2010.

Steckel, Richard and Jerome Rose. *The Backbone of History: Health and Nutrition in the Western Hemisphere*, Cambridge University Press: New York, NY, 2002.

Taubes, Gary. *Why We Get Fat, and What to Do about It*. Alfred A. Knopf: New York, NY, 2011.

Taubes, Gary. *Good Calories, Bad Calories: Fats, Carbs, and the Controversial Science of Diet and Health*, Anchor Books: New York, NY, 2008.

Ungar, Peter S., ed. *Evolution of the Human Diet: The Known, the Unknown, and the Unknowable*, Oxford University Press, Inc.: New York, NY, 2007.

Vonderplanitz, Aajonus. *The Recipe for Living without Disease*, Carnelian Bay Castle Press: Santa Monica, CA, 2002.

Vonderplanitz, Aajonus. *We Want to Live: Out of the Grips of Disease and Death*, Carnelian Bay Castle Press, LLC: Santa Monica, CA, 1997.

Weaver, Tara Austen. *The Butcher and the Vegetarian: One Woman's Romp through a World of Men, Meat, and Moral Crisis*, Rodale, Inc.: New York, NY, 2010.

Weissberg, Steven M., MD, and Joseph Christiano, APPT. *The Answer Is in Your Bloodtype: Research Linking Your Blood Type and How It Affects Your Life Span, Love and Compatibility, Your Likely Illness Profile, Diet, and Exercise for Maximum Life*, Personal Nutrition USA, Inc.: Lake Mary, FL, 1999.

Werner, Michael and Thomas Stockli. *Life from Light: Is It Possible to Live without Food? A Scientist Reports on His Experiences*, Clairview Books: Baden and Munich, Germany, 2007.

Westbrook, Gregory. *When Hallelujah Becomes "What Happened?": Crashing On the Vegan Diet*, E-book found at www.weighofwisdom.com.

Wharton, Charles Heizer, PhD. *Metabolic Man: Ten Thousand Years from Eden*, WinMark Publishing: Orlando, FL, 2001.

Wilson, James L, ND, DC, PhD. *Adrenal Fatigue: The 21st Century Stress Syndrome*, Smart Publications: Petaluma, CA, 2001.

Wolf, Robb. *The Paleo Solution: The Original Human Diet*, Victory Belt Publishing: Las Vegas, NV, 2010.

Wolfe, David. *Superfoods: The Food and Medicine of the Future*, North Atlantic Books: Berkeley, CA, 2009.

Wrangham, Richard. *Catching Fire: How Cooking Made Us Human*, Basic Books: New York, NY, 2009.

Zaidi, Sarfraz, MD. *Power of Vitamin D: A Vitamin D Book That Contains the Most Comprehensive and Useful Information on Vitamin D Deficiency, Vitamin D Level*, Outskirts Press, Inc.: Denver, CO, 2010.

Zavasta, Tonya. *Raw Food and Hot Yoga: From Severe Disability to Superior Health*, BR Publishing: Cordova, TN, 2009.

Zephyr. *Instinctive Eating: The Lost Knowledge of Optimum Nutrition*, Pan Piper Press: Pahoa, HI, 1996.

Index

Contact Information

I am available by phone for raw food coaching. I'll call you to make it easy for you, since I live in Ecuador. You can reach me for coaching requests, inquiries, comments, suggestions, and corrections at livefoodfactor@yahoo.com.

If you send me emotionally charged hate mail, I will not only block your e-mail, but might even use your letter as an example of how a vegan diet affects the emotions due to EPA deficiency.[*]

---

[*]See chapter 8.